Animal Models of Immunological Processes

Animal Models of Immunological Processes

edited by
JOHN B. HAY
Department of Pathology
University of Toronto
Canada

1982

ACADEMIC PRESS

A Subsidiary of Harcourt Brace Jovanovich, Publishers

LONDON NEW YORK
PARIS SAN DIEGO SAN FRANCISCO SÃO PAULO
SYDNEY TOKYO TORONTO

Academic Press Inc. (London) Ltd
24–28 Oval Road
London NW1

US edition published by
Academic Press Inc.
111 Fifth Avenue,
New York, New York 10003

British Library Cataloguing in Publication Data

Animal models of immunological processes.
1. Immunology
I. Hay, J. B.
591.2′95 QR186

ISBN 0-12-333520-5

LCCCN 81-68010

Phototypeset by Dobbie Typesetting Service, Plymouth, Devon
Printed by T. J. Press (Padstow) Ltd., Padstow, Cornwall

Contributors

A. O. ANDERSON[1]
United States Army Medical Research Institute of Infectious Diseases, Fort Detrick, Frederick, Maryland 21701, USA

N. D. ANDERSON
The Johns Hopkins University, Baltimore, Maryland 21205, USA

R. AUERBACH
Department of Zoology, University of Wisconsin, Madison, Wisconsin 53706, USA

A. D. BEFUS
Department of Pathology, McMaster University, Hamilton, Ontario, Canada L8N 4J9

J. BIENENSTOCK
Department of Pathology, McMaster University, Hamilton, Ontario, Canada L8N 4J9

R. N. P. CAHILL[2]
Basel Institute for Immunology, 487 Grenzacherstrasse, CH-4058 Basel, Switzerland

B. F. EDWARDS
Biology Department, Reed College, Portland, Oregon 97202, USA

J. B. HAY
Division of Experimental Pathology and Institute of Immunology, Medical Sciences Building, University of Toronto, Toronto, Canada M5S 1A8

†D. G. INGRAM
Ontario Veterinary College, Guelph, Ontario, Canada N1G 2W1

J. M. KEHOE
Department of Microbiology, Northeastern Ohio Universities, College of Medicine, Rootstown, Ohio 44272, USA

[1] *Present address: Departments of Pathology and Biology, University of Pennsylvania, Philadelphia, Pennsylvania 19104, USA*

[2] *Present address: Faculty of Veterinary Science, University of Melbourne, Parkville, Victoria 3052, Australia*

L. N. RUBEN
Biology Department, Reed College, Portland, Oregon 97202, USA
J. D. WHITE
The Johns Hopkins University, Baltimore, Maryland 21205, USA

Preface

Immunological reactions are a composite of multifactorial processes at the genetic, molecular, cellular and tissue levels of organization. A large number of phenomena have been described using *in vitro* models, particularly cell–cell interactions and molecule–cell interactions. In many instances very carefully defined criteria of cell numbers and culture conditions are necessary to observe certain biological consequences. Physiological concentrations of serum proteins, for example, inhibit many such test-tube interactions. Therefore, it is fundamental to delineate which of these interactions occur or are relevant in the complex, *in vivo* environment, and which are artificially contrived interactions. Animal models of immunological processes are indispensable in the final evaluation of the significance of *in vitro* processes. They are crucial to any physiological description of immune reactions. I believe that most of the information derived from inbred mice is likely to apply to outbred species and, conversely, that the biology of lymphocytes deduced from large animal experiments also applies to mice.

Some animal models are clearly superior to others for studying certain processes. This volume presents studies of *in vivo* models which facilitate the unique experimental analysis of different aspects of immunological reactions.

June 1981 J. B. HAY

Contents

Contributors v

Preface vii

1 *Selected Aspects of the Canine Immune Response*
J. M. KEHOE 1

I Introduction 1
II Fundamental nature of canine immune response 2
III Canine diseases with a significant immunological component 18
IV Immunodeficiency disorders 21
V Summary 21
References 22

2 *Lymphocyte Locomotion, Lymphatic Tissues and Lymphocyte Circulation in the Rat*
A. O. ANDERSON, N. D. ANDERSON and J. D. WHITE 25

I Introduction 25
II Intrinsic migratory behavior of "recirculating" lymphocytes 27
III Lymphocyte homing to HEV 36
IV Migration and differentiation of lymphocytes during development 44
V Lymphatic tissues in the adult rat 52
VI Circulation of lymphocytes during an immune response 86
References 90

3 *Lymphocyte Migration Patterns in Sheep*
J. B. HAY and R. N. P. CAHILL 97

I Introduction 97
II Blood lymphocytes 98
III Thoracic duct lymphocytes 100
IV Changes in the output of lymphocytes from antigenically challenged popliteal lymph nodes 101
V Effects of local and systemic anti-lymphocyte antibody on the cellular migration from popliteal lymph nodes 110

VI Changes in the lymph plasma from antigenically challenged popliteal lymph nodes 111
VII Lymph plasma proteins 112
VIII Cells from normal afferent lymph 116
IX Afferent lymph from pathological sites 121
X Similarities and differences between chronic inflammatory sites and lymph nodes 125
XI Intestinal lymph 126
XII Differences in lymphocyte migration patterns in lymph draining subcutaneous lymph nodes, mesenteric lymph nodes and chronic inflammatory sites 128
XIII Lymphocyte migration in the fetal lamb 130
References 130

4 Ontogeny of the Immune Response: Studies with Mutant Mice
R. AUERBACH 135

I Introduction 135
II Mouse mutations 138
III The major histocompatibility complex 148
IV Mouse strain variations 151
V Concluding comments 155
Acknowledgements 156
References 156
Addendum 162

5 The Mucosa-associated Immune System of the Rabbit
A. D. BEFUS and J. BIENENSTOCK 167

I Introduction 167
II Gut-associated lymphoid tissue (GALT) 169
III Lymphoid tissue at other mucosa-associated sites 193
IV The common mucosal immunologic system 203
Abbreviations 209
References 211

6 Comparative Aspects of Conglutinin and Immunoconglutinins
D. G. INGRAM 221

I Introduction 221
II Conglutinin 223
III Immunoconglutinins 229
IV Biological significance of conglutinin and immunoconglutinins 236

V Conglutination as a serological tool 245
VI Summary 249
References 250

7 *Aspects of Amphibian Immunity*
B. F. EDWARDS and L. N. RUBEN 255

I Introduction 255
II Serum immunoglobulin class heterogeneity 257
III Immunoglobulin as antigen receptor on amphibian lymphocytes 260
IV Physiology of antigen-binding cells 263
V Effects of mitogens and anti-immunoglobulin on lymphocyte activities 267
VI Specificity of antigen binding 270
VII The role of the thymus in amphibian immunity 273
VIII Metamorphosis as a model for self-sufficiency 280
References 282

Subject Index 287

1 *Selected Aspects of the Canine Immune Response*

J. M. KEHOE

1. Introduction

Immunological research in the last few years has shown that the biological foundation of the immune response is very similar in the various higher mammalian species. Thus, the lymphocyte, in its different functional varieties, is the key immunologically relevant cell in all species studied. Also, the distinct types of immunological responses varying from the cell mediated (CMI) to the humoral, from delayed hypersensitivity to anaphylaxis, *all* seem to be represented in all species studied. Nonetheless, there are some unique variations on these commonalities that are discernible in different species which are significant both for their possible effects on immune function *per se* and also for what such variations can tell us about the phylogenetic origins of adaptive immunity. One example of such a variation would be the occurrence of distinct *subclasses* of immunoglobulin proteins in most individual species. Structural analyses of the heavy chain constant regions of immunoglobulins from a number of species have shown that the different subclasses have arisen relatively recently in evolutionary time and that they have developed within, or close to, the individual species themselves. This pattern stands in contrast to the closer cross species relationships of immunoglobulin subclasses that would exist if the subclasses had arisen at a common point in evolutionary time prior to the divergence events that have led to the different species available for study today. The discernment of patterns such as this has required detailed and comparative examinations of the characteristic features of the immune response of individual species.

This chapter will consequently be concerned with the immune response of the dog in the hope that both its unique and shared features will be of use in more fully appreciating the nature of the vertebrate immune response.

II. Fundamental nature of the canine immune response

The dog, like man, is subject to a very large array of disease-producing processes against which an adaptive immune response can be active. These processes include infectious diseases caused by bacteria, viruses, protozoa, or helminths, and combinations thereof; and a large variety of neoplastic syndromes. Although immunodeficiency diseases have only recently begun to be characterized in the dog, there is every reason to believe that an insufficient, or compromised, immunological responsiveness will lead to marked increases in both the incidence of, and fatality from its infectious and neoplastic diseases. Some relevant support for this can be found in the fatal infections that occur in dogs that are given immunosuppressive drugs, as in organ transplantation studies or in animals being treated with antimetabolites for cancer chemotherapy. Thus there is every indication that a highly developed adaptive immune response exists in the canine species.

A. THE LYMPHOCYTE – THE KEY IMMUNOLOGIC CELL

As in other species, the lymphocyte, in its various functional categories, is clearly the central cell. Canine lymphocytes are broadly divisible into the two general populations known in other species: T (thymus-derived) cells and B (bursal equivalent) cells. Available information concerning the nature of the cell types in the dog is summarized below.

1. *T cells*

As is well known, the distinction between T and B lymphocytes was originally worked out in mice. All normal members of other mammalian species that have been examined to date also show both T and B cells in their lymphoid tissues and blood. The dog is no exception. The rosetting process with sheep red blood cells that has proved to be so useful for identifying human and murine T cells is not as useful for canine T cells since it evidently is specific for only a subpopulation of T cells from this species (Schultz, 1978). Nonetheless, other studies, including the specific blastogenic effects of the mitogens phytohemagglutinin (PHA) and concanavalin A (Con A), have shown that a T cell population does exist in the dog. Other studies by Schultz and his associates (1978) have suggested the presence of a canine T cell associated cell surface antigen which can be found in the brain as well as on the T cell surface membrane. This is formally analogous to the situation in mice with the Thy-1 T cell antigen which is found on brain cells as well as on murine T cells.

Since this canine T cell-brain tissue specific marker is present in approximately 65% of peripheral canine lymphocytes (approximately the number of peripheral T cells found in other species) and since a much lower percentage of these cells shows red blood cell rosetting, it would appear that in dogs the rosetting technique is measuring only a subpopulation of T cells. Such further subcategorizations of the T cell population could be very significant functionally and are consistent with similar observations made in other species, especially the mouse and man. Further study will be required to completely discern the T cell subcategory: specific function relationships for the dog.

2. *B cells*

Mammalian B cells have also been most intensively studied in two species, the mouse and man. Two surface immunoglobulin receptor molecules, IgM and IgD, have been identified as B cell specific markers in these species. IgG molecules are also seen on occasion as surface immunoglobulin. Approximately 15 to 20% of peripheral canine lymphocytes display immunoglobulins on their surface. IgM is the most common class shown, but IgG is also represented on about 10% of these cells. No IgD equivalent has yet been identified in the dog. Schultz *et al.* (1978) have also reported a receptor for the third component of complement on canine B cells. Canine B lymphocytes thus seem to correspond to comparable cells in other species.

3. *Null cells*

A certain subpopulation of lymphocytes of the dog does not show the characteristics of either T or B cells. While this subpopulation has not yet been studied intensely, it is believed to correspond to the "null" or K cell category that has been shown to participate in the antibody dependent cell mediated cytotoxicity (ADCC) reaction. This reaction requires the presence of an active cell membrane associated receptor for the Fc region of an IgG immunoglobulin. Such a receptor is present on the canine null cell population. It is thus likely, although not yet formally established, that the dog's host defense mechanism includes the ADCC reaction.

B. THE CELL MEDIATED IMMUNE (CMI) RESPONSE IN THE DOG

The presence of numerous T cells in its lymphoid organs and peripheral blood suggests that the dog has an active cell mediated immune system. However, the classical clinical manifestation of the CMI response, the delayed hypersensitivity (DTH) reaction elicited in the skin, has proven difficult to demonstrate and interpret in this species. The reason for this difficulty in the dog has not yet been worked out and represents a significant and interesting problem for future investigation. It does appear that, in contrast to the situation in man, neutrophils rather than monocytes are the principal recruited cell in the canine DTH reaction.

An especially definitive representation of the CMI response is the phenomenon of allograft rejection. This process has been studied extensively in the dog, especially in the kidney transplantation studies that preceded the extension of this procedure to man. These studies, and other related experiments, have shown unequivocally that the dog possesses a very active CMI response. The general subject of transplantation immunology and the current status of knowledge concerning the canine histocompatibility system has been recently reviewed (Vriesendorp, 1979). As in other species, skin allografts can be readily used as an index of the status of the canine CMI response.

Taken together, the combined data suggest that the dog possesses a highly active CMI system. While further study of specific syndromes in this species is necessary, this branch of the immune arm is undoubtedly very active against a variety of infectious diseases and cancer. Specific *in vitro* techniques useful for the assay of the canine CMI system have been described by Schultz and Adams (1978). Basically, these procedures are modifications of techniques that have been established in other species and serve to affirm the degree to which the dog shows the capacity for the various CMI manifestations that have been noted in these other animals. The mitogen-induced lymphocyte blastogenesis procedures and the demonstration of lymphokine production (e.g. migration inhibition factor) by canine lymphocytes are especially noteworthy in this regard.

C. THE HUMORAL IMMUNE RESPONSE OF THE DOG

More detailed information is currently available concerning the canine humoral response than is known concerning the CMI. This is partially because of the long-standing interest in the dog's humoral response by veterinary medical scientists interested in the care and prevention of infectious diseases and cancer. However, our understanding of the basic characteristics and unique features of the structure of canine antibodies has also been greatly aided by the availability of the pure homogeneous paraproteins often produced in animals affected with lymphoid tumors, especially multiple myeloma. In this respect, the resulting elucidation of some of the more subtle details of the structure of canine immunoglobulins is comparable to the way similar advances have been made previously with human immunoglobulins. Thus, the studies of the pure myeloma paraproteins have confirmed the identity of a number of classes and subclasses that are observable in whole serum. A representative, but not exhaustive, tabulation of canine myeloma paraproteins is presented in Table 1. To date, proteins of the IgM, IgG, and IgA classes have been identified in the serum of individual animals with monoclonal gammopathies. In addition, further study of the canine IgG population has demonstrated the presence of four subclasses of IgG molecules termed IgG1, IgG2a, IgG2b, and IgG2c (Reynolds and Johnson, 1970; Schultz, 1978). The dog thus corresponds to a number of other species in producing subclasses of a given immunoglobulin class.

1. *Immunochemical studies of canine myeloma paraproteins*

Some of these canine paraproteins have been studied immunochemically to provide more detailed information on their molecular characteristics. For example, Hurvitz *et al.* (1971) studied three canine immunoglobulins isolated from three separate animals with plasma cell dyscrasias. Antigenic and physicochemical analyses showed that one of these proteins was an IgM macroglobulin, another an IgA protein, and the third a canine Bence-Jones protein. Another canine IgM protein similar to the first of this series had previously been characterized by Capra and Hurvitz (1970).

The fundamental characteristics of these two IgM proteins were very similar. These characteristics included sedimentation coefficients ($S^{\circ}_{20,w}$ = 18·8 for protein Co; $S^{\circ}_{20,w}$ = 17·6 for protein Le), electrophoretic migration on cellulose acetate or polyvinyl copolymer (Pevikon) and immunologic cross reactivity. The immunologic studies were of particular interest. It was possible to show, for example, that cross-reactions occurred not only between the two canine IgM proteins but also between the canine protein and *human* IgM myeloma paraproteins. This relationship was demonstrated in a reciprocal manner. First, antisera prepared in rabbits to the canine proteins were shown to react with human myeloma macroglobulins. In addition,

TABLE 1
Representative canine monoclonal gammopathies

Case	Breed	Sex	Age at diagnosis	Total protein	A/G	Bence Jones proteinuria	M-component	Bleeding diathesis	Radiologic Bone lesions	Diagnosis
CO	Mixed	M	8	9·8	0·42	-	γM	+	-	Macroglobulinemia with hyperviscosity syndrome
LE	Mixed	M	9	11·8	0·25	-	γM	+	-	Macroglobulinemia with hyperviscosity syndrome
AG	Mixed	F	7	10·4	—	-	γM	+	-	Macroglobulinemia with hyperviscosity syndrome
FR	Poodle	F	10	4·9	0·40	ND	γM	-	-	Lymphosarcoma
GA	Mixed	M	10	13·0	0·11	-	γG	-	+	Multiple myeloma
CB	Dachshund	M	7	11·0	0·21	-	γG	+	-	Nonmyelomatous monoclonal gammopathy
HO	Cocker	F	10	9·4	0·24	-	γG	-	+	Multiple myeloma
Kl	Mixed	M	9	10·6	—	+	γG	-	+	Multiple myeloma
SI	Boxer	F	5	8·1	0·23	-	γG	-	-	Multiple myeloma
BU	German shepherd	F	6	10·4	0·25	+	γG	-	-	Multiple myeloma
AB	German shepherd	F	9	11·4	0·30	-	γG	-	+	Multiple myeloma
PI	Golden retriever	F	10	12·5	0·17	-	γG	-	+	Multiple myeloma

BO	German shepherd	M	8	9·6	0·25	-	γG	-	-	Nonmyelomatous monoclonal gammopathy
JO	Mixed	M	7	10·2	0·15	-	γG	+	-	Multiple myeloma
GM	Airedale	M	10	12·5	0·19	-	γA	-	+	Multiple myeloma
DU	Mixed	M	15	10·0	0·30	-	γA	-	+	Multiple myeloma
LO	Standard poodle	M	13	9·2	0·28	-	γA	+	+	Multiple myeloma
ST	Mixed	M	6	12·5	0·19	-	γA	+	-	Plasma-cell leukemia
CP	Airedale	M	10	8·2	0·41	-	γA	-	-	Nonmyelomatous monoclonal gammopathy and malignant melanoma
AS	Mixed	F	14	10·9	0·28	+	γA	-	-	Multiple myeloma
BL	Coonhound	F	5	7·4	0·35	+	γA	+	-	Multiple myeloma
FO	Scottish	M	×	7·6	0·52	+	γA	-	+	Multiple myeloma
PR	Mixed	F	10	6·9	0·92	+	Lchain	-	+	Light-chain disease

Slightly revised from Hurvitz (1974).
ND, not determined

comparable antisera to the human proteins reacted with the canine proteins. An example of such reactions is shown in Fig. 1. A detailed inspection of the patterns illustrated here reveal further interesting

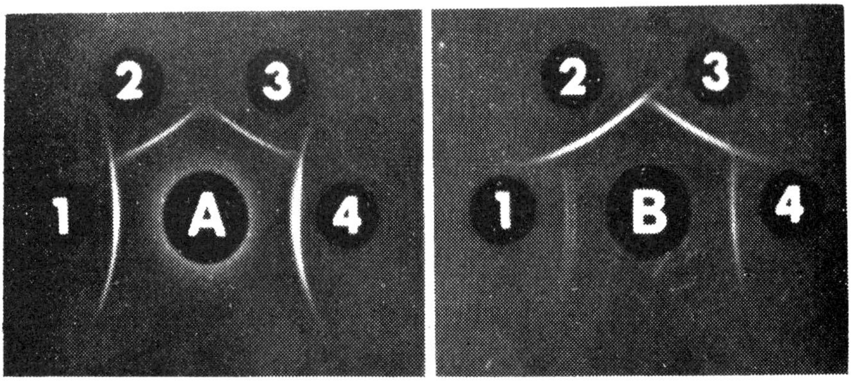

FIG. 1 Immunodiffusion analyses of canine and human myeloma paraproteins. Well A contains a specific anti-human IgM antiserum while well B contains a specific anti-canine IgM antiserum. Well 1 contains a human IgM myeloma paraprotein with kappa light chains, wells 2 and 3 different canine IgM myeloma paraproteins (Le and Co), and well 4 a human IgM paraprotein with lambda light chains. The patterns shown here are discussed further in the text. (Reproduced from Hurvitz *et al.*, 1971, with permission of the publisher.)

relationships. The pattern on the left of Fig. 1 shows that the canine protein, although reactive with the anti-human IgM serum, is antigenically deficient relative to the homologous system. This is indicated clearly by the "spur" of the human macroglobulin precipitin line over that involving the canine protein. A comparable, but reciprocal, effect is shown on the right where an anti-canine IgM serum has been employed. The pattern on the right also shows the "individual" specificity (idiotypic) of a particular canine protein since, when reacted with its own antiserum (anti-Le in this case), the homologous canine system definitely spurs over the precipitin line produced with the second canine protein (protein Co). As in all other species examined to date, no definitive evidence for IgM subclasses has yet been found in the dog. Clear immunologic evidence for a structural relationship between canine and human IgM proteins was thus found soon after the discovery of canine myeloma paraproteins. As is described below, subsequent amino acid sequence analyses confirmed and defined the exact extent of the heavy chain constant region relationship.

A novel canine monoclonal protein of unusual interest has been described by Hurvitz *et al.* (1977) and Middaugh *et al.* (1978). This IgM protein, which was produced by a dog with a lymphoid gammopathy, was clearly classifiable as a cryoimmunoglobulin. These proteins comprise a heterogeneous group long known in human medicine whose common characteristic is the propensity to precipitate as the plasma temperature drops below 37°C. The biophysical studies of Middaugh *et al.* (1978) showed neither unique features of the canine cryoglobulin as compared with its human counterparts nor a clear indication of why this protein comes out of solution in the cold. Undoubtedly, other such proteins are produced by dogs so additional searches and detailed study of canine cryoimmunoglobulins should be possible. As in man, these proteins not only show their peculiar chemical behavior in the laboratory but also have *in vivo* consequences that lead to disease, especially when the ambient temperature is low. These consequences are particularly reflected in such organs as the skin and the tongue where the cryoglobulin-induced vascular stoppages affect normal function.

2. *Amino acid sequence studies of canine immunoglobulins*

As has been the case with other proteins, studies of the primary structure of dog myeloma paraproteins have revealed important relationships which would not be discernible by other means. Differences in primary structure can shed light on evolutionary patterns and divergence from other proteins as well as providing supporting information for purely immunological studies such as those described above. Although the amount of amino acid sequence information available for dog immunoglobulins does not approach that known for man and the mouse, important data on both heavy and light chains has been obtained. This information and some possible interpretations it supports are presented below.

a. *Canine immunoglobulin variable region sequences*

i. *Light chains.* Wasserman and Capra (1978a) reported the amino acid sequence of a kappa chain prepared from a canine IgA myeloma paraprotein. The occurrence of a kappa chain produced by a dog is, in itself, of considerable interest since normal dog serum immunoglobulin shows a great preponderance of lambda chains (Hood *et al.*, 1967). The expression of canine kappa chain genes would thus seem to be a relatively rare event.

										10										20					
GOM	ASP	ILE	VAL	MET	THR	GLN	THR	PRO	LEU	SER	LEU	SER	VAL	SER	PRO	GLY	GLU	PRO	ALA	SER	ILE	SER	CYS	ARG	SER
ROY	—	—	GLN	—	—	—	SER	—	SER	—	—	—	ALA	—	VAL	—	ASP	ARG	VAL	THR	—	THR	—	GLN	ALA
CUM	—	—	—	—	—	—	—	—	—	—	—	PRO	—	THR	—	—	—	—	—	—	—	—	—	—	—
TI	GLU	—	—	LEU	—	—	SER	—	GLY	THR	—	—	LEU	—	—	—	—	ARG	—	THR	LEU	—	—	—	ALA

					30										40										50
GOM	SER	GLN	SER	ASN	LEU	ASP	TYR	LEU	ASN	TRP	TYR	LEU	GLN	LYS	ALA	GLY	GLN	SER	PRO	ARG	LEU	LEU	PRO	GLU	GLN
ROY	—	—	ASP	ILE	SER	ILE	PHE	—	—	—	—	GLN	—	—	PRO	—	LYS	ALA	—	LYS	—	—	ILE	TYR	ASP
CUM	—	—	—	LEU	ASN	THR	—	—	—	—	—	—	—	—	—	—	—	—	—	GLN	—	—	ILE	TYR	THR
TI	—	—	—	VAL	ASN	SER	PHE	—	ALA	—	—	GLN	—	—	PRO	—	—	ALA	—	ARG	—	—	ILE	TYR	VAL

										60										70					
GOM	ASP	SER	GLN	ARG	ALA	SER	GLY	VAL	PRO	ASP	ARG	PHE	SER	GLY	SER	GLY	SER	GLY	THR	ASP	PHE	THR	LEU	ARG	ILE
ROY	ALA	—	LYS	LEU	GLU	ALA	—	—	—	SER	—	—	—	—	THR	—	—	—	—	—	—	—	PHE	THR	—
CUM	LEU	—	TYR	—	—	—	—	—	—	—	—	—	—	—	—	—	—	—	—	—	—	—	—	LYS	—
TI	ALA	—	SER	—	—	THR	—	ILE	—	—	—	—	—	—	—	—	—	—	—	—	—	—	—	THR	—

					80										90										100
GOM	GLY	ARG	VAL	GLU	ALA	GLU	ASP	ALA	GLY	ILE	TYR	TYE	CYS	MET	GLN	ARG	SER	PHE	TYR	PRO	TYR	THR	PHE	GLY	GLN
ROY	SER	GLY	LEU	GLN	PRO	—	—	ILE	ALA	THR	—	—	—	GLN	—	PHE	ASP	ASN	LEU	—	LEU	—	—	—	GLY
CUM	SER	—	—	GLN	—	—	—	VAL	—	VAL	—	—	—	—	—	—	LEU	GLU	ILE	—	—	—	—	—	—
TI	SER	GLY	LEU	GLN	PRO	—	—	PHE	ALA	VAL	—	—	—	GLY	—	TYR	GLN	SER	SER	—	SER	—	—	—	—

GOM	GLY	THR	ARG	LEU	GLU	VAL	ARG	ARG
ROY	—	—	LYS	VAL	ASP	PHE	LYS	—
CUM	—	—	LYS	—	—	ILE	—	—
TI	—	—	LYS	VAL	—	LEU	LYS	—

FIG. 2 The amino acid sequence of a canine kappa light chain as determined by Wasserman and Capra (1978a). This sequence is compared with three human kappa chain sequences of distinct subgroups. (Reproduced with permission of the publisher.)

The sequence of the canine kappa chain studied by Wasserman and Capra (1978a) is illustrated in Fig. 2 together with representative human light chains of the V_KI, V_KII, and V_KIII subgroups chosen by these authors. As the authors point out, the close relationship of this canine kappa chain to members of the V_KII subgroup of human light chains, together with the fact that kappa chains isolated from other non-human species have all corresponded to the V_KI subgroup, indicates that the divergence of kappa chains occurred at least prior to mammalian speciation in evolutionary time. This finding thus corroborates a similar conclusion previously reached by Milstein and Svasti (1971) on the basis of the study of mouse kappa chains. This pattern thus stands in contrast to the previously mentioned subclass divergence which is believed, also on the basis of amino acid sequence data, to occur *subsequent* to speciation. The study of the canine protein has thus provided an important verification of this significant pattern in the evolutionary development of immunoglobulins. Little other canine light chain sequence information has been reported to date.

ii. *Heavy chains.* Canine heavy chains from myeloma paraproteins were initially sequenced by Kehoe and Capra (1972). This work, which included proteins of the IgM, IgG, and IgA classes, gave the initial indication of the prominence of the V_HIII subgroup among canine immunoglobulins. In addition, this study highlighted the presence and implications of certain amino acid residues which appeared to be associated with certain phylogenetic groupings, including that of the dog. Fig. 3 shows representative amino terminal sequences of dog myeloma paraprotein heavy chains compared with comparable sequences from man and the cat (reproduced with the permission of the publisher from Kehoe and Capra, 1972). Note, in particular, the residues at positions 10, 21, and 23. The presence of these "phylogenetically associated" residues in the heavy chains of these three species indicated that constraints on the number of genes in the immunoglobulin heavy chain variable region pool were very likely and that formal "germ line" bases for the origin of antibody diversity (i.e. a separate germ line gene for each variable region gene expressed) were unlikely to apply, at least to some heavy chain variable regions. Some recent work in nucleic acid biochemistry involving the direct assay of the number of V_HIII genes present in the genome of the mouse and man (Rabbits *et al.*, 1980) tends to formally establish this fact since an upper limit of 10 and 20 V_HIII genes respectively were found for these two species. The basic idea is thus suggested that the various "phylogenetically associated" residues reflect the limited duplication and expansion on a species level of certain sets of genes which code for

										10										20										30
Arbitrary $V_h$iii Prototype	GLU	VAL	GLN	LEU	VAL	GLU	SER	GLY	GLY	GLY	LEU	VAL	GLN	PRO	GLY	GLY	SER	LEU	ARG	LEU	SER	CYS	ALA	ALA	SER	GLY	PHE	THR	PHE	SER
Ga Canine γ										ASP					ALA								VAL							
Le Canine μ										ASP										VAL			VAL							
Co Canine μ										ASP													VAL							
Lo Canine α										ASP		ALA	VAL										VAL				LEU			
St Canine α										ASP					ALA			ILE	GLY				VAL							
Tei Human γ1																														
Was Human γ1					LEU																							SER		
Jon Human γ3	ASP												LYS																	
Zap Human α										ALA									GLY											
Ben Human μ												ALA									ALA									
Lay Human μ	ALA				LEU																									
Pom Human μ					LEU																									
Di Feline γ	ASP									ASP						ASP					THR		VAL							
Gr Feline γ	ASP									ASP											THR		VAL							
Sc Feline γ										GLU											THR		VAL							

FIG. 3 Representative amino terminal amino acid sequences of canine myeloma paraprotein heavy chains compared with comparable sequences from man and the cat. (Reproduced from Kehoe and Capra, 1972, with permission of the publisher.)

segments of heavy chain variable regions. Thus, even these limited amino-terminal sequence analyses of the canine proteins, when compared with comparable segments of polypeptide chains from other species, have provided useful information on the biological processes involved in the synthesis of antibody proteins in general.

The similar framework region structures (FR1 of Kabat *et al.*, 1976) observed in this series of canine myeloma protein sequences was also striking, especially given their origin in individual dogs of assuredly diverse genetic background. The similarity of this region of the heavy chain variable region in different canine antibodies becomes even more noteworthy when compared with the same region of heavy chains from other species (Fig. 3). The same degree of similarity is observed among these distinct species as among the individual proteins of the dog (or either of the other two species shown, for that matter). This marked similarity led to the study of the comparable region of pooled *normal* IgG immunoglobulins in the dog and other species (Capra *et al.*, 1973). By and large, the observed sequence of the *total* IgG pool of the dog corresponded to that observed with the myeloma proteins described above. This obviously indicates that the individual antibodies of widely differing specificity had very similar structures in the FR1 segment of their heavy chains. The significance of this pattern was heightened even further when careful analyses of the yields of the pooled proteins being degraded indicated that essentially *all* of the antibodies present were being detected (Capra *et al.*, 1973). In other words, the highly similar antibody proteins being examined did not represent a unique *subpopulation* of the dog's pool but rather were reflective of the *totality* of the humoral immune response to the composite of antigens to which the various individual animals had been exposed up to that point. This observation was one of several that have led to the concept that, especially in heavy chains, the covalent structure (and thus genetic control) of mammalian antibodies is under much more constraint than had been originally anticipated. The recent work analyzing immunoglobulin genes directly and carried out in species other than the dog have more precisely defined the detailed nature of the genetic constraints involved (Rabbits *et al.*, 1980).

Two complete canine heavy chain immunoglobulin variable region sequences have been reported by Wasserman and Capra (1977). These sequences are displayed in Fig. 4. The two proteins were of different class (IgA and IgM) and were from two unrelated, genetically outbred dogs. The initial most striking feature of this data is the overall degree of similarity in sequence. Of the 113 positions comprising the V_H segment, 76 show the same amino acid in both proteins. In the

10 — 20 — 30

Gom GLU VAL GLN LEU VAL GLU SER GLY GLY ASP LEU VAL LYS PRO GLY GLY SER LEU ARG LEU SER CYS VAL ALA SER GLY ILE THR PHE SER
Moo GLU VAL LYS LEU VAL GLU SER GLY GLY ASP LEU VAL LYS PRO GLY GLY SER LEU ARG LEU SER CYS VAL ALA SER GLY PHE THR PHE SER

40 — 50 — 60

Gom GLY TYR ASP MET GLN ( ) TRP VAL ARG GLN ALA PRO GLY LYS GLY LEU GLN LYS VAL ALA TYR PHE ASN ASP ALA LEU SER ALA GLN
Moo SER ASN GLY MET SER ( ) TRP VAL ARG GLN ASP PRO GLY GLU GLY LEU GLN TRP VAL ALA ASP ILE SER SER SER GLY GLN THR ( )

70 — 80 — 90

Gom GLY TYR ALA ASP ALA VAL LYS GLY ARG PHE THR ILE SER LYS ASP ASN ALA LYS ASP SER LEU TYR LEU GLN MET ASN SER LEU ARG ALA
Moo TYR TYR ALA ASP ALA VAL LYS GLY ARG PHE SER ILE SER ARG ASP ASN ALA LYS ASN THR LEU TYR LEU GLN MET GLU ASP LEU ARG VAL

100 — 110

Gom GLU ASP THR ALA VAL TYR TYR CYS ALA PRO ( ) TRP GLN PHE GLU TYR TRP GLY GLN GLY THR LEU
Moo GLU ASP THR ALA VAL TYR TYR CYS ALA THR GLU GLY ASP ILE GLU ILE PRO ARG TYR PHE GLY GLN GLY THR ILE

FIG. 4 Complete amino acid sequences of two canine heavy chain variable regions as determined by Wasserman and Capra (1977). (Reproduced with permission of the publisher.)

framework (non-hypervariable region) segments of these two polypeptide chains, only 14 differences were observed. A comparison with the framework region of a human V_HIII subgroup prototype sequence showed that the canine proteins were 78% homologous to those of the human species. Thus, this study indicates that the high degree of framework region preservation previously observed with the amino-terminal sequences holds for the entire canine V_H segment. The significance of these similarities is heightened by recent findings concerned with the organization of the genes involved in the formation of mammalian heavy chains (Early *et al.*, 1980).

The detailed structural analysis of the variable region of selected canine immunoglobulins has therefore helped elucidate not only important aspects of the dog's humoral immune response itself, but also has provided useful comparative information concerning the general nature of the antigen binding mechanism used by the mammalian immune system. This has been especially true when the characteristics of the canine proteins are compared with related proteins from the mouse and man.

b. *Canine immunoglobulin constant region sequences*

i. *Light chains.* No sequence information on canine light chain constant regions has yet been published. On the basis of studies of pooled canine light chains, Hood *et al.* (1967) concluded that normal dogs produced a preponderance of lambda light chains and very few kappa chains. The limited number of canine myeloma proteins analyzed to data is consistent with this pattern but, as indicated above, a canine kappa chain has been isolated and studied by Wasserman and Capra (1978a). However, the constant region sequence of this protein has not yet been published.

ii. *Heavy chains.* The only canine constant region for which complete, or even extensive, amino acid sequence information is available involves the mu (IgM) chain (Wasserman and Capra, 1978b; McCumber and Capra, 1979). These studies showed that the overall homology between the canine mu chain and the previously reported human mu chain (Watanabe *et al.*, 1973; Putnam *et al.*, 1973) was 81%. It was of particular interest that the individual constant region domains (i.e. the C_H1, C_H2, C_H3, and C_H4 mu chain domains) varied from a low of 72% homology to a high of 85% between these two species. This very likely represents differential selection pressures on these IgM constant region domains that are presently only incompletely understood. It would be especially interesting to know if there are some unique functional capacities of the canine

IgM protein compared with that of other species, including man.
Further analyses and interpretations of the primary structure of canine heavy chains from other isotypes will have to await additional amino acid sequence determinations.

3. *Additional canine immunoglobulin polypeptide chains*

For some time after the initial discovery of the two constituent polypeptides (heavy and light, or H and L) of the IgG molecule (Edelman and Gall, 1969), it was thought that these two types comprised the only native polypeptides that would be found in any immunoglobulin protein. However, an additional component termed the "J", or joining, polypeptide chain was subsequently found in the two "polymeric" classes of immunoglobulin, first IgA and then IgM (Halpern and Koshland, 1970; Mestecky *et al.*, 1970; O'Daly and Cebra, 1971). The "J" chain was first identified in rabbit and human polymeric immunoglobulins.

TABLE 2
Amino acid composition of isolated polypeptide chains of a canine IgA myeloma paraprotein (St). (Reproduced from Kehoe *et al.*, 1972, with the permission of the publisher.) The amino acid composition of the human IgA "J" chain used for comparison is reproduced from Mestecky *et al.*, 1973, with permission of the publisher

	St-H	St-L	St-J	Human serum IgA-J
Lysine	26	12	6	12
Histidine	10	4	2	2
Arginine	11	6	17	19
Half-cystine	11	5	11	13
Aspartic acid	43	18	42	38
Threonine	30	17	21	19
Serine	24	19	19	12
Glutamic acid	55	20	32	29
Proline	20	17	15	18
Glycine	36	24	10	6
Alanine	32	16	12	12
Valine	46	24	22	19
Methionine	8	0	5	2
Isoleucine	17	4	12	17
Leucine	44	13	15	17
Tyrosine	12	6	7	12
Phenylalanine	18	6	2	3
	443	211	250	250

Shortly thereafter, Kehoe *et al.* (1972) detected a "J" component in a canine IgA myeloma paraprotein that was under study. As shown in Table 2, this protein showed a similar amino acid composition to that reported for purified human "J" chain. In addition, the intact canine IgA myeloma paraprotein containing "J" chain showed a positive immunodiffusion reaction with a human "J" chain specific antiserum as demonstrated in Fig. 5. This study thus showed that a canine polymeric immunoglobulin possessed a third type of polypeptide chain corresponding to that seen in comparable proteins from man and the rabbit.

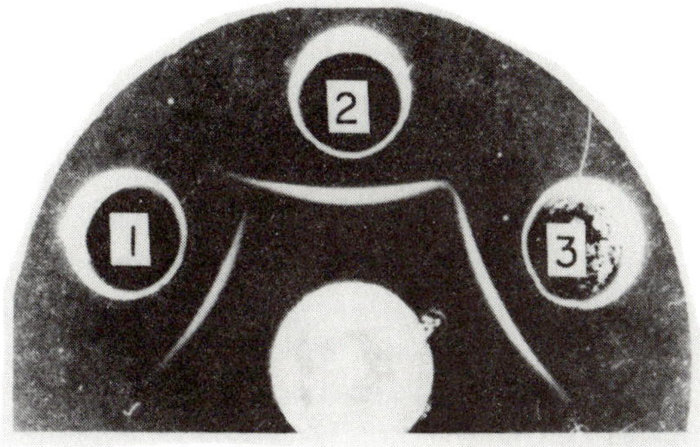

FIG. 5 Serologic reactivity of immunoglobulins and an anti-human "J" chain antiserum. The antiserum is in the center well. A *canine* IgA myeloma paraprotein (St) that contains a reactive "J" chain is in well 1 and a human IgM and a human IgA protein are in wells 2 and 3 respectively. (Reproduced from Kehoe *et al.*, 1972, with permission of the publisher.) See text for additional details.

An additional polypeptide chain, termed secretory component (SC), has also been associated with immunoglobulins of the IgA class in a wide variety of species (Tomasi and Bienenstock, 1968; Heremans, 1974). IgA from the dog has proved to be no exception. A thorough discussion of the immunochemical aspects of canine secretory component has been provided by Vaerman (1973) and by Thompson *et al.* (1979). The latter authors studied the structural aspects of free canine secretory component in detail including its molecular weight, electrophoretic and antigenic properties, and amino-terminal sequence. These latter studies showed unambiguously that the canine protein is closely related to the secretory components of man and the cow. This is illustrated formally in Fig. 6 where the available amino-terminal sequences of the dog, the cow, and man are shown. The close homology in at least this section of these three proteins is obvious. The dog secretory component, in fact, shows some uniqueness in positions 11 and 12.

	5	10
Canine	Lys-Ser-Pro-Ile-Phe-Gly-Pro-Glu-Glu-Val-Asn-Ile	
Bovine	Lys-Ser-Pro-Ile-Phe-Gly-Pro-Glu-Glu-Val-Asp-Ser	
Human	Lys-Ser-Pro-Ile-Phe-Gly-Pro-Glu-Glu-Val-Asp-Ser	

FIG. 6 Available amino-terminal amino acid sequences of secretory component from the dog, the cow, and the man. (Reproduced with permission of the publisher from Thompson *et al.*, 1979.)

Another publication by Thompson and Reynolds (1977) describes the association of canine secretory component with secretory IgM. In addition, this article described the results of chemical cleavages (by cyanogen bromide) of isolated secretory component, which studies have led to the suggestion of the possible existence of two subpopulations of this canine polypeptide chain. Additional immunochemical studies are required to definitively clarify this latter possibility.

Secretory component is believed to play a similar or identical role in the dog as other species, namely, to protect secretory IgA against rapid or excessive proteolytic degradation by the many proteolytic enzymes present in secretions (milk, tears, saliva, etc.). Notably, this protein is not synthesized by the lymphocytes responsible for the other polypeptide chains making up the IgA molecule, but rather is manufactured by neighboring epithelial cells and attached to the IgA molecules as they pass through the epithelium on their way to the secretions (Tomasi and Bienenstock, 1968). In other respects as well, the IgA system of the dog appears to correspond closely to that of the other species that have been studied to date.

III. Canine diseases with a significant immunological component

Immunological reactions of various types are now understood to be so commonly and intimately involved with disease processes that there can be difficulties in characterizing specific syndromes as more or less purely "immunologic" in nature. Nonetheless, a number of conditions in various species have been shown to be predominantly, if not exclusively, immunologic in character. The dog is no exception to this and no discussion of the canine immune response would be complete without at least some reference to such syndromes. Thus a representative, but not exhaustive, series of such canine diseases is outlined below.

A. MULTIPLE MYELOMA

The existence of multiple myeloma in the dog has been alluded to previously. Proteins produced by animals with this syndrome have been very useful in defining the characteristics of canine antibodies (Hurvitz *et al.*, 1971), as shown above. In addition, although rare, these conditions occur with sufficient frequency to be a potential clinical problem that must be anticipated in veterinary medicine.

B. AUTOIMMUNE DISEASE

Autoimmune disease can be defined as an active immune response to self components and consequently represents a breakdown of self tolerance. Both the cell mediated and humoral arms of the immune response can be involved. There can be some problem in unambiguously defining whether an observed anti-self product represents a cause or an effect. For example, anti-DNA antibodies are found in systemic lupus erythematosus. In principle, these could be either a direct consequence of the autoimmune reaction itself or, alternatively, could be due to another autoimmune reaction that has already destroyed cells thus releasing the DNA to stimulate the individual's immune reactivity secondarily. This circularity is a potential consideration in many instances of possible autoimmune disease.

Specific autoimmune diseases that have been identified in the dog include:

1. *Autoimmune hemolytic anaemia (AIHA)*

Numerous instances of this syndrome have been described in dogs (Lewis *et al.*, 1963; Jain, 1975). The anti-red blood cell antibodies, in conjunction with the complement system, lead to extensive intravascular hemolysis with hemoglobinemia and hemoglobinuria. Autoagglutination of erythrocytes also occurs and the Coombs antiglobulin test can be used to confirm the diagnosis. The syndrome thus qualifies as a true autoimmune disease.

2. *Systemic lupus erythematosus (SLE)*

This disease, known for some time in both man and the mouse, is now a clearly established clinical entity in the dog (Lewis and Schwartz, 1971; Quimby *et al.*, 1978). As reported by the latter authors, it has been possible to inbreed a colony of dogs with a very high incidence of SLE. Significantly, these animals also show *other* autoimmune syndromes including autoimmune hemolytic anemia, rheumatoid arthritis, and a Sjogren's-like syndrome. This might imply that some central regulatory process (e.g. suppressor cells) is being affected by the inbreeding process.

3. *Rheumatoid arthritis*

This syndrome is a progressive polyarthritis in which autoantibodies to IgG are commonly present (Halliwell *et al.*, 1972). These autoantibodies, which are generally, although not exclusively, of the IgM class occur in the blood and synovial fluids. As in man, the pathogenesis of the disease involves, at least in part, the activation of the classical complement cascade by the IgG-anti-IgG complexes. The resultant generation of chemotactic factors through this cascade brings in neutrophils which generate joint damage by the release of lysosomal enzymes.

4. *Immunologically mediated nephritis*

It has been known for some time that immunologic mechanisms play a role in a variety of nephritic syndromes in man and other species (McCluskey and Klassen, 1973). Classically, two general processes have been described whereby immune mediated kidney damage can occur. In the first, an authentic autoimmune reaction, anti-glomerular basement membrane antibodies are produced. In the second process, antigen-antibody complexes of a variety of types (e.g. virus-antibody complexes) are trapped in the capillary walls of glomeruli. Both processes involve activation of the classical complement cascade with consequent attraction of inflammatory cells to the kidney followed by tissue damage. There is good reason to believe that such mechanisms participate in certain forms of kidney disease in the dog (Krohn *et al.*, 1971).

5. *Thrombocytopenic purpura*

This syndrome, also known in man and some other species, occurs when anti-platelet antibodies (usually IgG) severely reduce the level of circulating platelets. This may occur when antibodies are directed toward some surface antigen of the platelets themselves (true autoimmune disease) or are directed toward platelets that have been altered to some degree by an infectious agent (e.g. virus) or a drug (e.g. sulfonamides, salicylates). As could be expected, a variety of bleeding problems is associated with this immunologically mediated disease.

IV. Immunodeficiency disorders

It seems very likely that primary immunodeficiency disorders, due to inherited genetic defects, occur in the dog. However, relatively few have been formally described as yet. One report by Farrow *et al.* (1972) suggested the existence of such a syndrome. In this study, six male miniature Dachshunds nine to twelve months of age died of pneumonia induced by *Pneumocystis carinii.* The dogs were not siblings but were closely related and the invocation of a sex-linked genetic condition thus seems plausible, if not established. Unfortunately, a detailed analysis of the immune status of these animals was not made available. Hopefully, extensive studies of comparable syndromes in this species can be made in the future.

V. Summary

Considerable knowledge has accrued in recent years concerning the canine immune response. Currently, more detailed information is available concerning the humoral arm of this response than is known for the cell-mediated component. In this, the dog mirrors the present situation for a number of other species including man.

The detection and study of the paraproteins produced in the multiple myeloma syndrome has significantly aided the advancement of knowledge concerning the structure of canine antibodies. Such studies have also provided for comparative analyses of these proteins with those of other species and have consequently aided our understanding of the phylogenetic bases of the mammalian immune response.

The most acute requirement for additional information in canine immunology may well be the need for knowledge about T cell subsets and their functional correlates. Such information would provide both sorely needed information concerning the detailed workings of cell-mediated immunity in this species and, potentially, the possibility of profitable intervention (for either augmentation or suppression) of both the humoral and cell-mediated components of the canine immune response. Such information might also further point up important unique features of this adaptive biological response in this species.

References

CAPRA, J. D. and HURVITZ, A. I. (1970). *J. Immun.* **105**, 949-956.

CAPRA, J. D., WASSERMAN, R. L. and KEHOE, J. M. (1973). *J. exp. Med.* **138,** 410-427.

EARLY, P., HUANG, H., DAVIS, M., CALAME, K. and HOOD, L. (1980). *Cell,* **19**, 981-992.

EDELMAN, G. M. and GALL, W. E. (1969). *A. Rev. Biochem.* **39**, 415-466.

FARROW, B. R. H., WATSON, A. D. J., HARTLEY, W. J. and HUXTABLE, C. R. R. (1972). *J. comp. Path. Ther.* **82**, 447-453.

HALLIWELL, R. E. W., LOVELLE, R. B. and BUTT, K. M. (1972). *J. small anim. Pract.* **13**, 239.

HALPERN, M. S. and KOSHLAND, M. E. (1970). *Nature,* **228**, 1276-1278.

HEREMANS, J. F. (1974). *In* "The Antigens" (M. Sela, ed.), vol. II, pp. 365-522. Academic Press, New York and London.

HOOD, L., GRAY, W. R., SANDERS, B. G. and DREYER, W. J. (1967). *Cold. Spring Harb. Symp. quant. Biol.* **XXXII,** 133-146.

HURVITZ, A. I. (1974). *In* "Current Veterinary Therapy" (Ed. R. W. Kirk), vol. V. W. B. Saunders, Philadelphia.

HURVITZ, A. I., KEHOE, J. M. and CAPRA, J. D. (1971). *J. Immun.* **107**, 648-654.

HURVITZ, A. I., MACEWEN, E. G., MIDDAUGH, C. R. and LITMAN, G. W. (1977). *J. Am. vet. med. Ass.* **170**, 511-513.

JAIN, N. C. (1975). *Canine Practice* **2**, 30-36.

KABAT, E. A., WU, T. T. and BILOFSKY, H. (1976). "Variable Regions of Immunoglobulin Chains", pp. 1-130. Bolt, Beranek, and Herman, Inc., Cambridge, Massachusetts.

KEHOE, J. M., TOMASI, T. B., ELLOUZ, F. and CAPRA, J. D. (1972). *J. Immun.* **109**, 59-64.

KEHOE, J. M. and CAPRA, J. D. (1972). *Proc. natn. Acad. Sci. U.S.A.* **8**, 2052-2055.

KROHN, K., MERO, M., OKSANEN, A. and SANDHOLM, M. (1971). *Am. J. Path.* **65**, 157-172.

LEWIS, R. M., HENRY, W. B., Jr., THORNTON, G. W. and GILMORE, C. E. (1963). Proc. 100th Ann. Mtg., AVMA, pp. 140-163.

LEWIS, R. M. and SCHWARTZ, R. S. (1971). *J. exp. Med.* **134**, 417-438.
McCLUSKEY, R. T. and KLASSEN, J. (1973). *New Engl. J. Med.* **288**, 564-570.
McCUMBER, L. J. and CAPRA, J. D. (1979). *Molec. Immun.* **16**, 565-570.
MESTECKY, J., ZIKAN, J. and BUTLER, W. T. (1971). Science, **171**, 1163-1165.
MIDDAUGH, C. R., GERBER-JENSEN, B., HURVITZ, A., PALUSZEK, A., SCHEFFEL, C. and LITMAN, G. W. (1978). *Proc. natn. Acad. Sci. U.S.A.* **75**, 3440-3444.
MILSTEIN, C. and SVASTI, J. (1971). *Prog. Immun.* **1**, 33.
O'DALY, J. A. and CEBRA, J. J. (1971). *Biochemistry,* **10**, 3843-3850.
PUTNAM, F. W., FLORENT, G., PAUL, C., SHINODA, T. and SHIMIZU, A. (1973). *Science,* **182**, 287-291.
QUIMBY, F. W., JENSON, C., NAWROCKI, D. and SCOLLIN, P. (1978). *Vet. Clin. N. Am.* **8**, 665.
RABBITS, T. H., MATTHYSSENS, G., and HAMLYN, P. H. (1980). *Nature,* **284**, 283-243.
REYNOLDS, H. Y. and JOHNSON, J. S. (1970). *J. Immun.* **105**, 608-703.
SCHULTZ, R. D. (1978). *Vet. Clin. N. Am.* **8**, 555-583.
SCHULTZ, R. D. and ADAMS, L. S. (1978). *Vet. Clin. N. Am.* **8**, 721-753.
THOMPSON, R. E. and REYNOLDS, H. Y. (1977). *J. Immun.* **118**, 323-329.
THOMPSON, R. E., REYNOLDS, H. Y. and WAXDAL, M. J. (1975). *Biochemistry,* **14,** 2853-2860.
TOMASI, T. B. and BIENENSTOCK, J. (1968). *Adv. Immun.* **9**, 1-96.
VAERMAN, J.-P. (1973). *Res. Immunobiol. Immunochem.* **3**, 91.
VRIESENDORP, H. M. (1979), *Adv. vet. Sci. Compar. Med.* **23**, 229-265.
WASSERMAN, R. L. and CAPRA, J. D. (1977), *Biochemistry,* **16**, 3160-3168.
WASSERMAN, R. L. and CAPRA, J. D. (1978a). *Immunochemistry,* **15**, 303-305.
WASSERMAN, R. L. and CAPRA, J. D. (1978b), *Science,* **200**, 1158-1161.
WATANABE, S., BORNIKOL, H. Y., HORN, J., BERTRAM, J. and HILSCHMANN, N. (1973). *Hoppe-Seyler's Z. physiol. Chem.* **354**, 1505-1510.

2 *Lymphocyte Locomotion, Lymphatic Tissues and Lymphocyte Circulation in the Rat**

A. O. ANDERSON, N. D. ANDERSON, and J. D. WHITE

I. Introduction

Gowans and his collaborators (1957, 1959) provided the first convincing evidence that lymphocytes constantly travel from the blood stream into lymphatic tissues and return to the circulation via major efferent lymphatics. Success of the rat model depended upon the availability of highly inbred strains (Heslop and Hardy, 1971), small animal surgical techniques for thoracic duct cannulation (Bollman *et al.*, 1948), and radionucleotide labeling methods for tracing tagged lymphocytes *in vivo* (Gowans, 1959). The phenomenon of recirculation is now regarded as representative of normal lymphocyte behavior in most mammals, including man.

Lymphocytes can be divided into two classes with distinctly different functions. In birds, cellular immunity is dependent upon thymus-derived lymphocytes, while humoral antibody responses are mediated by lymphocytes originating in the bursa of Fabricius (Glick, 1956). The analogue for the bursa has not been identified in other species, but it is generally believed that the liver and bone marrow serve this function in immature and adult mammals, respectively (Cooper *et al.*, 1973). This division of labor is not so rigid as originally believed. Miller (1962a, b) found that neonatal thymectomy in rodents impaired both cellular

*The views of the authors do not purport to reflect the positions of the Department of the Army or the Department of Defense.

and humoral responses, and infusions of thoracic duct lymphocytes or thymic grafts (Osoba and Miller, 1964) corrected these defects. The T cell contribution to humoral immunity was revealed by subsequent observations that both thymus and bone marrow cells were needed to restore humoral antibody responses in irradiated mice (Mitchell and Miller, 1968; Claman and Chaperon, 1969). The demonstration by karyotype analysis that Jerne plaque-forming cells from such mice were of bone marrow and not thymic origin (Nossal *et al.*, 1968b) promoted the concept that T cells played important "helper cell" functions in humoral immunity. It is currently believed that T cell help is required for most humoral antibody responses (Mitchison, 1971; Jacobson and Herzenberg, 1972; Herzenberg *et al.*, 1973; Kishimoto and Ishizaka, 1973), but some repeating-polymer antigens, such as pneumococcal polysaccharide, may directly stimulate B cells. T cell help is also believed to be important in the triggering and differentiation of cytotoxic T cells, nonspecific suppressor cells, and antigen-specific suppressor cells (Shevach, 1981).

Since soluble factors released by immunoregulatory cells can mediate amplification or suppression of immunity, it is not clear whether helper or suppressor T cells need to directly contact the respective effector cell in order to produce their effects. In the case of B cell responses, antigens are bound to the surfaces of specifically reactive cells via immunoglobulin molecules which are inserted in the membrane; such antigen-binding activity has been difficult to demonstrate for T cells. Apparently the T cell antigen receptor is not an immunoglobulin and is either secreted into the surrounding environment (Binz and Wigzell, 1975a, b) or is weakly held by the lymphocyte membrane. Since T cells depend heavily on Ia-antigen-bearing macrophages for antigen reactivity, it is possible that macrophages serve an antigen-binding role for T cells by nonspecifically absorbing onto their surfaces the released T cell receptor–antigen complexes as predicted by Feldman (1973) in his IgT model. Nonphagocytic dendritic (Steinman *et al.*, 1975; Stenman and Vaheri, 1978) and Langerhans cells (Katz, 1977) apparently serve this antigen-binding presentation role as well.

Indications of functional heterogeneity among the classes of lymphocytes and evidence that various kinds of cellular interactions were highly restricted contributed to rather than weakened the status of lymphocyte recirculation as an immunological phenomenon. Considering the tremendous diversity of antigens in the environment and the "one-cell one antigenic determinant" tenet of the clonal selection theory of immunity (Burnet, 1959), it is difficult to see how the appropriate cells would be in the same place at the same time as antigen without a dynamic process-like lymphocyte recirculation. This constant flux and sorting of immunocompetent lymphocytes guarantees that a significant portion of the total uncommitted lymphocyte population will traffic past antigen/macrophage depots in lymphatic tissues. Studies by Gowans (1959) and Ford (1969) indicate that the tempo of recirculation is sufficient to replace the blood pool of lymphocytes ten times daily and up to 20% of the lymphocytes in each lymph node in the same period. It was initially believed that only T cells recirculated but recent studies by Howard *et al.* (1972), Ford and Simmonds (1972), and Sprent (1977) have indicated that both T and B lymphocytes recirculate from blood to lymph; however, B cells incorporated ^{3}H-uridine less intensely than T cells; B cells transit lymphatic tissues more slowly than T cells. Radioautographic evidence of differential uptake of tritiated uridine by T and B cells has been useful in enumerating and tracing the migratory populations of these respective cells in lymphatic tissues (Howard *et al.*, 1972; Anderson and Reynolds, 1979). Human T cells also label more heavily than B cells, thereby contributing to the model characteristics of the rodent immune system for similar phenomena in humans.

Given these vital functions of recirculating lymphocytes in immunity, what mechanisms control the homing, emigration, and recirculation of immunocompetent cells *in vivo*? This chapter will attempt to answer this question by discussing: (a) factors which are intrinsic to the migrating cells, such as spontaneous locomotory behavior, cytoskeleton-mediated intrinsic motility, and ability to exhibit chemotaxis; (b) factors which control *in vivo* distribution, such as regional blood flow and cell-surface recognition phenomena; (c) effects of the development and differentiation of lymphocytes and lymphatic tissues on lymphocyte migration and distribution; and (d) mechanisms controlling the migration patterns and tissue distribution of lymphocytes in normal and antigenically stimulated adult lymphatic tissues.

II. Intrinsic migratory behavior of "recirculating" lymphocytes

It has been known for nearly 50 years that lymphocytes are motile cells which exhibit cycles of spontaneous movement interrupted by resting stages of variable length (Lewis, 1931). However, migration is executed by lymphocytes only with great difficulty because of a relative deficiency of the cytoplasmic machinery for locomotion (McCutcheon, 1946). The high nuclear:cytoplasmic ratio is probably responsible for

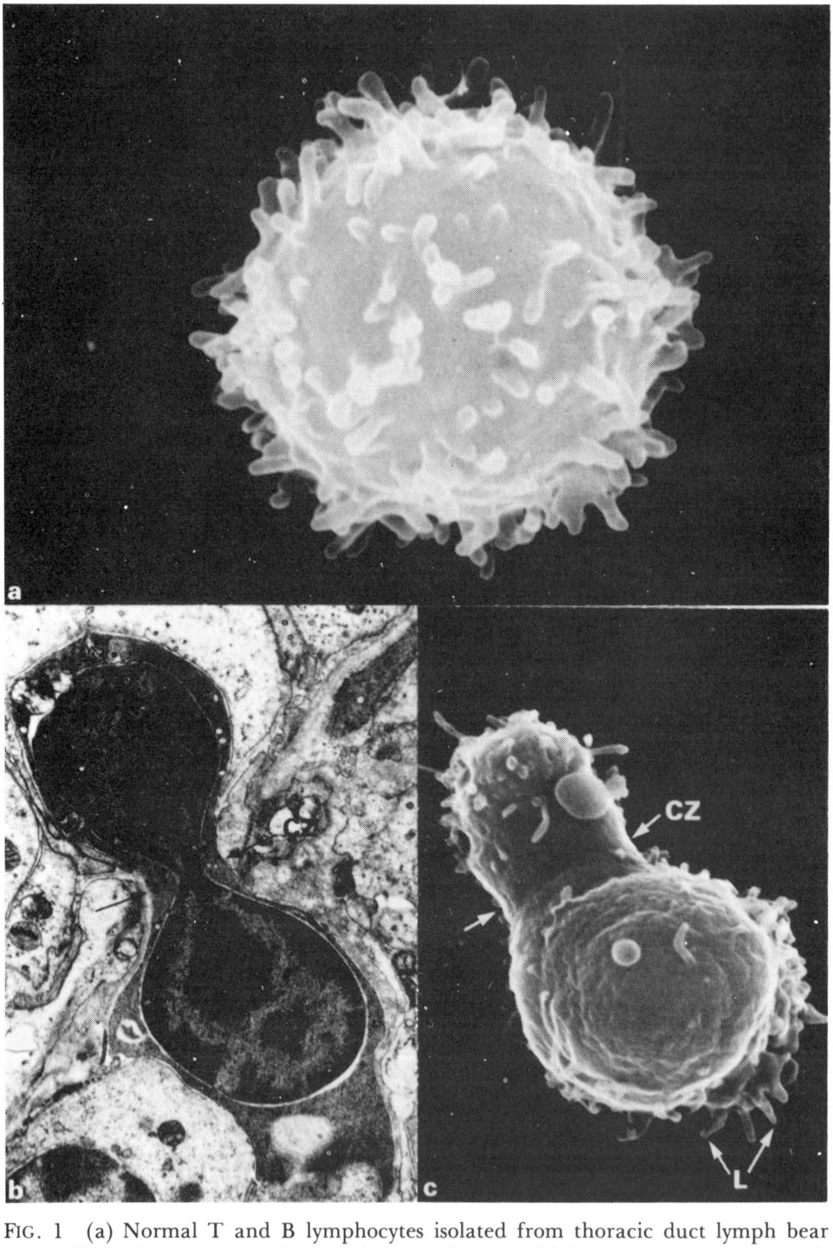

FIG. 1 (a) Normal T and B lymphocytes isolated from thoracic duct lymph bear microvilli on their surfaces. (b) and (c) Lymphocytes which are locomoting lose their microvilli over the zone of constriction (CZ) as lamellipodia (L) form anteriorly and microvilli cluster at the end of the uropod (arrow).

the characteristic morphology of locomoting lymphocytes observed by Lewis (1931), Harris (1954), and others. Resting lymphocytes isolated from thoracic duct lymph or peripheral blood are spherical cells with uniformly distributed microvilli on their surfaces (Fig. 1). Between 15·6 and 30% of these cells spontaneously move during 10 min of observation of coverslip preparations warmed to 37°C. As migration begins, the lymphocyte probes its surroundings by extending and retracting villous projections and lamellipodia. Adhesion of a lamellipodium to the substratum causes the cell to elongate into the characteristic "hand-mirror" shape with anterior nucleus and posterior uropod. The lymphocyte continuously extends lamellipodia anteriorly and appears to drag its uropod like a "ball and chain" as it contracts and relaxes through cycles of translocation. Waves of cytoskeletal contraction constrict the nucleus and squeeze it into the anterior end of the cell as each contraction propagates from front to rear. The constriction zone, which contains a circumferentially thickened sub-plasmalemmal microfilament network, remains stationary with respect to the substratum as the rest of the cell moves forward (Fig. 1). The cell surface overlying the constriction zone is devoid of microvilli when examined by scanning electron microscopy (Anderson *et al.*, 1979). Both T and B lymphocytes exhibit spontaneous motility, although rates of locomotion vary. Small T lymphocytes from thoracic duct lymph travel at a mean velocity of 11·9 μm min^{-1} while B cells move more slowly (5·3 μm min^{-1}), if at all. B cells appear to require some stimulation before they move. Exposure of B cells to anti-immunoglobulin induces capping, which is followed by translocation (Schreiner and Unanue, 1975). B cells also begin to move after they have been fondled by a migrating T cell. Blast cells of either class move faster than small lymphocytes, their average speed being 24 μm min^{-1}. While the migration characteristics of lymphocytes do not appear to be as great as those of neutrophils and monocytes, which move at rates between 30 and 70 μm min^{-1}, what movement lymphocytes can manage is obviously sufficient to transport these immumocompetent cells across the vascular barrier into the reticular meshworks and lymphatic channels of lymph nodes, Peyer's patches and spleen (Fig. 2). Global redistribution of ligands bound to surface receptors ("capping") is another manifestation of lymphocyte motility (Schreiner and Unanue, 1976). Most capping phenomena appear to involve participation of the cytoskeleton, protein synthesis and cellular respiration, since drugs which affect these activities inhibit capping. However, in rare instances, capping may also result from passive diffusion and aggregation of cross-linked receptors within the fluid

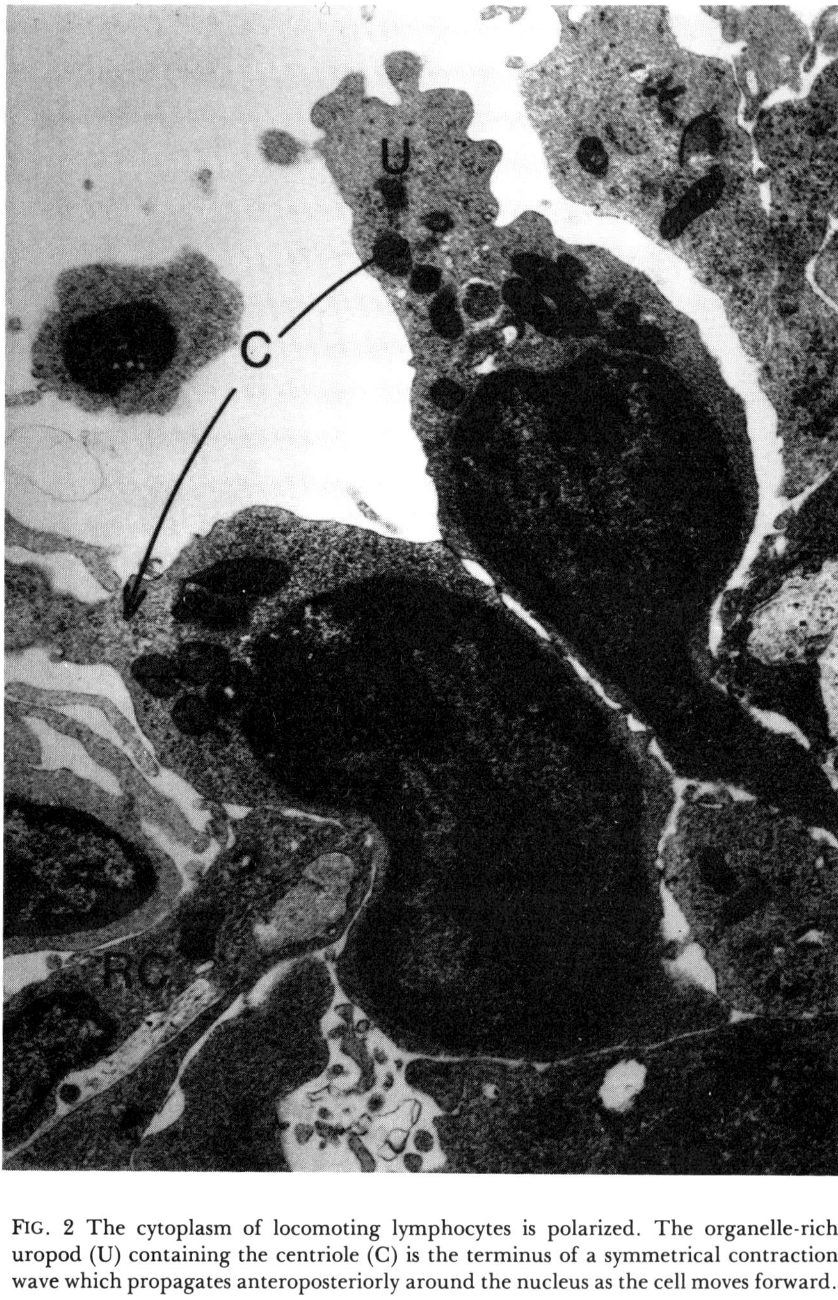

FIG. 2 The cytoplasm of locomoting lymphocytes is polarized. The organelle-rich uropod (U) containing the centriole (C) is the terminus of a symmetrical contraction wave which propagates anteroposteriorly around the nucleus as the cell moves forward.

membrane. The capping of membrane-associated immunoglobulin molecules by multivalent anti-immunoglobulin antibodies apparently is an inductive signal, which precipitates B cell locomotion, because it frequently is followed by translational movement. Regardless of whether the B cell caps or locomotes first, the anti-Ig cap is usually found at the end of the uropod of migrating cells. This is also true of the red cells stuck to locomoting human T cells, which had been incubated with sheep erythrocytes (Fig. 3). These phenomena suggest that oriented movement of surface receptors occurs from front to rear during locomotion. This is not necessarily true during all cases of capping, since certain ligands form caps which are not localized over

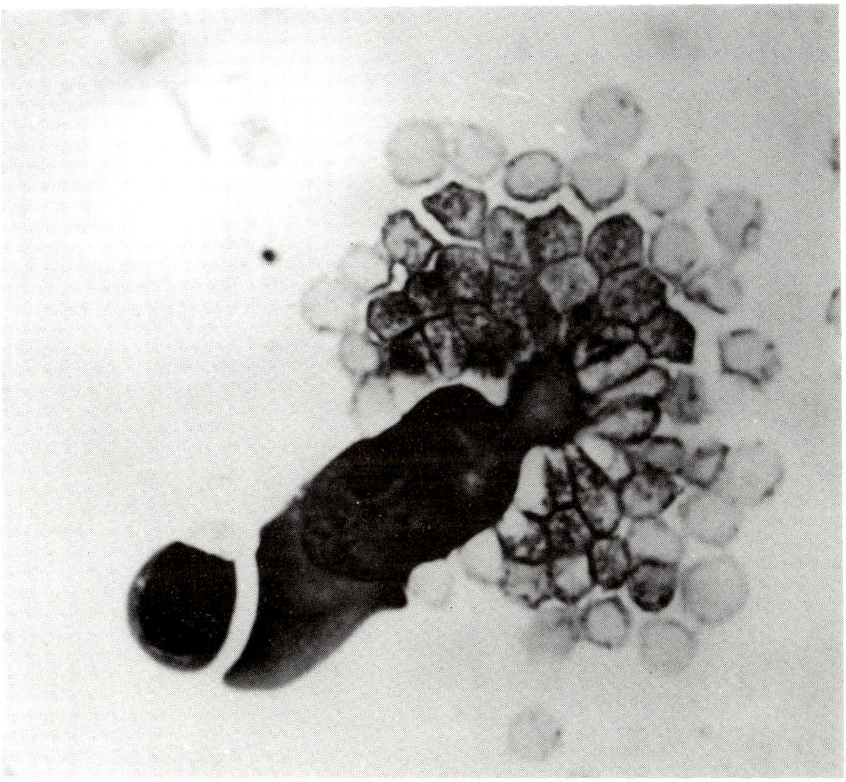

FIG. 3 Human lymphoblasts (generated during 7-day culture in 5% fetal calf serum) avidly bind and cap sheep erythrocytes (Michalski *et al.*, 1980).

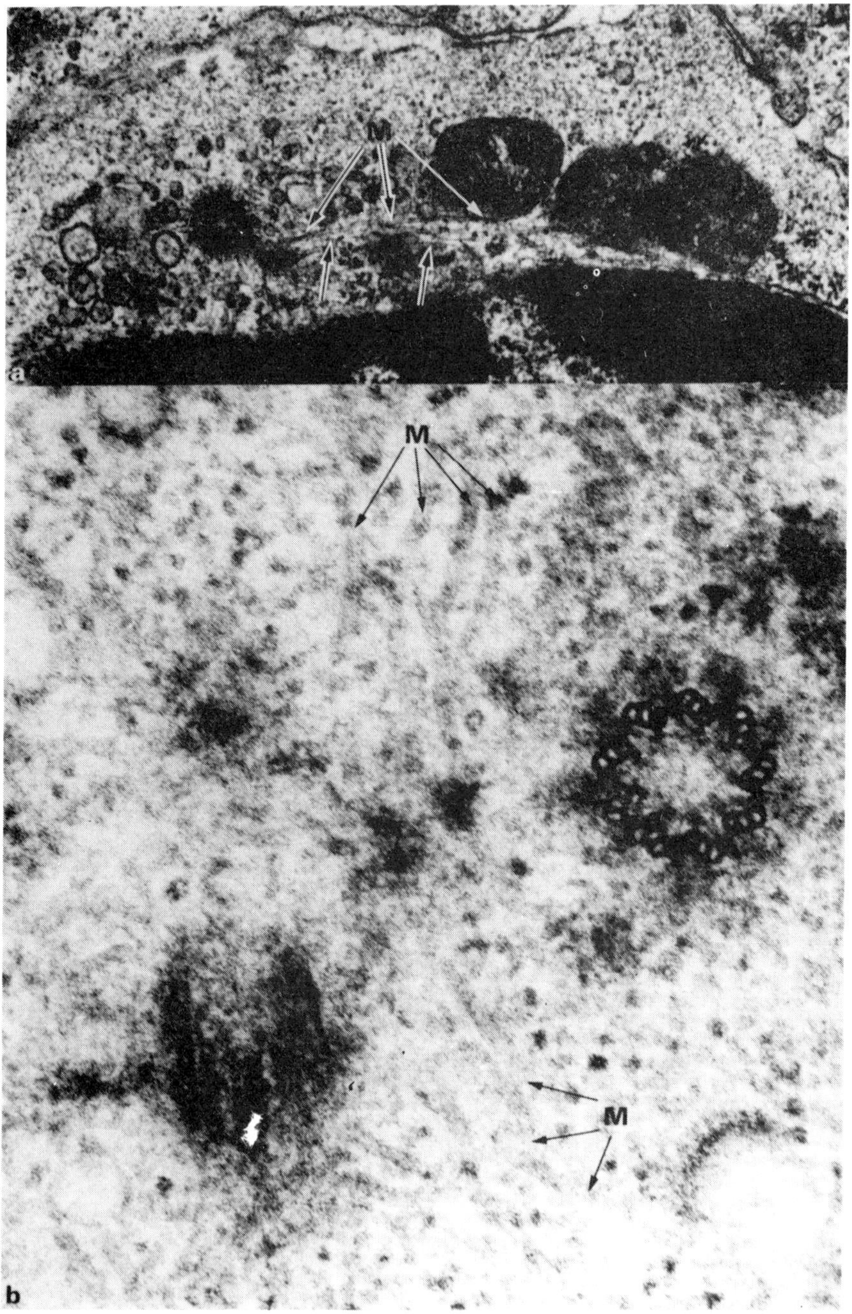
M
a
M
M
b

the centriole or Golgi zone of the cell. Since the centriole is always found in the uropod end of locomoting and capping lymphocytes, it is likely that this structure is responsible for the cytoplasmic and cytoskeletal polarization necessary for these motile functions. A primary cilium generated by the centriole appears to serve this orienting function in other types of eukaryotic cells. The organization of the lymphocyte cytoskeleton is still uncertain, but an umbrella-like network of microtubules (Fig. 4) may be seen radiating from the centriole around the nucleus toward the lamellipodia of lymphocytes which have become polarized prior to locomoting (Anderson *et al.*, 1978a, b). A network of 5-nm filaments forms a continuous mat beneath the plasmlemma and is arranged within the core of microvilli as longitudinally oriented fibers. Ten-nanometer filaments appear to extend anteriorly beside the microtubules and can be seen forming loops in the lamellipodia of motile cells. The complex interrelationships of these fibers during various biological activities remain to be determined.

The directed migration of leukocytes along a chemical gradient is generally accepted as playing an important *in vivo* role in regulating cellular traffic and promoting the accumulation of inflammatory cells at sites of tissue injury. Historically, lymphocytes were not regarded as being capable of chemotaxis, because of their erratic behavior in crude coverslip chambers (McCutcheon, 1946; Harris, 1954). Recent evidence indicates that mitogen-stimulated T lymphoblasts and some lines of transformed lymphocytes display chemotaxis toward casein hydrolysates, denatured albumin, endotoxin-activated serum, submitogenic doses of plant and microbial lectins (Russell *et al.*, 1975; O'Neill and Parrott, 1977; Wilkinson *et al.*, 1977). In addition, supernatants isolated from mixed lymphocyte cultures, mitogen-stimulated lymphocytes and activated macrophages have been said to evoke chemotaxis by spleen and lymph node cells (Ward *et al.*, 1971, 1977). Many of these studies were conducted in systems which cannot distinguish between chemotaxis (directed migration of cells which are oriented by a gradient) and chemikinesis (increased random migration which is greatest on the side facing the gradient), and each of these factors are equally chemoattractive to other leukocytes. Therefore, it is possible that true chemotaxis cannot be demonstrated using single-

FIG. 4 (a) and (b) Microtubules (M) and 10-nm filaments (arrows) radiate from the centriole, around the nucleus, in polarized lymphocytes. The thin section shown in (a) is oriented longitudinally from left to right, while (b) is a coronal section through the centriolar region.

parameter assays. Preliminary observations using a "three-chamber" agarose system (Anderson and Warren, 1979) suggest that thoracic duct lymphocytes (TDL) are inefficient in their ability to orient in a gradient of endotoxin-activated serum presented to them by diffusion

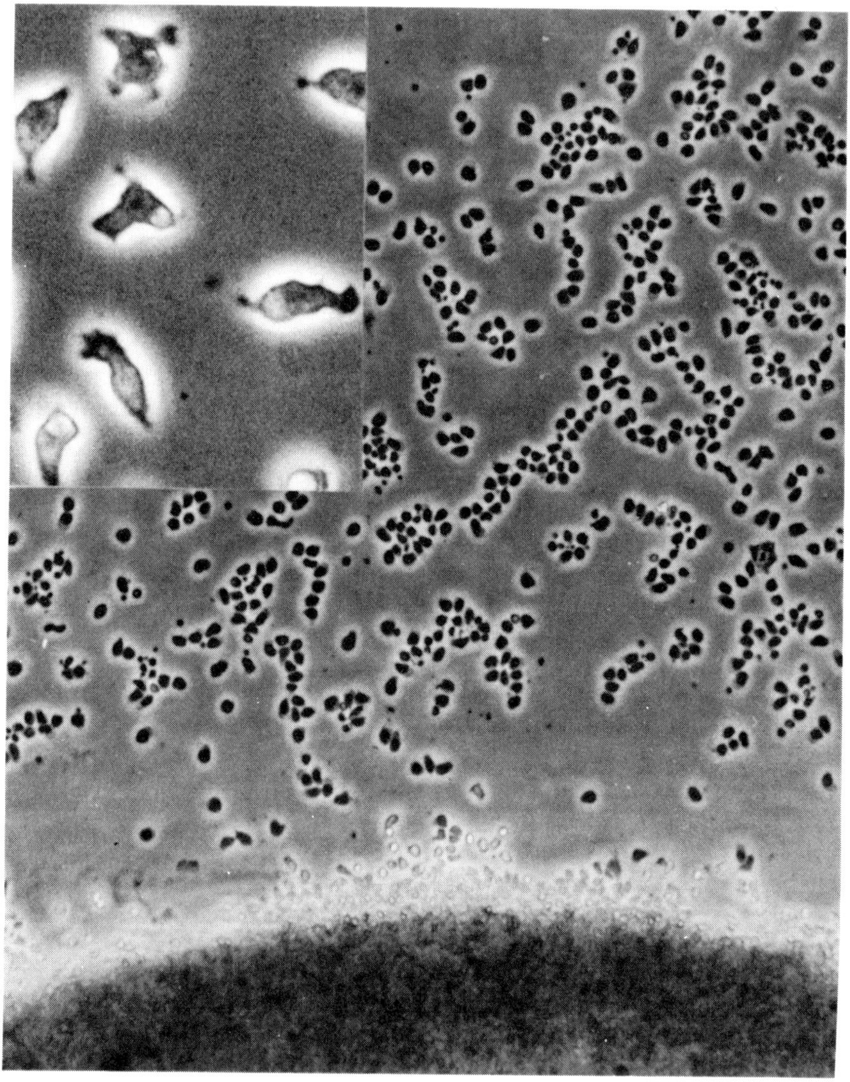

FIG. 5 Thoracic duct lymphocytes crawl beneath agarose for distances ranging from 80 to 60 μm during 18-24 hours' incubation at 37°C in 5% CO_2. *Insert:* high-power view of locomoting live lymphocytes.

through agarose. However, TDL populations show significant net orientation and directional migration toward such a gradient when compared to random migration controls (Fig. 5). Closer examination of the cellular interactions among these slightly heterogeneous populations indicates that T lymphocytes appear to be about as attracted to nearby B lymphocytes and small macrophages as they are to the artificial gradient (Anderson and Warren, 1980). This local interference in gradient-sensing by cellular chemotaxins is probably responsible for the highly erratic migration patterns of lymphocytes moving into chemotactic gradients (Fig. 6). Since directed lympho-

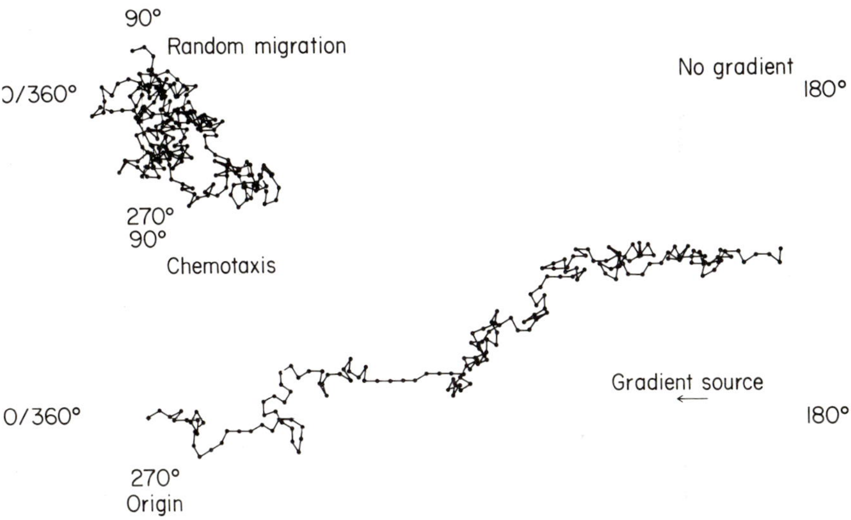

FIG. 6 Randomly migrating lymphocytes and lymphocytes which show directed movement toward a "chemotactic" gradient exhibit erratic migration paths. Lymphocytes are capable of correcting enough of the erroneous orientations to make progress toward a gradient of endotoxin-activated serum. The deviations in the course appear to be caused by locally released "factors" generated by the B cells and/or macrophages present in TDL. (Anderson and Warren, 1980.)

cytes frequently reverse or change orientations by 90° increments, while making net movement toward the gradient source, the chemotropism index for chemotaxing lymphocytes is 0·45-0·50. This is what one would expect of a randomly moving neutrophil. However, lymphocytes moving in the absence of a gradient, reverse direction so often that they fail to accumulate any net forward movement and produce chemotropism indices between 0·09 and 0·12. Further studies are needed to determine whether chemotaxis plays any role in regulating the characteristic traffic patterns displayed by lymphocytes *in vivo*. Specialized microvascular structures at lymphatic tissue/blood interfaces may have developed during evolution to compensate for the relative inability of lymphocytes to display efficient "goal-directed" forward movement. Diffusion of small quantities of factors produced by macrophages, antigens, immunoblasts and concentrations of other lymphocytes into vascular lumens may be all that is needed to provoke the emigration of a circulating lymphocyte. Once inside, other factors and interactions with other cells apparently determine its ultimate tissue distribution (Curtis and de Sousa, 1973).

III. Lymphocyte homing to HEV

It has been widely observed that the proportion of lymphocytes to other blood elements is incredibly high in the lumens of high endothelial venules of lymph nodes (Zimmerman, 1923; Schulze, 1925). Early anatomical studies attributed this accumulation to movement of lymphocytes generated in the node into the blood stream at these sites. However, numerous radiolabel tracer studies by Gowans and collaborators clearly indicated that the traffic was from blood to lymph. Since uridine strongly labels T cells but only weakly B cells, it is possible that some cells (perhaps a population which goes unlabeled) could migrate in opposite directions or return to the blood directly after a rapid sojourn in the connective tissue sheath of the HEV (Sainte-Marie and Sin, 1970). Other mechanisms were proposed to explain the accumulation of lymphocytes in HEV lumens, however. Schulze (1925) postulated that stagnation of blood flow produced by the sudden transition in vascular diameter as narrow capillaries emptied into wide HEV lumens could result in concentration of circulating lymphocytes within these venule lumens, while others concluded that lymphocytes in the circulation bumped into HEV endothelial cells which protruded into the lumen.

A. THE HOMING RECEPTOR

There seems to be little reason for doubting that slowing of venous flow through HEV might facilitate lymphocyte endothelial cell interactions, since lymph nodes contain a microvasculature which is capable of rather extreme changes in hemodynamics (Anderson *et al.*, 1975; Hay and Hobbs, 1977). Attempts to dislodge adherent lymphocytes by flushing with arterial perfusates revealed that 75% of the luminal lymphocytes remained attached to endothelial surfaces (Van Ewijk *et al.*, 1975; Anderson and Anderson, 1976). *In vivo* studies of leukocyte sticking in other vascular beds (Atherton and Born, 1972) indicated that luminal adhesion depends upon the net forces of cellular adhesion and hemodynamic shearing. Under these conditions accelerated blood flow through HEV might prevent homing, while sluggish flow might facilitate surface interactions. Since other blood leukocytes rarely are found adhering to HEV surfaces or emigrating across their walls, several investigators (Gowans and Knight, 1964; Marchesi and Gowans, 1964; Goldschneider and McGregor, 1968; Sordat *et al.*, 1971; Schoefl, 1972) suggested that selective movement of lymphocytes across these venules was dependent on cell-surface recognition mechanisms. Although HEV possess characteristic structural and metabolic features (Anderson *et al.*, 1976), none of these has been directly shown to regulate cellular traffic. However, scanning electron microscopy (SEM) studies demonstrated that the luminal surface of HEV was studded with shallow pits which morphologically resembled so-called "coated pits" on transmission electron microscopy (TEM) sections. While these structures might be seen on other vascular surfaces, their size and distribution on HEV were more prominent. Lymphocytes attached to these surface foci via microvilli which deeply indented the endothelial surface (Fig. 7, 8). Since EM preparations using mordants which preserved surface oligosaccharides revealed membrane specializations and electron-dense cross-bridging between lymphocyte and endothelial cell membranes, it is proposed that this represented some form of homing "receptor" complex. The presence of complementary surface receptors for homing on lymphocytes was first suggested by Gesner and Ginsburg (1964) and Woodruff and Gesner (1968), when they found that removal of membrane glycoproteins by *in vitro* trypsin digestion prevented treated lymphocytes from homing to HEV. Subsequent studies by Woodruff (1974) indicated that 24 h later these cells had resynthesized their receptors and thus were able to home normally to HEV. Reciprocal studies (Anderson and Anderson, 1976) where the lymph node microvasculature was perfused with 0·1% trypsin indicated that all adherent lymphocytes could be dislodged without affecting HEV surface coat or structural integrity. These studies did not take into consideration the cytoplasmic effects of external trypsin treatment (i.e. release of microfilament attachments to membrane by digestion of alpha actinin and "activation" of the cyclic AMP system by trypsin treatment); nevertheless, it seemed likely that both cellular recognition and attachment were dependent upon interactions between membrane glycoproteins on lymphocytes and endothelial cells. Perfusion studies also indicated that an EDTA-chelatable divalent cation was important in lymphocyte adhesion, possibly by forming cationic bridges between negatively charged carboxyl or sulfate groups on apposing membranes (Bangham, 1964). Since strongly anionic linear polymers, such as heparin or dextran

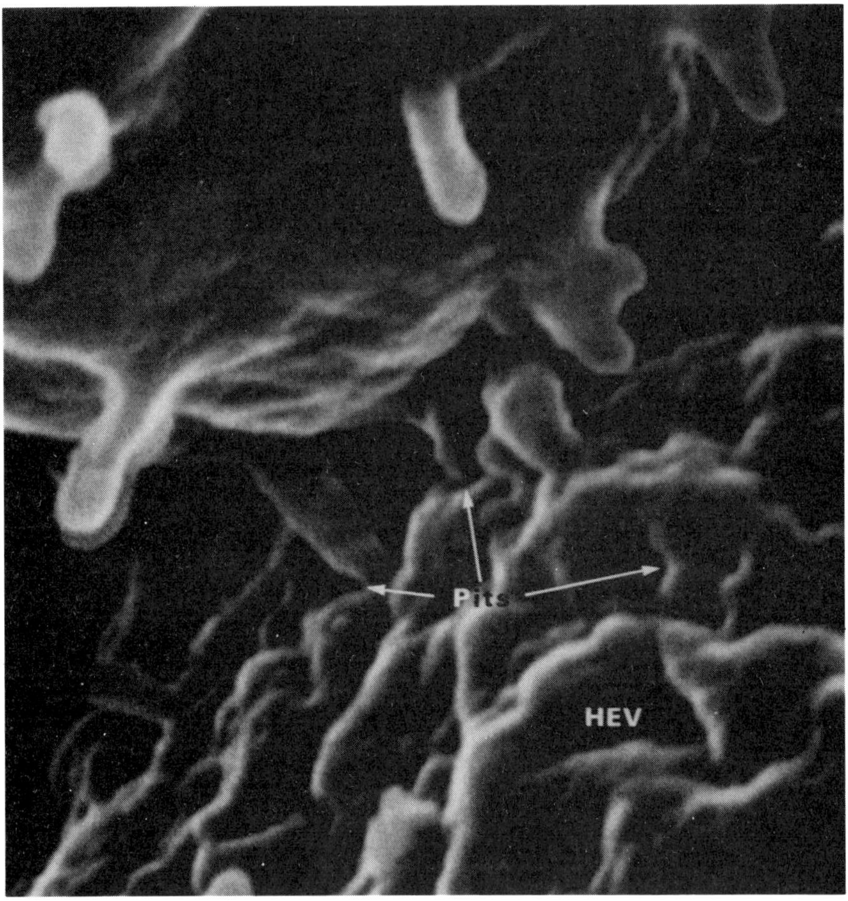

FIG. 7 In perfusion-fixed scanning electron microscopic preparations of lymph node high endothelial venules (HEV), lymphocytes remain adherent to endothelial surfaces via microvilli which interact with "pits" on the endothelial cells.

sulfate, appear to block lymphocyte homing without damaging these cells or resulting in sequestration in RE organs, it is possible that electrostatic linkages (Ford *et al.*, 1978) between "selective" oligosaccharide groups may be one mechanism for lymphocyte homing, but the issue remains open for the time being.

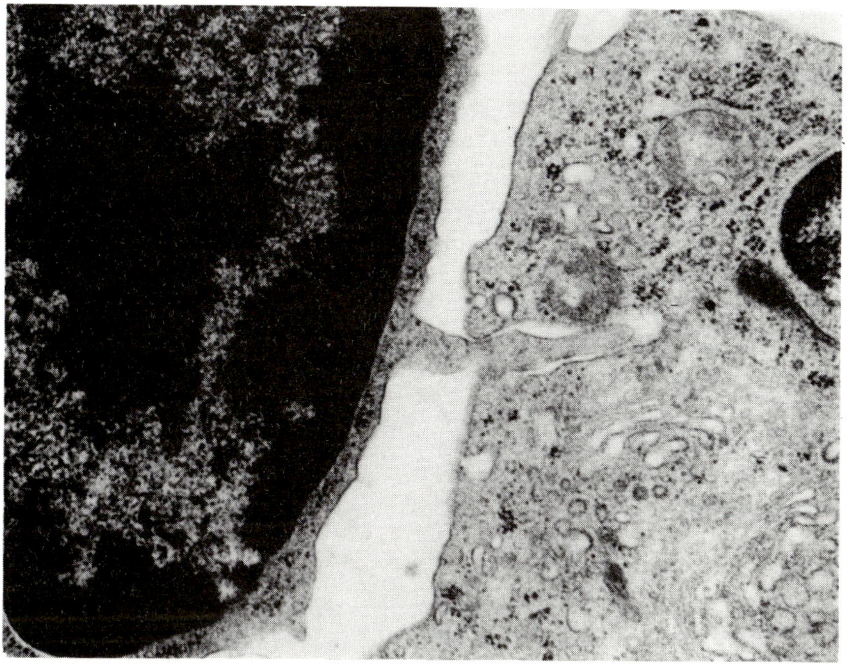

FIG. 8 Transmission electron microscopy studies indicate that this villus-pit interaction provides sufficient interdigitation to prevent the hydrodynamic shear forces of perfusates from dislodging the cells.

B. ROLE OF ACTIVE MOTILITY IN LYMPHOCYTE HOMING AND EMIGRATION *IN VIVO*

Recirculating lymphocytes emigrate from the blood into lymph nodes by selectively adhering to the endothelial surfaces of HEV and crossing the walls by active translocation. This process depends on the existence of membrane receptors for attachment to endothelium and on the capacity of the lymphocytes to propel themselves across HEV. Microfilaments and microtubules may be involved in both of these aspects of

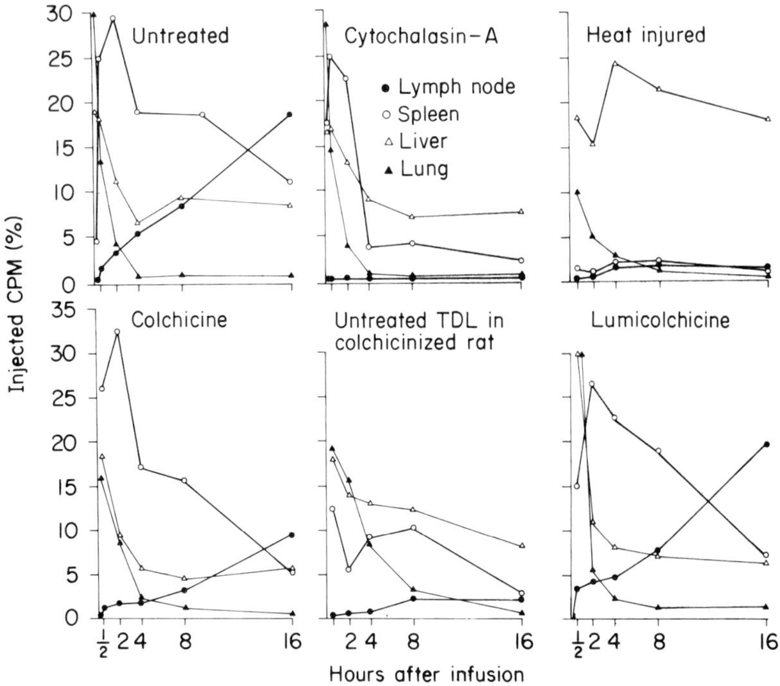

FIG. 9 There is a rapid accumulation of label in the lung, liver and spleen immediately after transfusion of 4 × 10^8 normal ^{3}H-uridine-labeled lymphocytes. The magnitude of initial accumulation of label is proportional to the percentage of the cardiac output flowing through each organ. The spleen normally skims off large numbers of lymphocytes within its blood-filtering reticulum and the cell accumulation naturally peaks early. The radioactivity in the spleen after 2 hours represents semi-selective migration of lymphocytes into the periarteriolar lymphatic sheath (PALS). Some lymphocytes are returned without ever coming into contact with the PALS. The progressive accumulation of label in lymph nodes is generally regarded as an indication of "selective emigration" from the blood. TDL treated with 4·0 μg ml^{-1} CA failed to accumulate in lymph nodes in appreciable numbers, and splenic uptake was also reduced. Liver uptake of CA-treated lymphocytes was not different from normal, which attested to the viability of CA-treated TDL. Heat-killed lymphocytes were sequestered in the liver by Kupfer cells at the expense of all other tissues. Lymphocytes treated with 10^{-4} M colchicine showed depressed accumulation in lymph nodes, which was signficantly reduced until 8 hours after infusion. When untreated TDL were infused into rats given intraperitoneal colchicine at 1·0 μg g^{-1} body weight, both lymph node and splenic uptake was depressed. In contrast, 10^{-4} M lumicolchicine-treated TDL migrated normally when infused into untreated rats.

emigration, since the receptors for homing may depend upon transmembrane linkages to cytoskeletal structures for clustering or distribution of these receptors on microvilli or in patches of specialized membrane, and receptor complexes may be transported through the membrane along the longitudinal axis of the cell during translocation. Doses of cytochalasin A and colchicine which disrupt lymphocyte microfilaments and microtubules were used in studies by Anderson *et al.* (1978a, b, 1979) to show that emigration was dependent upon a functional cytoskeleton (Fig. 9). Those studies provided additional information. Cytochalasin A (CA) clearly blocked lymphocyte locomotion without preventing homing. Despite the absence of microvilli, some of these treated lymphocytes recognized and attached to HEV surfaces via membrane segments associated with clusters of microfilaments which remained anchored to the inner leaflet of the membrane.

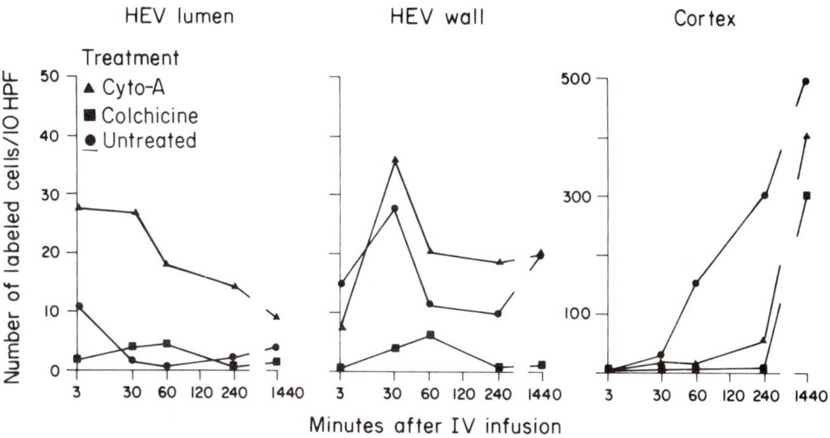

FIG. 10 Autoradiography of lymphocyte entry into lymph nodes after intravenous infusion was quantitated. Untreated TDL were rapidly cleared from the vascular lumen by 30 min post-infusion. Migrating labeled cells accumulated in the surrounding parenchyma in a nearly linear fashion. Lymphocytes treated with 4·0 $\mu g\ ml^{-1}$ CA persisted in significant numbers along luminal surfaces of HEV. Increases in interendothelial cells were also seen, and a small percentage of the CA-treated TDL gained access to the lymph node cortex. Lymphycytes treated with 10^{-4} M colchicine showed reduced luminal accumulation at 3 min post-infusion, failed to accumulate appreciably in the node parenchyma during the 4-hour study, and remained in the circulation.

Residual motility in cells treated with intermediate doses of CA resulted in eccentric and markedly distorted emigration morphologies by cells which bore similar aggregated filament-rich adhesion sites. Colchicine treatment resulted in accumulation of treated cells in the circulating blood, and these cells failed to stick to HEV surfaces in radioautographic studies (Fig. 10). Other studies of the effects of metabolic inhibitors and agents which activate cytoplasmic cyclic AMP lymphocyte homing and recirculation *in vivo* tended to support the above observations (Smith and Ford, 1979; Freitas and Bognacki, 1979).

C. GENETIC FACTORS IN LYMPHOCYTE HOMING AND RECIRCULATION

Genetic identity has long been known to be a basic requirement for successful cellular transfer of immunity (Landsteiner and Chase, 1942). This is apparently due to the requirement of identity of major histocompatibility gene-determined surface receptors for immune cells to cooperate for the production of antibody or cellular cytotoxicity (Katz, 1977). The early studies of lymphocyte recirculation were performed in inbred species as insurance against introducing artifacts caused by genetic differences, for examples, graft-versus-host or host-versus-graft phenomena. As a result of this precedent, almost all studies of lymphocyte recirculation have been performed using autologous lymphocytes or lymphocytes collected from snygeneic donors. A few recent studies compared the homing capacity of syngeneic and allogeneic lymphocytes and concluded that homing was impaired in allogeneic combinations (Heslop and Hardy, 1971). Later studies in mice (Viklický *et al.*, 1976) and sheep (Frost *et al.*, 1975) provided additional evidence that products of the major histocompatibility complex may be involved in lymphocyte homing to lymph nodes. Most recently, non-identity of both H-2K and H-2D determinants in mice were shown to significantly impair homing and localization of labeled lymphocytes in lymph nodes after intravenous infusion (Degos *et al.*, 1979; Viklický and Micková, 1979). In these genetic studies, congenic mice with identical H-2 determinants but different backgrounds and recombinant strains carrying different H-2 haplotypes on the same B10 background were used to obtain controlled, quantitative data about the genetic determinants controlling lymphocyte homing and accumulation in lymph nodes. They found that complete H-2 identity, or at least identity of the K and/or D region genes, would result in optimal homing regardless of whether these haplotypes were on the same or different backgrounds. I-region identity did not seem to be relevant unless it was in combination with at least a K or D identity. A problem in interpreting these observations is whether decreased lymph node homing resulted from the failure of allogeneic or semi-allogeneic lymphocytes to recognize lymph node homing sites or from elimination of these cells from the blood circulation by another mechanism, such as sequestration on RE cells in the liver or spleen. Because of the relatively small uptake of labeled lymphocytes in lymph nodes (12% of the injected dose in 24 h) compared to the combined uptake in the liver and spleen (30-35% of injected dose), a minor incremental increase in RE organ uptake would result in major deprivation of circulating cells available to enter lymph nodes. Degos *et al.* (1979) admitted that there was a large splenic and hepatic uptake, but did not show the data. Since T cell antigen receptors with specificity for foreign MHC determinants have been demonstrated in the serum of rats which have never been immunized (Binz and Wigzell, 1975a, b, 1976; Binz *et al.*, 1979), it is possible that a cellular immune phenomenon analogous to the humoral ABO blood group system may exist. If this is true, then the MHC non-identical lymphoid cells would bind the circulating T cell alloantigen receptor causing them to alter their homing characteristics either because their MHC-determined homing receptors are masked or because the homing receptor/T cell alloantigen receptor complex causes a new affinity for Ia-bearing RE cells in the liver and spleen. Feldmann (1973) proposed a mechanism for immune cell cooperation, where antigen-specific T cell receptor (he called it Ig-T) bound to macrophage surfaces after complexing with antigen and release from the T cell surface. In light of current knowledge of the T cell receptor for antigen, Feldmann's Ig-T, which had affinity for macrophage surfaces is identical to the T cell receptor removed from normal rat serum by anti-idiotypic immunoadsorbent columns (Binz *et al.*, 1979). There is also a possibility that preformed T cell alloantigen receptor might be directly injurious or might activate natural killer cell aggression toward the foreign cells, as indicated by data showing increased urinary excretion of ^{51}Cr label in recipients of labeled allogenic cells (McNeilage and Heslop, 1980). However, simple or multiple minor H-2 disparities (which could be sufficient to cause graft rejection) did not prevent homing as long as one or both K or D regions were identical. The K and D regions apparently code for surface molecules, which are important for antitumor or antiviral cellular cytotoxicity, where adhesion to the target cell is necessary for killing (Zinkernagel and Doherty, 1975). It may be that K and D region-determined molecules regulate high avidity cellular adhesion, and non-K- or non-D-determined molecules affect adhesion so minimally that differences in these genes are inconsequential. Studies of specific positive and specific negative selection of H-2 reactive cells (Wilson *et al.*, 1976) have taken advantage of the observation that allogeneic and/or alloreactive cells can be deleted from the recirculating pool by filtration through a recipient of the appropriate genetic composition (Howard and Wilson, 1974; Sprent and Miller, 1976). However, allogeneic and xenological lymphocytes show normal patterns of recirculation in thymus-less nude mice lacking auto-antiallotypic T cell receptors. These data suggest that MHC surface antigenic identity is a requirement for unimpeded recirculation in normal animals, but the defect in lymph node homing described by Degos *et al.* (1979) was due to depletion of homing cells from the circulation and not failure of these cells to recognize migration sites.

IV. Migration and differentiation of lymphocytes during development

Studies of the ontogeny of the immune system in rats and other animal models indicate that lymphocyte diversity results from proliferation and differentiation of precursor cells within various developing tissues; ultimately this differentiation continues during extrauterine life within the thymus, bone marrow and peripheral lymphatic tissues. The resultant immunocompetent cells are committed to a particular cell lineage and effector or regulator function which can be established by the phenotypic markers expressed on their membranes. Rat models are useful in studying the end-stages of ontogeny, since the development and population of peripheral lymphatic tissues occurs during the first three or four days after birth. The intrauterine development of primary lymphoid organs and populations of lymphocytes in rat fetuses parallels in much shorter time intervals the development of human lymphoid tissue, as indicated by the tissue studies of Bailey *et al.* (1975a, b).

A. T CELL DIFFERENTIATION AND MATURATION

In rat embryos pluripotential stem cells for erythrocytes and leukocytes are present in the yolk sac early in gestation. The stem cells for lymphocytes resemble large blast cells, but lack immunocompetence and typical lymphocyte surface markers. These cells migrate into hepatic sinusoids and produce lymphoid, myeloid and erythroid colonies. The liver remains the major site of fetal hemopoiesis until shortly before birth. Since venous blood returning from the placenta flows through the liver before being mixed with the circulating fetal blood, it is likely that developing lymphoid cells are exposed to maternal antigens, cells and antibodies which may have passed the placental barrier. The liver may thus be functioning as a bursal-equivalent, since the bursa of Fabricius also develops from yolk sac tissue, which is privy to environmental antigens crossing the shell of developing fowl eggs. Colonies of T cell precursors are programmed to display some T cell characteristics even before thymic development begins, since fetal liver cells stimulated by allogeneic lymphocytes will proliferate and express T cell surface markers.

The thymus develops fron endoderm derived from the third and part of the fourth branchial pouches and its epithelial cells differentiate under the inductive stimuli provided by mesenchymal components. Primitive T lymphocytes infiltrate the gland by wedging themselves between adjacent epithelial cells. Proliferation and entry of new precursors distend the interepithelial spaces, resulting in densely packed clusters of lymphoid cells surrounded by an epithelial cell reticulum linked together by desmosomes. Macrophages and macrophage-like cells also infiltrate the thymus; recent *in vitro* studies indicate that factors released by these cells also influence thymic cell maturation (Beller and Unanue, 1978; Oppenheim, 1981).

Following birth and continuing until long after sexual maturity, stem cells originating in the bone marrow, move through the blood stream, pass through the walls of blood vessels in the outer cortex of the thymus, and infiltrate the epithelial reticulum. These cells proliferate rapidly and exhibit population turnover times of 24-36 h. Many of these lymphocytes may die *in situ*, but they are endocytosed and degraded by parenchymal macrophages so quickly that morphological evidence of cell death in normal thymuses is difficult to demonstrate by light microscopy. The surviving cells leave the thymus by migrating across the corticomedullary junction and exit to the blood via post-capillary venules or pass directly into efferent lymphatics in interlobular septae. The emigrant cells then pass into the blood and seed peripheral lymphatic tissues, where they carry out the various T cell functions in immune responses. Recent studies indicate that short-lived thymic cortical cells preferentially accumulate in the spleen, while long-lived thymic medullary cells recirculate and accumulate in lymph nodes. Studies of cell-surface differentiation markers in mice indicate that the cells bearing these proteins have important functional differences. In mice, some marrow stem cells exhibit faint staining for the T cell specific Thy-1 (theta) antigen. These cells appear to be prepared for T cell differentiation, since mitogens or thymic factors can induce them to display the surface markers of mature T cells *in vitro*. The surface marker changes of these cells as they infiltrate the thymus include: (a) loss of surface TL (thymic-lymphoma) antigen; (b) secretion of addition Thy-1 surface antigens; and (c) acquisition of new differentiation antigens from the Ly system described by Cantor and Boyse (1972), which define additional functions of T cell subpopulations. About 50% of peripheral blood thymocytes express all three Ly antigens [$Ly^{(1+,2+,3+)}$]. These cells may be precursor cells which will differentiate into specific accessory T cells after exposure to antigens and/or help from T cells. T cells expressing the $Ly^{(1+)}$ determinant are long-lived and recirculate and function as helper cells for both humoral and cellular immune responses. The subpopulation of T cells excressing $Ly^{(2+,3+)}$ determinants function as suppressor cells and/or mediate cellular cytotoxicity against foreign target cells. $Ly^{(1+,2+,3+)}$ cells appear to be short-lived, since they rapidly disappear from the circulation after adult thymectomy; $Ly^{(1+)}$ and $Ly^{(2+,3+)}$ cells persist for relatively long periods.

Early studies indicated that the primary function of the thymus was to confer immunocompetence upon developing and peripheralized T cells (Miller, 1975); relatively recent studies suggest that this function is equally shared with the more important service of maintaining immunological tolerance to self-antigens and beneficial molecules which must be able to persist in the body, such as food substances en route to centers of bodily assimilation. This may be underscored by the relatively heavy traffic of $Ly^{(2+,3+)}$ suppressor cells to the Peyer's patches and perifollicular mantels of lymph node germinal follicles described by de Sousa *et al.* (1979).

B. B CELL DIFFERENTIATION AND MATURATION

The germ-line genes presumably carry the full complement of genes required for making every possible antibody, but due to random selection processes during early maturation each primordial B cell expresses only the very limited portion of this information required to react with a single antigenic determinant. B cell differentiation and proliferation begin in the liver and continue in the bone marrow as maturation continues. These lymphocytes contain cytoplasmic immunoglobulin, but for unknown reasons do not express this protein on their surfaces. Shortly before birth, lymphocytes with detectable surface IgM are present in bone marrow and this is followed by the appearance of other cells bearing IgD or both IgD and IgM on their surfaces. Thereafter, B cells bearing all the mature immunoglobulin isotypes can be detected and these cells proliferate and populate lymphatic tissues without maturing into plasma cells. The B cell system appears to be more susceptible to tolerance induction in the early phases of neonatal differentiation (Nossal, 1979). Moreover, the injection of antibodies directed against isotypic, allotypic or idiotypic immunoglobulin determinants can lead to long-lasting inactivation of antigen-reactivity of B cells bearing these proteins on their membranes. This tolerant state is readily produced when the maturing B cells express only IgM, and is more difficult to achieve after the IgD marker is expressed. Further, anti-immunoglobulin can induce idiotype-specific T-suppressor cells which may induce tolerance of another sort.

Studies of the life-span of T and B lymphocytes (Sprent and Basten, 1973; Sprent, 1977) suggest that B cells live shorter lives than T cells. This may actually be an artifact of the radiolabel methods used to quantitate the life span. B cells, or their progeny, may live on after antigen-induced proliferation which breaks the train and scores as a loss of ^{3}H-thymidine-bearing interphase B cells. If the life span of the average B cell is actually shorter, then a greater degree of antigen-independent proliferation must be present in order to maintain adequate numbers of clonal precursor cells to react with the 10^6-10^7 various antigenic specificities. The bone marrow most obviously serves this purpose; but is it also possible that germinal follicles dispersed among all the lymphoid tissues of the body might also function to turn out precursor progeny. Recent evidence suggests that this might be the case; but, environmental antigens may be the stimulus for the continued production of precursor B cells which require an additional hit by antigen and/or accessory cell factors for final proliferation, differentiation and maturation into antibody-secreting plasma cells (Cebra *et al.*, 1977).

C. DEVELOPING LYMPHATIC TISSUES

The peripheral lymphatic tissues of the rat complete their structural development and are populated by lymphocytes during the first few days of extrauterine life. Since certain microenvironments in these peripheral tissues apparently depend upon the cellular or hormonal contributions of the thymus, it is possible to impede the development of these regions in newborn rats and mice by removing the thymus immediately after birth (Parrott *et al.*, 1966). However, other structures in lymphatic tissues develop normally in the absence of a thymus, but thymus engraftment or infusion of thymic lymphyocytes restores the total tissue, thereby indicating that local mesenchymal structures are also vitally important in the formation of lymphatic tissue microenvironments.

1. *Lymph node*

The earliest lymph node to develop in the newborn rat is the mesenteric. Immediately after birth this node is a lymphatic sac lying near the neurovascular bundle in the mesentery. Reticular cells are present, but the sac is not yet partitioned into lymphatic sinusoidal spaces and reticulum. Development of lymphatic channels occurs first; by the second day a subcapsular sinus and some medullary sinuses appear. Lymphocytes are present in the peripheral blood, but none have entered the lymph nodes. Between days 2 and 3 the small venous vessels in the developing lymph nodes undergo proliferation and segments of vessel appear, which have plump endothelial cells capable of reacting positively in nonspecific esterase histochemical preparations. Concomitant with the development of these new vessels, small lymphocytes begin to populate the mesenteric lymph node. Diffuse lymphoid tissue lacking germinal follicles and plasma cell cords is present by day 7; by 14 days the lymph node appears almost fully formed. A network of nonbranching HEV can be seen deployed vertically between the subcapscular sinus and the hilum in lymph nodes perfused intraarterially with alcian blue dye (Fig. 11). By 12 weeks of age, most of the lymph nodes in the rat contain diffuse collections of lymphocytes, cords of plasma cells and germinal follicles.

2. *Spleen*

The architecture of the rat spleen is apparently more developed than the lymph node at birth. The red pulp reticulum is a functional RE filter and also maintains some extramedullary hematopoiesis. The white pulp is fairly well developed. The periarteriolar lymphatic sheath (PALS) is delimited from the red pulp by a marginal zone rich

FIG. 11 These are alcian blue dye perfusion preparations of lymph nodes from 7-day old (a) and 84-day old (b) rats. Note the relatively simple arrangement of blood vessels in (a) compared to (b). The adult rat lymph node has networks of HEV (arrows); germinal follicles (GF) interrupt the cortical vascular arcades (A) and the subcapsular lymphatic sinus (SCS).

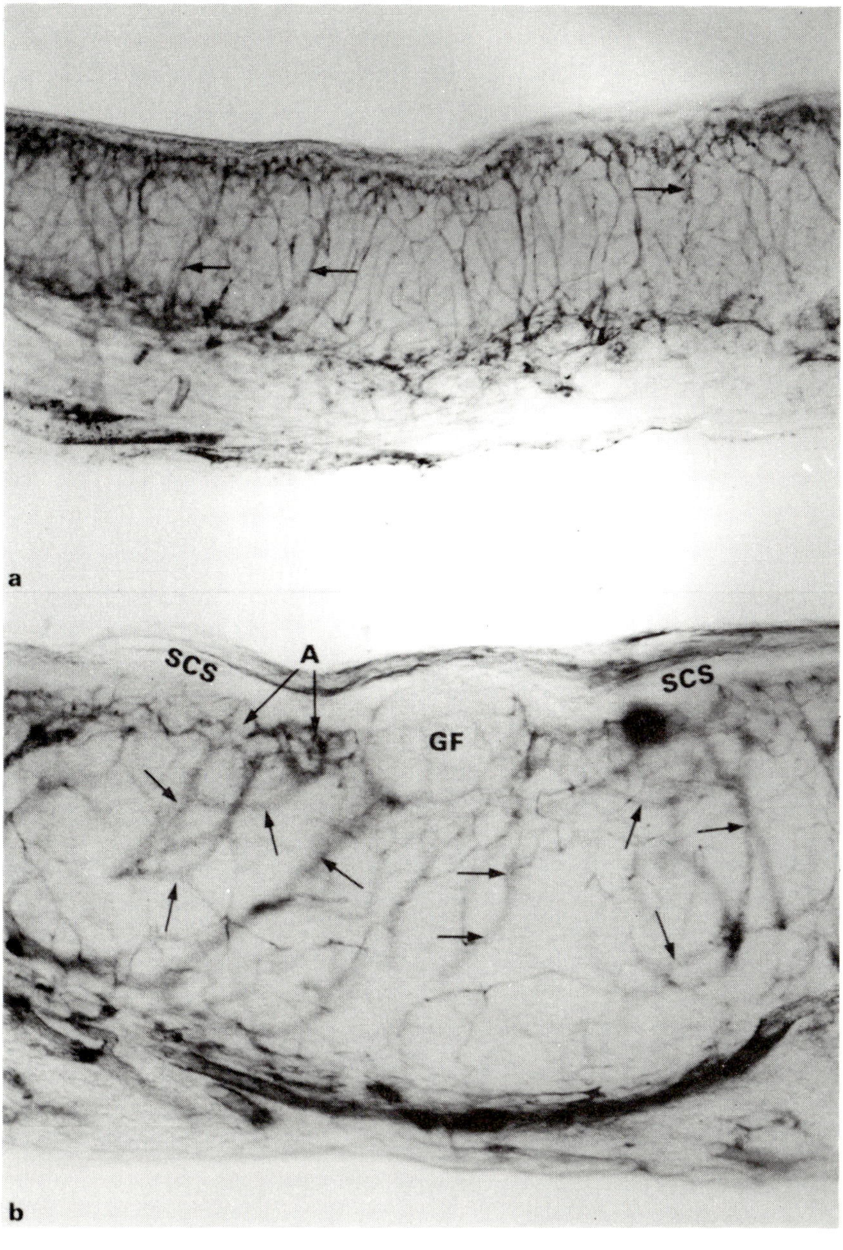
a
SCS
A
SCS
GF
b

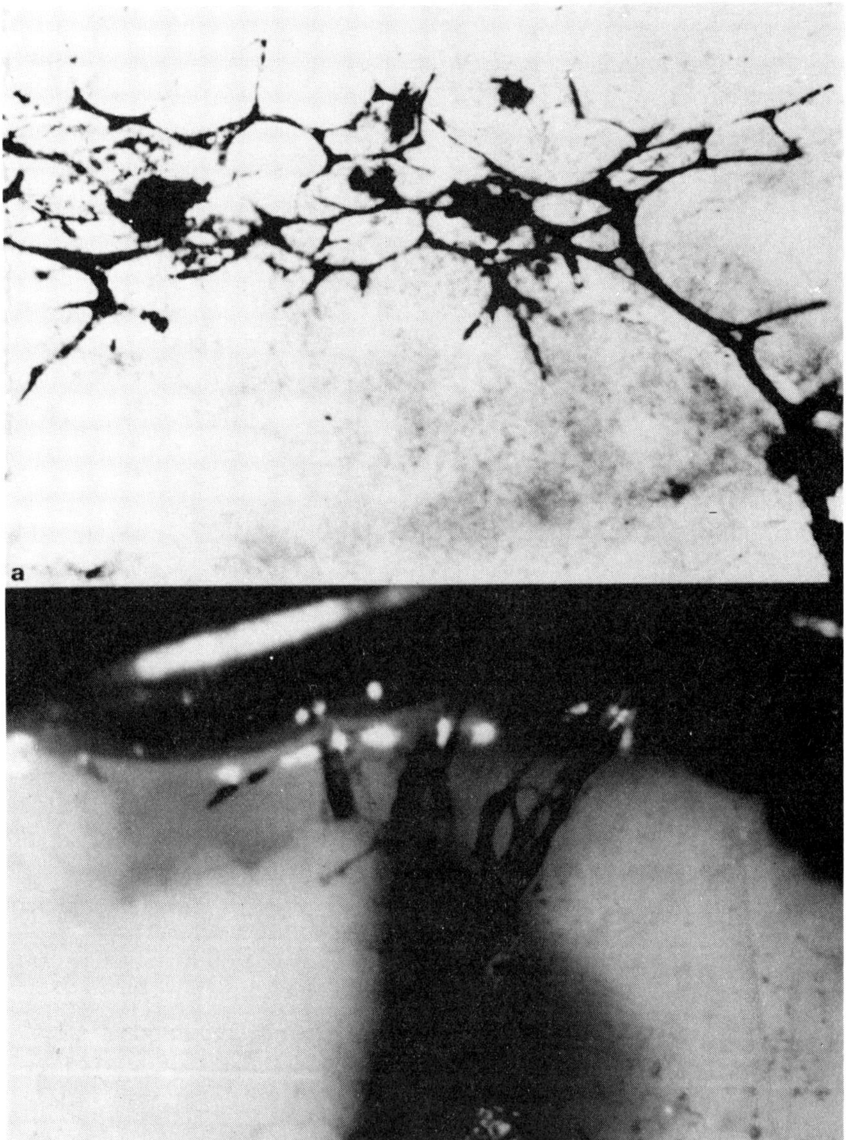

FIG. 12 Retrograde perfusion of the thoracic duct with India ink delineates the network of lymphatic channels present within (a) and draining from (b) the newborn rat spleen. These lymphatic channels connect PALS regions through anastomoses which are perpendicular to the PALS, similar to that described for the bridging zones of Mitchell (1973).

in esterase-positive moncytic cells. There are clusters of small lymphocytes in the periarteriolar lymphatic sheath; some cells can be seen lining up in what appear to be networks of lymphatic capillaries which bridge PALS regions in a "chicken wire" network. Retrograde infusions of India ink from the thoracic duct to the spleen parenchyma reveal these lymphatics (Fig. 12). The newborn rat spleen appears to be completely organized, with respect to the partitioning of lymphoid and red pulp tissues, by the end of the first week of extrauterine life.

3. *Peyer's patches*

Peyer's patches do not appear to be morphologically recognizable in the intestines of late fetal and newborn rats. However, Parrott (1976) has shown that an environment exists which subsequently becomes populated with lymphoid cells when these loops of intestine are grafted beneath the renal capsules of mature syngeneic rats. In addition, unpublished studies of Anderson and Anderson (1974) indicate that an epithelial and connective tissue site which is predestined to become a Peyer's patch exists in these immature rats. By retrograde infusion of

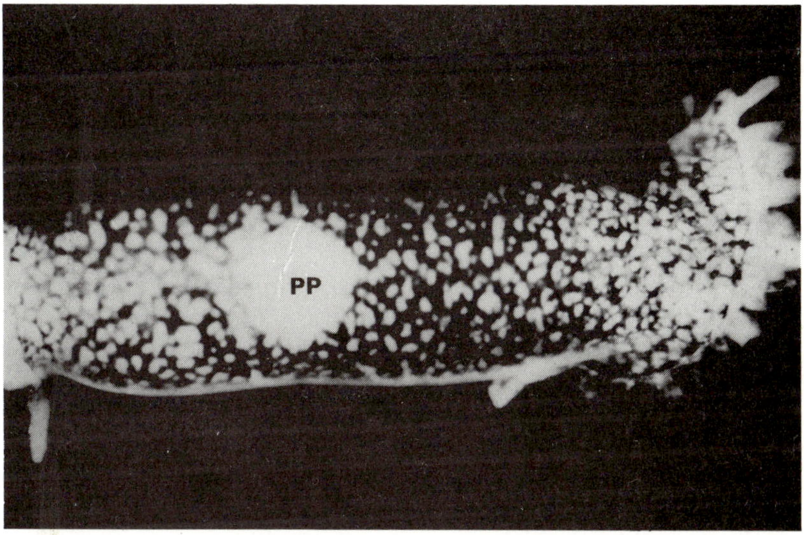

FIG. 13 The connective tissue stroma of the developing Peyer's patch (PP) excludes collateral lymph flow from the submucosal and subserosal lymphatic plexuses. When these spots are examined by electron microscopy, they are devoid of lymphocytes, but possess reticular meshworks and an overlying epithelium which is very endocytic.

India ink into the mesenteric lymphatics, nonstaining patches on the antimesenteric border of the intestine can be discerned because the ink blackens the subserosal lymphatic network up to, but not through, these sites (Fig. 13). Plastic, 1-nm thick sections and ultrastructural examination of these patches reveals that they lack germinal follicles and small lymphocytes, but contain reticular cells, lymphatic channels and an overlying epithelium, which exhibits extensive endocytic activity. Again, small lymphocytes do not begin to populate Peyer's patches until extrauterine day 2, when esterase-positive HEV develop. Germinal follicles begin to appear in Peyer's patches by days 14 to 28, which is paralleled by the population of the interfollicular areas with recirculating T cells.

V. Lymphatic tissues in the adult rat

The lymphatic tissues in adult rats may be grouped into central and peripheral lymphoid organs, as are found in most mammalian species. The central lymphoid organs, consisting of the bone marrow and the thymus, are where antigen-independent proliferation and differentiation of B and T lymphocytes continue into adult life. The peripheral lymphatic tissues include the lymph nodes, spleen and submucosal lymphoid nodules of the respiratory and gastrointestinal systems. While some antigen-independent lymphocyte development might occur in peripheral lymphoid tissue, most of this activity is usually related to antigen exposure.

A. CENTRAL LYMPHATIC TISSUES

1. *Bone marrow*

The bone marrow serves as a protected environment where lymphocyte precursors undergo the antigen-independent proliferative steps and genetic recombinations necessary for the continued generation of diverse repertoires of immune cells. The bone marrow's aggregate mass is about equal to that of the liver. It is a vascular organ composed of central and radiating venous sinuses which surround and separate wedge-shaped interstitial compartments containing hematopoietic cells. These compartments are separated from the vascular spaces by a thin endothelium, which forms an irregular sandwich with the adventitial cells of the interstitium. The granular basement membrane between endothelium and adventitia shares many morphological characteristics with reticular fibers found in peripheral lymphatic tissues. The adventitial cells face the hematopoietic areas and extend cytoplasmic processes into the cellular compartment. The white cell components generated within the interstitium traverse the sinus endothelium by actively migrating between endothelial and adventitial cells. Since the sinus endothelium is very attenuated, intravasating leukocytes might pass through parts of the endothelial cell cytoplasm, but this point is controversial. The sinus lining-cell complex is thought to bear some regulatory influence upon circulating leukocyte levels by controlling which cells enter the blood (Weiss, 1972). Apparently, only cells of sufficient maturity are capable of crossing this vascular barrier.

Lymphocytes and their precursors are usually scattered among the other hematopoietic cells, but occasionally are found in discrete nodules. Up to 20% of the nucleated cells in marrow may be lymphoid cells, but in hyperimmunized animals or following corticosteroid treatment, the marrow concentration of small lymphocytes is much higher. Macrophages are frequently found among clusters of rapidly dividing lymphocytes. These cells may encourage continued proliferation by removing effete or aberrant lymphocytes, and releasing recycled proteins and nucleic acids along with lymphocyte-activating factors (LAF).

2. *Thymus*

The thymus is a pale, lobulated organ which is largest, relative to total body weight, at birth. It gradually increases in size until sexual maturity, after which it involutes slowly. Each lobule is composed of a cortex and medulla. The densely populated cortex forms the periphery, while the more sparsely populated medulla branches to form the central portion of each lobule. Inside the cortex, large numbers of rapidly dividing lymphocytes form multicellular nests which stretch and distort the desmosome-linked epithelial cells into a honey-combed reticulum. These epithelial cells display major histocompatibility antigens, including Ia, H-2K and H-2D (Rouse *et al.*, 1979). The presence of these "self" antigens within the thymus may be an underlying microenvironmental feature responsible for self-tolerance and nonself-recognition by T cells.

a. *Special cells in the thymus*

At the corticomedullary junction, a thin basal lamina and specialized mesenchymal cells separate the cortical from the medullary lymphoid populations. Macrophages and interdigitating cells which resemble Langerhans' cells (Oláh *et al.*, 1975) are found within the epithelial stroma of the thymus. The macrophages contain large phagolysosomes filled with nuclear debris and periodic acid Schiff-positive membrane glycoproteins. These macrophages may also exert a stimulatory or differentiating effect on surrounding thymocytes by releasing LAF or other factors (Beller and Unanue, 1978). Thymic "nurse" cells derived from the epithelial reticular cells have also been isolated *in vitro* (Wekerle *et al.*, 1980). These large cells appear to encase clusters of proliferating and differentiating lymphocytes. Since they display Ia antigens, they may serve an instructive role in self-tolerance or self-recognition. "Special cells", with distinctive electron-lucent cytoplasm, striated cytoplasmic granules and multiple interdigitating extensions and processes, have been found at the corticomedullary border. These cells resemble novel dendritic cells of peripheral lymphatic tissues (Steinman *et al.*, 1975; Steinman and Witmer, 1978) and Ia antigen-bearing Langerhans' cells (Silberberg-Sinakin *et al.*, 1976; Stingl *et al.*, 1978), which have been shown to be effective presenters of skin-sensitizing antigens to T cells. Whether these corticomedullary "special cells" present antigen or tolerogen to maturing T cells, which migrate past *en route* to the medulla and the circulation, remains to be shown.

There are fewer lymphoid cells in the thymic medulla, which causes the epithelial cells to appear more polygonal and glandular. Some of these cells form concentric whorls and become keratinized. These unusual structures are called Hassel's corpuscles. Their function remains obscure, despite their distinctive appearance. Some morphologists feel that these structures provide for the destruction and turnover of epithelial reticular cells, since the centers of the Hassal's corpuscles frequently contain acid hydrolases.

b. *The blood-thymus barrier*

A blood-thymus barrier was initially proposed because of differences in immune responsiveness to antigens injected directly into the thymus versus intravenously (Marshall and White, 1961). Since intrathymic injection of antigen resulted in local development of germinal follicles and other structures associated with B cell immune responses, the differences in immune responsiveness observed after immunization by these routes could be attributed to changes in the thymic micro-environment, rather than a blood-thymus barrier. Horiuchi and Waksman (1968) used a different antigen, but a similar experimental design and found that intrathymic inoculation with antigen resulted in the induction of tolerance. This apparently contradictory result lead to reexamination of the blood-thymus barrier, since systemic antigens may produce subtle effects on thymus lymphoid populations.

A number of anatomical studies, which specifically addressed the question of blood vessel permeability within the thymus, showed that cortical thymocytes, in contrast to those of the medulla, are protected from circulating macromolecules (Chapman and Bopp, 1970; Raviola and Karnovsky, 1972). Blood vessels (Fig. 14) in the thymic cortex were

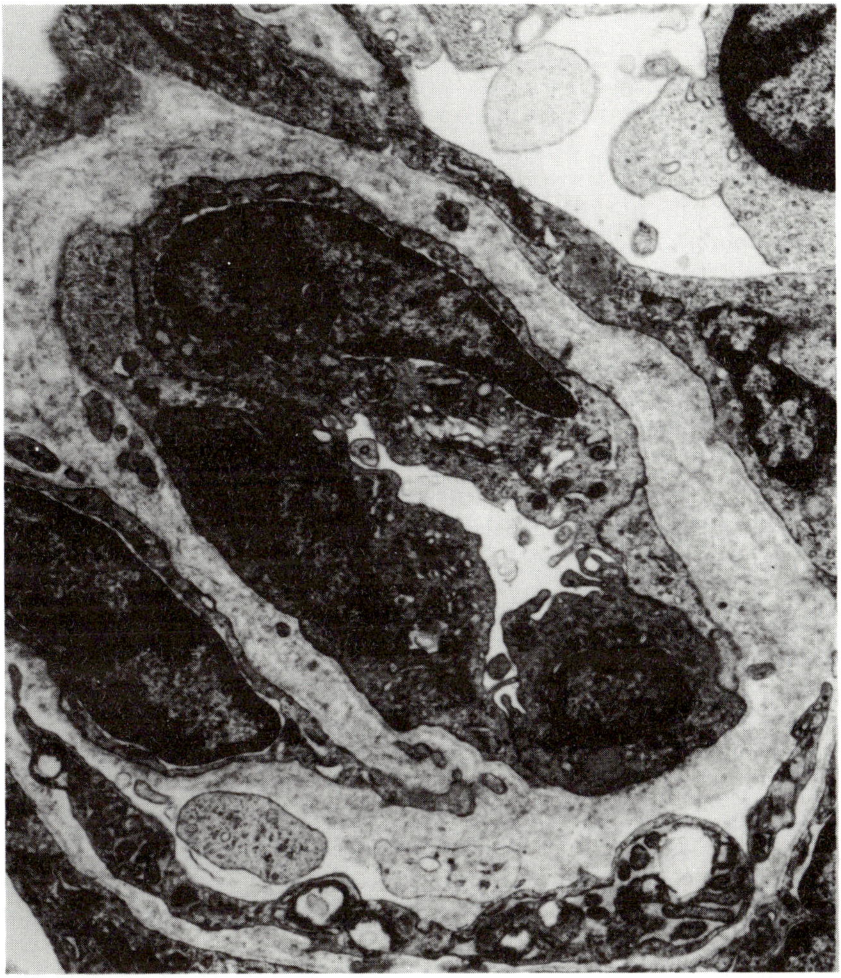

FIG. 14 This is a blood vessel located in the cortex of the thymus. Note the thick basement membrane and complex perivascular sheath.

not permeable to the physiologic tracers, but the postcapillary venules of the thymic medulla permitted tracers to leak along the clefts between migrating lymphocytes and endothelial cells. The tracers which crossed medullary venule walls had limited distribution in the thymic parenchyma because macrophages in the perivascular space ingest and retain much of the leaked tracer. The tissue distribution of the small amounts of antigenic tracer which escaped endocytosis was further limited to the medulla by the phagocytic cells and basal lamina at the corticomedullary border.

B. PERIPHERAL LYMPHOID ORGANS

The peripheral lymphoid organs are encapsulated and nonencapsulated reticular structures which provide sites for the interaction of immune cells with antigen by way of their afferent lymph and blood vascular connections and their constant access to circulating immunocompetent cells. Variations in the structure and location of these organized lymphatic tissues appear to represent specific adaptations, which assist the host in mobilizing immune responses against pathogens invading distant tissue sites, the blood stream and mucous membranes.

1. *Lymph nodes*

Lymph nodes are complex filters which interrupt the current of afferent lymph draining specific regions of the body. The lymph is forced to percolate through a reticulum containing lymphoid cells before gaining access to more recognizable efferent lymphatic channels.

Reticular cell meshworks provide a microenvironment which is conducive to: antigen trapping, adhesion and locomotion of lymphocytes and monocytes and dynamic sorting and functional grouping of cells which participate in immune responses. Reticular cells display fibronectin on their surfaces, which may contribute to establishing a lymphatic microenvironment (Stenman and Vaheri, 1978). Fibronectin is an important cell-surface glycoprotein which participates in such diverse processes as coagulation (Mosher, 1975), particle opsonization (Blumenstock *et al.*, 1978) and contact inhibition of proliferation and locomotion (Vaheri *et al.*, 1976). Reticular cells are said to be phagocytic, but they primarily provide anchoring sites for macrophages which do the bulk of the phagocytosis. These cells may selectively endocytose and recycle complex molecules secreted by

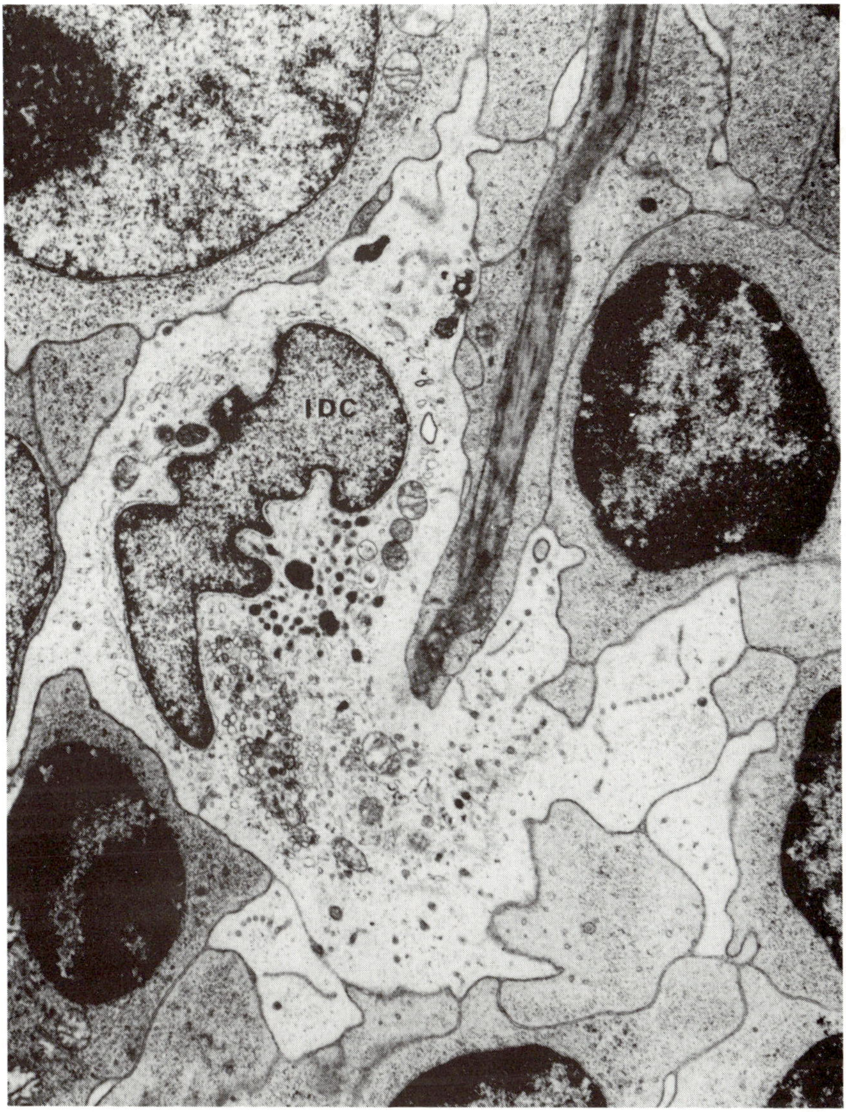

FIG. 15 This is an interdigitating (IDC), or novel dendritic cell (Steinman *et al.*, 1978) located in the paracortex of a rat lymph node. These cells are virtually identical in morphology to the "special cell" found in the corticomedullary junction of the thymus and is similar to descriptions of Langerhan's cells found in regional lymph nodes. They display Ia antigens on their surfaces and prime T cells for mixed lymphocyte reactivity.

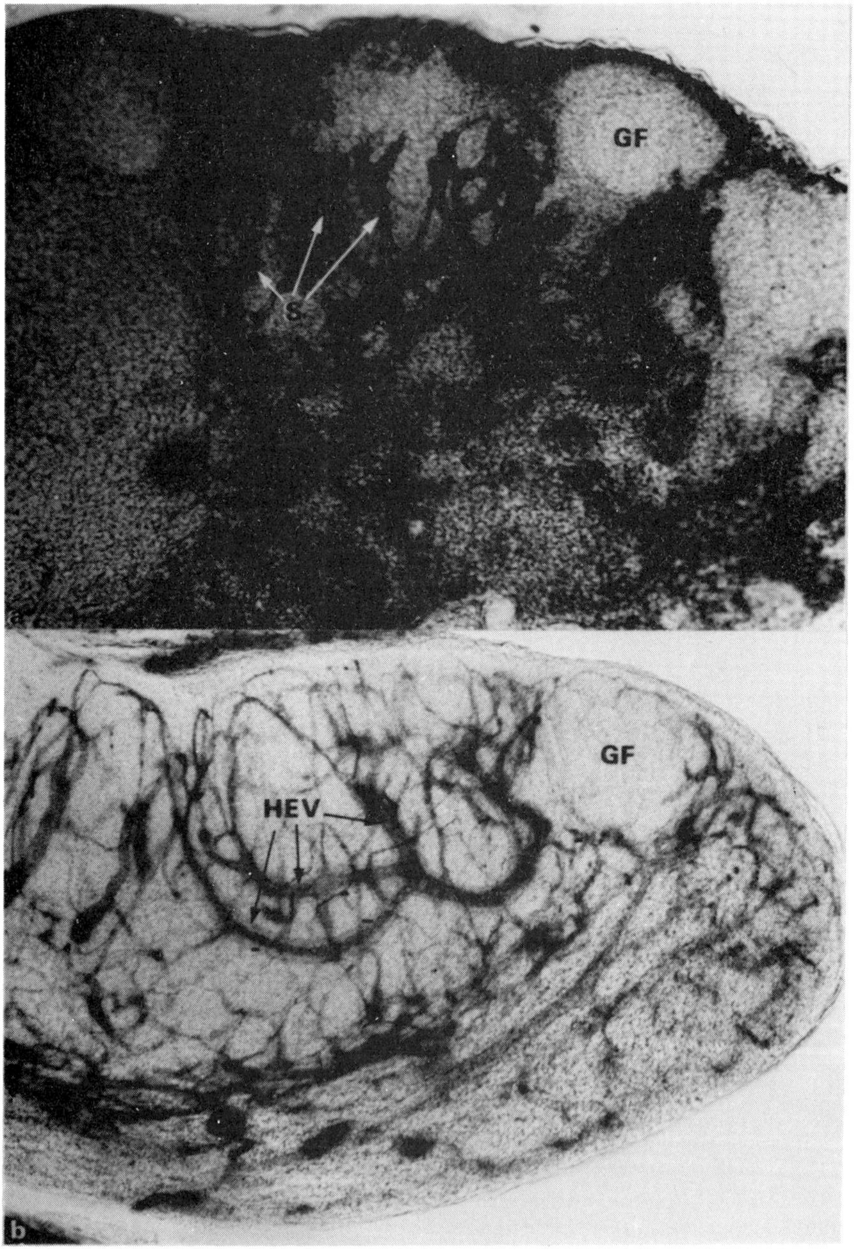

GF
S
a
GF
HEV
b

neighboring cells. This is illustrated by the observation that reticular cells engulf the heparin-rich stroma of secreted mast-cell granules (Fig. 17). The antigen-trapping function of these cells is related to the ability of meshworks of them to cause turbulence in lymph flow, which impacts particles against the surfaces of reticular cells and sinus macrophages. In addition, immunofluorescence studies indicate that immunoglobulins and antigens bind nonspecifically to reticular cell surfaces, possibly by utilizing intermediary molecules, such as heparin, fibronectin, and serum complement components.

a. *Passage of lymph through lymph nodes*

Afferent lymphatic vessels originate in delicate plexuses beneath the epithelium of the skin, gut and urogenital tract and within the connective tissues of all organs. These capillaries merge into larger lymphatics which drain into lymph nodes (Yoffey and Courtice, 1956). Efferent lymph from regional nodes may drain into one or two additional nodes before flowing into the large lymphatics which join the thoracic duct (from the lower part of the body) or the right lymphatic ducts (from the upper thorax and head). These major efferent ducts return lymph to the blood by emptying into the great veins at the base of the neck. The lymph nodes which are interspersed along this network of channels serve as filtering chambers and are constructed of a meshwork of reticular cells and fibers, macrophages and specialized blood vessels enclosed in a tough connective tissue sac. Since all lymph passes through at least one lymph node before returning to the blood, any environmental antigens, such as bacteria, viruses or virus proteins expressed on host cell membranes, protein antigens and tumor cells, will be trapped; under normal conditions these materials would not enter the blood. Any antigens which might escape lymph node entrapment will ultimately be removed from the blood by macrophages in the spleen, liver or bone marrow. Sophisticated tracer and EM studies were needed to show that subcapsular sinuses are connected to medullary sinuses by delicate plexuses of intermediary sinuses (Fig. 16), and by channels created by vertically

FIG. 16 (a) Lymph flowing into the subcapsular lymphatic sinuses of a lymph node via afferent lymphatics is broken up into anastomosing smaller networks of lymph channels as it passes through the paracortex. (b) These intermediary sinuses (S) surround HEV so that the lymph node interstitium between the blood and lymph interfaces need not be wider than 10 or 20 lymphocytes. This is vitally important to the immunological schema, since recently emigrated lymphocytes will lie in parenchyma, which is close to the antigen-carrying lymph stream. Note also that germinal follicles are neither highly vascular nor infiltrated by lymph.

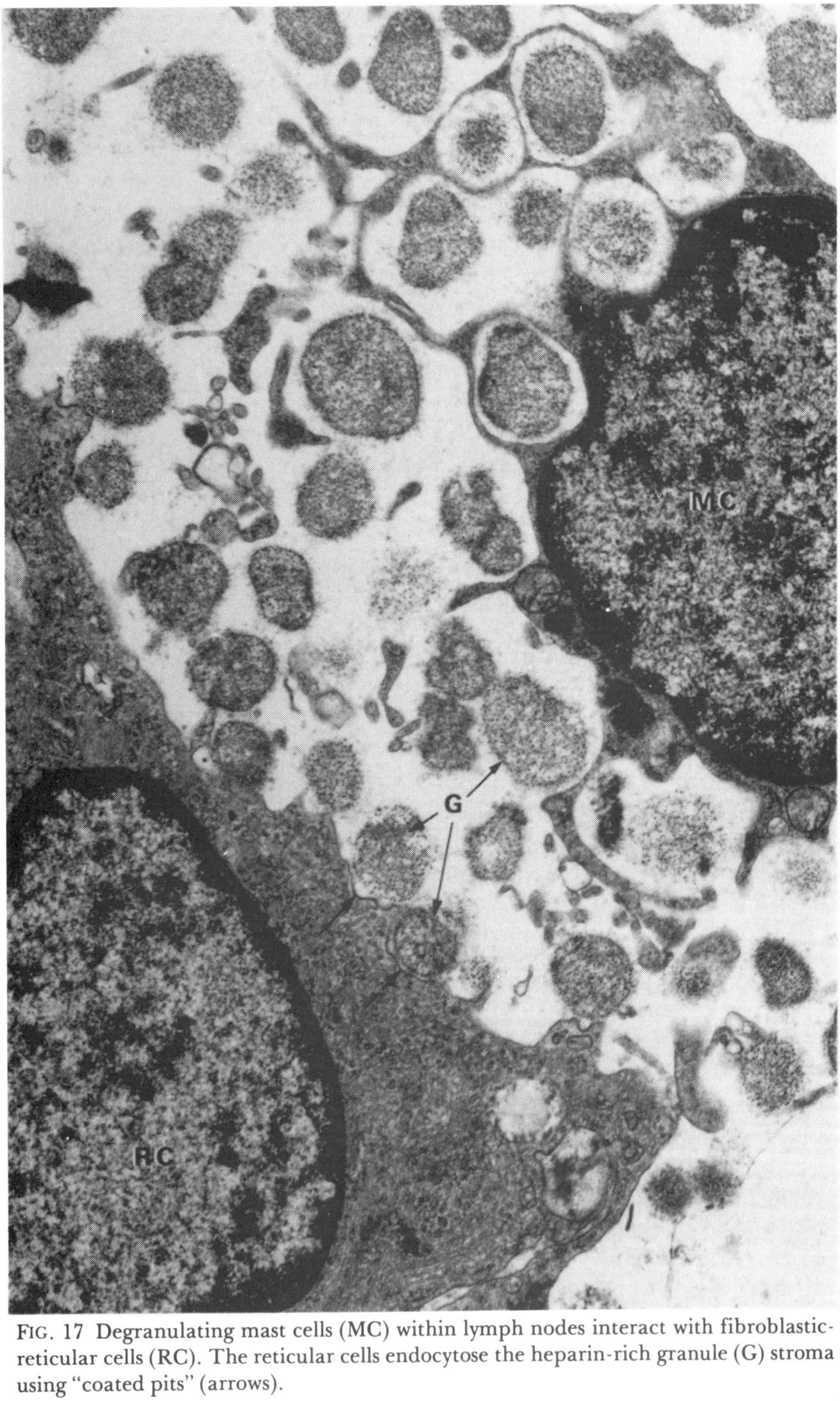

FIG. 17 Degranulating mast cells (MC) within lymph nodes interact with fibroblastic-reticular cells (RC). The reticular cells endocytose the heparin-rich granule (G) stroma using "coated pits" (arrows).

oriented reticular meshworks, which communicate with the floor of the subcapsular sinus through pores (Fig. 18). Macrophages cling to reticular cell processes inside lymph sinusoidal spaces. Antigens entering a lymph node for the first time will be bound to the surfaces of portal-guarding macrophages which endocytose most of the antigen, but leave some remaining on their surfaces (Nossal and

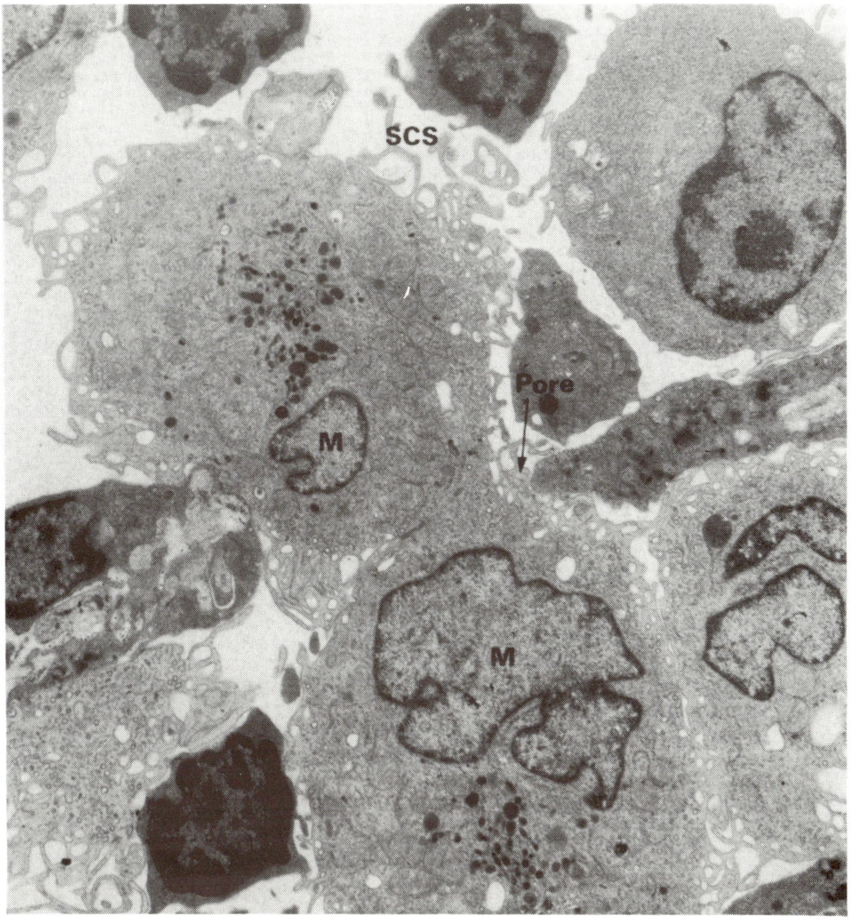

FIG. 18 Macrophages (M) guard every portal of lymphatic tissues. Here, two macrophages protrude through a pore in the floor of the lymph node subcapsular sinus (SC).

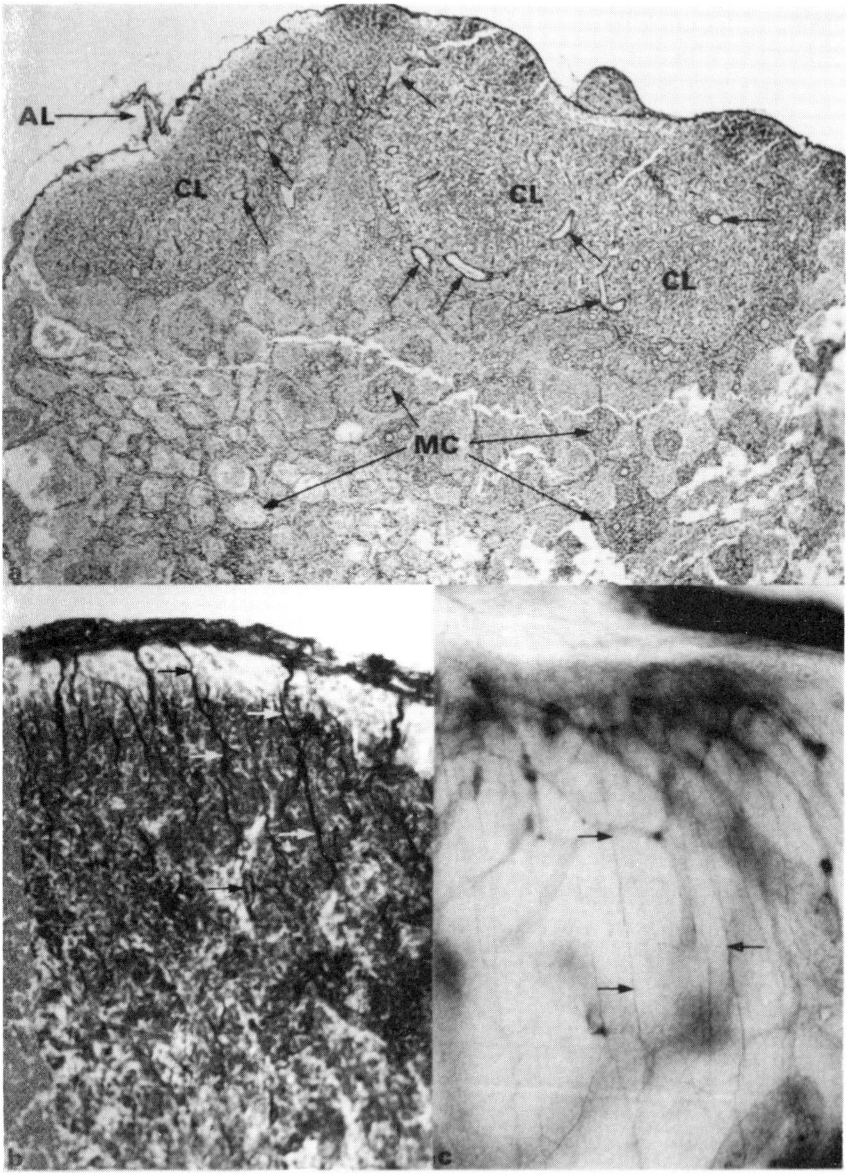

FIG. 19 The lobular architecture of the rat lymph node cortex is defined by the transitions in the organization of reticular cell meshworks at corticomedullary borders. (a) Silver impregnation methods reveal the dense meshwork of reticulum in cortical lobules (CL) and medullary cords (MC). Note how reticular fibers condense the

Ada, 1971). Reticular cells also bind antigen without phagocytosing. Langerhans' cells from epidermal skin sites (Stingl *et al.*, 1978) and/or novel interdigitating dendritic cells (Fig. 15) localize in the paracortex and serve an antigen-presenting role, which appears to affect T cells selectively. After 3 or 4 days, cytophilic antibody and complement facilitate binding of antigen by the dendritic cells within germinal follicles (Humphrey, 1976). Antigen remains bound to follicular dendritic cells for a fairly long period of time and the same antigen will bind to these cells with greater avidity on secondary exposure (Hanna and Szakal, 1968). The molecular mechanisms of antigen-binding during primary antigenic exposure may be related to natural antibody or to non-specific opsonins, such as fibronectin, displayed on macrophage and reticular cell surfaces or to absorption of inflammatory products, such as complement components, present in the antigen-containing afferent lymph (Pryjma and Humphrey, 1975). Antigen-binding after a secondary immune response is much more efficient, due to specific recognition provided by cytophilic antibodies bound to macrophage membranes at Fc receptors. The phagocytosis of antigens within the node may provide the antigen-processing and facilitate the macrophage helper functions for immune responses to thymus-dependent antigens.

b. *Lymph node structure*

Lymph nodes can be divided into cortex and medulla, based on the relative density of small lymphocytes. In large lymph nodes, cortical tissue is distributed as rounded lobules densely packed lymphocytes which are delimited on one side by the floor of the subcapsular sinus and on the other by the terminations of vertically oriented reticular fibers at the origins of medullary cords (Fig. 19). Germinal follicles in the superficial cortex partially interrupt the subcapsular sinus. These structures are generated by proliferating lymphocytes which displace the cortical reticulum to form a basket-like enclosure (Fig. 16). Inside the enclosure are lymphoblasts, intermediary lymphocytes, dendritic cells (Nossal *et al.*, 1968a, b) and "tingible-body" macrophages. On the outside is a mantel comprised almost entirely of small B

sheaths of HEV (arrows). (b) and (c) The parenchyma of cortical lobules is at a relatively uniform thickness (with respect to the subcapsular sinus) by vertically oriented fibers (arrows). In the rat, enlargement of the cortex induced by antigen usually results from lateral expansion of each lobule.

lymphocytes. Immunofluorescence (Weissman, 1975) and antibody-coated erythrocytes (Dukor *et al.*, 1970) delineate the follicular mantel as a B cell zone. The lymphocytes within the internodular areas and the deeper cortex are largely T cells (the thymus-dependent zone). Since both B and T cells enter the lymph node parenchyma by passing through the walls of specialized venules in the deep cortex, the thymus-dependent zone should be thought of as a transient-cell zone containing about the same proportions of T and B cells presented to it by the blood. In most cases, this is 75% T cells and 25% B cells, but antigenic stimulation (Gery *et al.*, 1977) or treatment with adjuvants (Anderson and Reynolds, 1979) can alter these ratios considerably by supplementing the normal cell traffic with additional T or B cells from the blood or from the injection site.

Beneath the cortex and filling all the spaces between cortical lobules of large lymph nodes is the medullary tissue composed of wide sinuses which surround cords of reticulum filled with antibody-forming B lymphocytes and plasma cells.

c. *Lymph node vasculature*

The circulatory system of the lymph node serves the special physiologic requirements of a tissue populated by transient cells with widely fluctuating metabolic activities which are capable of rapid changes in cellular traffic after antigenic stimulation. Recirculating cells depend on local blood flow, permeability and balances between vascular and tissue hydrostatic pressure for the capacity to settle onto surfaces and for the generation of diffusible chemotactic signals.

Arterial vessels enter lymph nodes at the hilus and branch once or twice as they cross into cortical lobules. These vessels give off capillary twigs and arteriovenous communications at arcades of capillaries in the superficial cortex and in medullary cords. Arteriovenous communications and short venules connect with vessels lined by large polygonal endothelial cells (Fig. 20(a)) called HEV.

The distal segments of HEV open into capacitance vessels with wide lumens and thin walls which drain segments of cortical lobules and merge to form lobular veins. At sites where these veins anastomose with each other and with the systemic circulation, muscular contractile structures are found which may serve to prevent dramatic intranodal circulatory changes from influencing the systemic blood flow (Fig. 20(b)).

Little information has been provided about vascular structures which regulate blood flow in regional lymphatic tissues. Generalizations about blood flow in lymph nodes were based on model systems

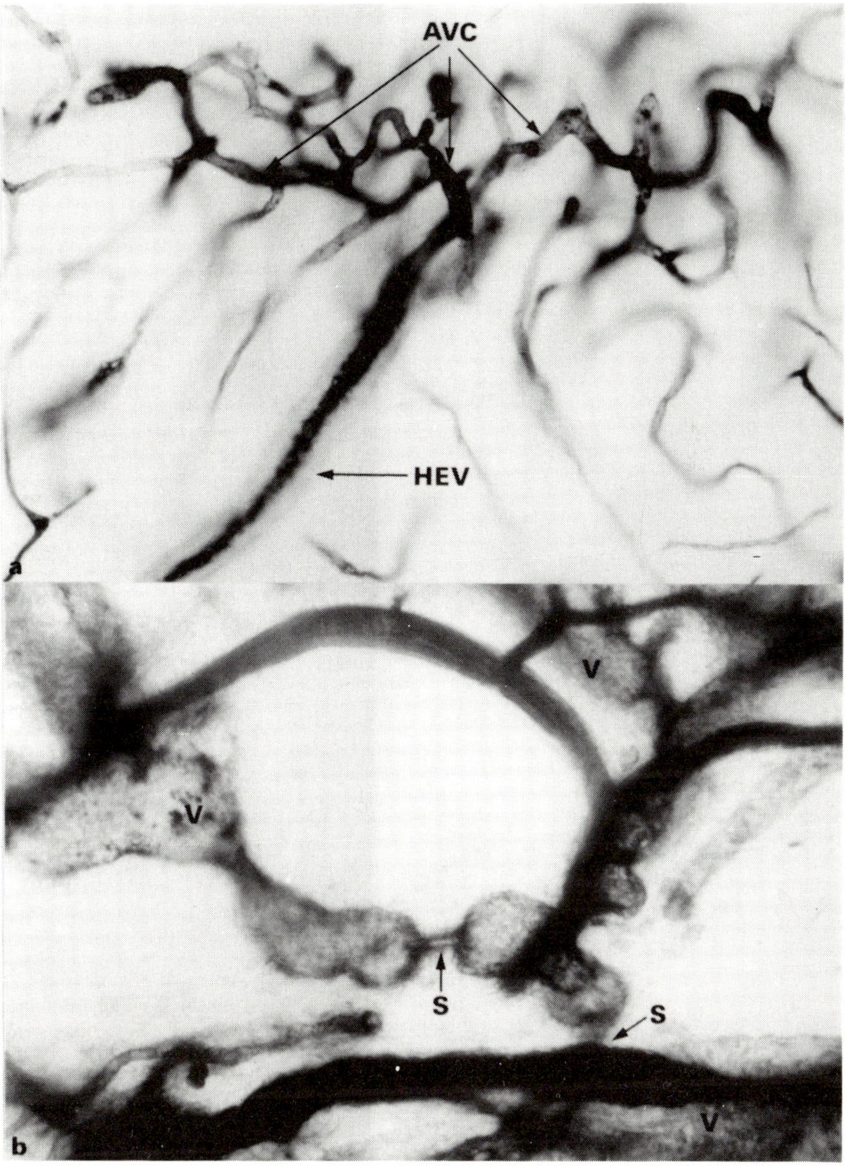

FIG. 20 These high magnification micrographs of an alcian blue preparation show the connections of arteriovenous communications (AVC) within the superficial cortex with a HEV (a) and venous sphincters (S) in lobular veins (V) located near the hilum (b).

where contraction of arterioles and precapillary sphincters regulated capillary flow (Calvert, 1897; Zimmerman, 1923; Schulze, 1925; Lundgren and Wallentin, 1964). Dabelow (1939) was the first to suggest that arteriovenous communications (AVC) were responsible for blood flow redistribution in lymph nodes, but he was unable to provide unequivocal anatomic demonstrations of arteriovenous anastomoses. Although some reports described AVC within mesenteric lymph nodes, these structures were not consistently found (Herman *et al.*, 1969;

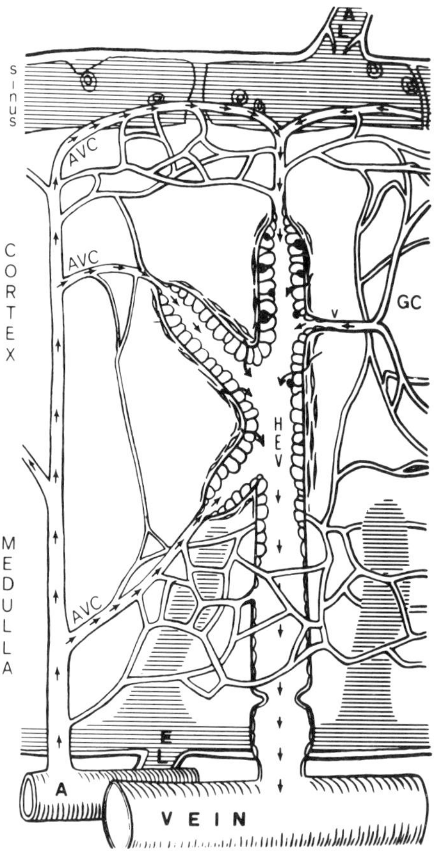

FIG. 21 The location of HEV between arteriovenous communications (AVC) and venous sphincters (VS) provides a unique system for regulating blood flow and pressure in lymph node venules. Afferent and efferent lymphatic connections are indicated by AL and EL and GC defines the displacement of AVC around germinal centers.

Davidson *et al.*, 1973). This difficulty in demonstrating AVC in routine perfusion preparations may be attributed to postexcisional constriction of the shunts (Baumel *et al.*, 1970). Direct intraarterial infusions with soluble alcian blue dye (Anderson and Anderson, 1975) demonstrated numerous AVC within the superficial cortex of axillary lymph nodes (Fig. 21). These vessels directly linked arterial circulation with HEV. Longitudinally deployed bundles of elastic tissue in the walls of the AVC permitted these vessels to remain intact during stretching and displacement by expanding germinal centers. The structure and distribution of AVC indicated that they participated in the shunting of blood past the cortical capillary arcades. Studies of regional blood flow through lymph nodes using double labeled 9- and 15-μm microspheres clearly demonstrated normally elevated arteriovenous shunting through nodal microvasculature, which increased dramatically along with total blood flow after antigenic stimulation (Herman *et al.*, 1978).

Little is known about the regulation of venous blood flow in lymph nodes. It is known from other systems that venous tone and segmented contraction or dilatation might influence efferent blood flow. In rat lymph nodes these types of control mechanisms would have to be located near the hilum, since HEV and lobular veins lack smooth muscle and their lumens are kept open by differences between vascular and tissue hydrostatic pressure. The existence of sphincteric structures, composed of circumferential bundles of smooth muscle, at terminal ends of thin-walled lobular veins suggested that the pressure and flow of efferent blood draining from individual cortical lobules could be regionally controlled. Lobular vein diameters ranging from 50 to 150 μm in "stimulated" lymph nodes indicated wide variability in the normal tone of those sphincters in a given node. These and other observations suggested that lobular vein/venous sphincter complexes serve as capacitance/resistance structures which accommodate the wide volume and pressure changes which occur within lymph node vessels.

Studies of circulation changes in stimulated lymph nodes have demonstrated a biphasic shift in blood flow following antigen inoculation. An early increase in flow up to 30 times normal is associated with hyperemic effects induced by antigen (Hay and Hobbs, 1977). This increased flow is also associated with increased shunting (Herman *et al.*, 1979) and increased lymphocyte traffic rates (Ottoway and Parrott, 1979). The gradual return to increased blood flow which occurs later in the response is thought to result from increased vascularity of the node. In morphological studies, this second phase of increased flow is associated with elongation and increased branching of the network of HEV; autoradiography (Fig. 22) following infusion of ^{3}H-thymidine revealed that the endothelial cells of HEV located nearest to primary follicles became labeled between 3 and 6 days

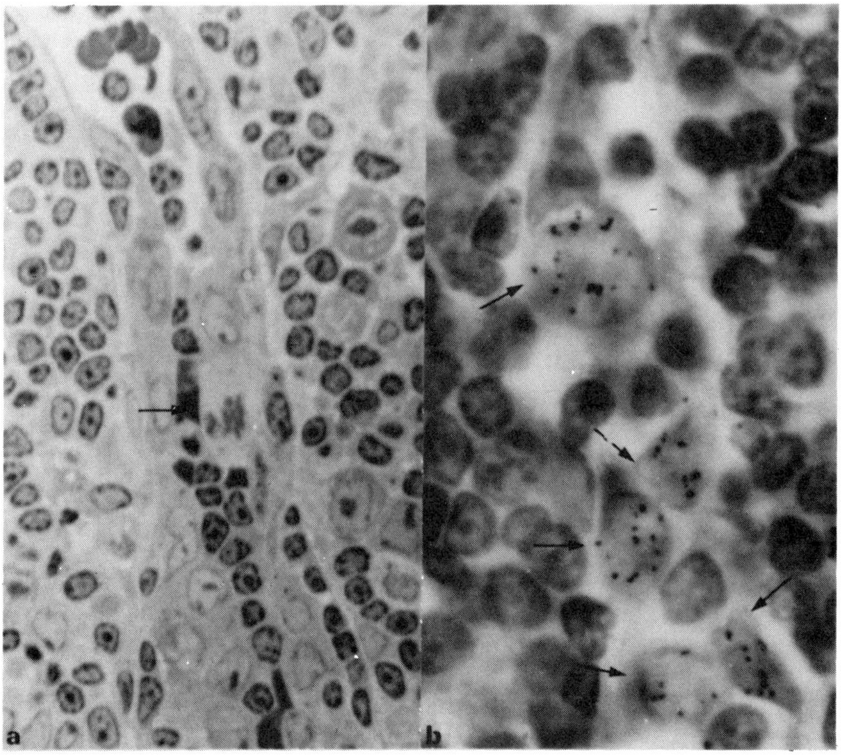

FIG. 22 Proliferation of high endothelial cells (arrows) in proximal segments of HEV 2 and 6 days after alloantigenic stimulation (Anderson *et al.*, 1975b). This endothelial proliferation was identified by appearance of mitotic figures (arrows) (a) and ^{3}H-thymidine incorporation (arrows) (b).

after alloantigenic stimulation (Anderson *et al.*, 1975). It is likely that these alterations in the microcirculation directly affect transvascular lymphocyte migration into antigen-stimulated lymph nodes initially by increasing the rate of migration across existing HEV and subsequently by enlarging the area of endothelium available for migration.

Several investigators proposed that HEV are specialized vascular units which regulate fluid and cellular exchange between lymphatic tissues and blood. Schulze (1925) described HEV as leaky vessels lined by an endothelium containing stomata for the passage of lymphocytes; Dabelow (1939) later demonstrated that HEV were not highly permeable to particulate dyes. He suggested that the plump endothelium of HEV permitted lymphocyte migration without extravasation because the soft endothelial cells would close around the contours of migrating lymphocytes, thereby permitting them to cross like "ships in canal locks" (Dabelow, 1939). This hypothesis was supported by numerous ultrastructural studies indicating intimate moulding of the highly plastic endothelial cells about lymphocytes migrating through intercellular pathways (Schoefl, 1972; Wenk *et al.*, 1974). Recent studies (Anderson *et al.*, 1976; Anderson and Anderson, 1976) suggested that the entire wall of HEV and their surrounding reticular cell sheaths should be regarded as a structural adaptation for controlling fluid and cellular transport. HEV endothelial cells are linked together by discontinuous macular junctional complexes. Lymphocytes may therefore migrate from blood to lymphatic tissue through potential spaces between adjacent endothelial cells. Since these junctional complexes are not broken by the transmigrating cells, the endothelial cell cytoplasm is displaced and moulded about them. As migrating lymphocytes crossed the basal lamina and entered the reticular cell sheath the HEV endothelial cells appeared to secrete new basal lamina to seal the gap. The overlapping plates of the reticular cell sheath were individually linked to structural members of the lymph node reticulum through anchoring filaments and cytoplasmic specializations analogous to those described in lymphatic capillaries by Leak and Burke (1968). This structure could provide additional valve-like functions which would be responsive to changes in intranodal tissue pressures. In nodes subjected to inflammatory stimuli, increased interstitial fluid pressure might cause these plates to separate and release a pulse of tissue fluid and macromolecules which would diffuse between the endothelial cells into the lumen. Such a mechanism permits the formation of an interendothelial "chemotactic" gradient which could induce lymphocytes to begin migrating into the node (Kelly *et al.*, 1972). Ultrastructural studies of the permeability of HEV suggest that this might occur (Anderson and Anderson, 1976), but other studies using slightly different methodologies concluded that HEV were generally leaky vessels (van Deurs *et al.*, 1976). Our study was conducted using Wistar/Furth rats, which are resistant to the altered permeability induced by horseradish peroxidase (HRP), which

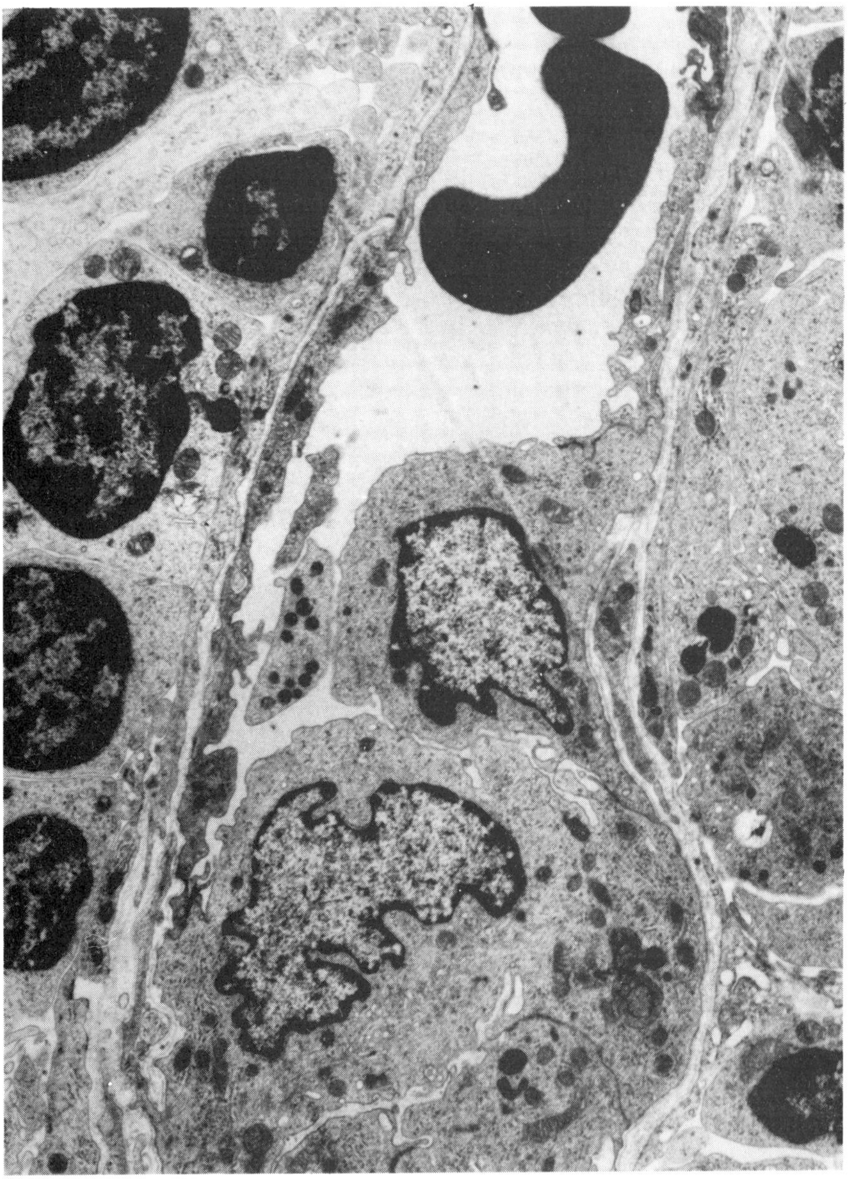

FIG. 23 This electron micrograph shows the abrupt transition from low to high endothelium in proximal segments of HEV.

was the tracer for both these studies (Cotran *et al.*, 1968), while van Deurs' study was conducted in BALB/c mice which may differ in resistance to the mast cell degranulating effects of HRP.

The endothelial cells of HEV are unlike those of normal venules anywhere in the body (Fig. 23). These cells characteristically exhibit diffuse nonspecific esterase activity in their abundant cytoplasm, almost reaching the staining intensity of monocytes. The presence of a prominent Golgi apparatus, multivesicular bodies, and phagolysosomes in the cytoplasm of HEV cells (which also appear to lack typical Weibel-Palade bodies) suggest that this endothelium may be composed of monocyte-like cells (Anderson *et al.*, 1976). Indeed, the analogy of HEV cells to monocytes can be carried further because the binding of lymphocytes to HEV endothelial cells is morphologically similar to that of cultivated mononuclear cells (Lipsky and Rosenthal, 1973). However, the observation that HEV cells form a continuous lining linked together by junctional complexes which lie upon a basal lamina secreted by these cells is more consistent with a uniquely specialized endothelium than a lining formed by modified monocytes.

d. *Lymphocyte emigration into lymph nodes*

High endothelial venules were shown by Gowans and Knight (1964) to be the site of large-scale blood-to-lymph emigration of recirculating lymphocytes. Other investigators proposed direct entry of nodal lymphocytes into the blood at these sites, because HEV lumens frequently contain high concentrations of lymphocytes. Subsequent studies indicated that cellular accumulation in HEV lumens was due to selective adhesion of lymphocytes to endothelial surfaces (Figs 7, 8, 24) presumably via receptor molecules located on the tips of microvilli (Anderson and Anderson, 1976). A specific "homing" receptor has not been isolated and characterized, but various studies (Goldschneider and McGregor, 1967) suggest that it may be a sialoglycoprotein, which requires divalent cations and transmembrane connections to a functional cytoskeleton (Anderson *et al.*, 1979) in order to mediate recognition and adhesion of lymphocytes to endothelial surfaces (Ford *et al.*, 1978). Gowans (1959) found that cell viability was essential for "homing", since heat-killed lymphocytes sequestered in the liver and spleen. Preincubation of lymphocytes in trypsin, crude glycosidases and neuraminidase altered the tissue distribution of these cells when infused into normal rates. These experiments were based largely on whole organ counting, and did not establish whether this enzymatic treatment destroyed specific receptor sites or simply made lymphocyte surfaces nonspecifically "sticky". Despite these limitations, Gesner's studies have been widely cited as evidence for specific membrane receptors on lymphocyte surfaces which "recognize" membrane constituents of high endothelial cells to promote selective emigration at this site. *In vitro* models of lymphocyte homing have recently been developed which may help in the chemical and biological characterization of the receptor (Stamper and Woodruff, 1976; de Bono, 1976).

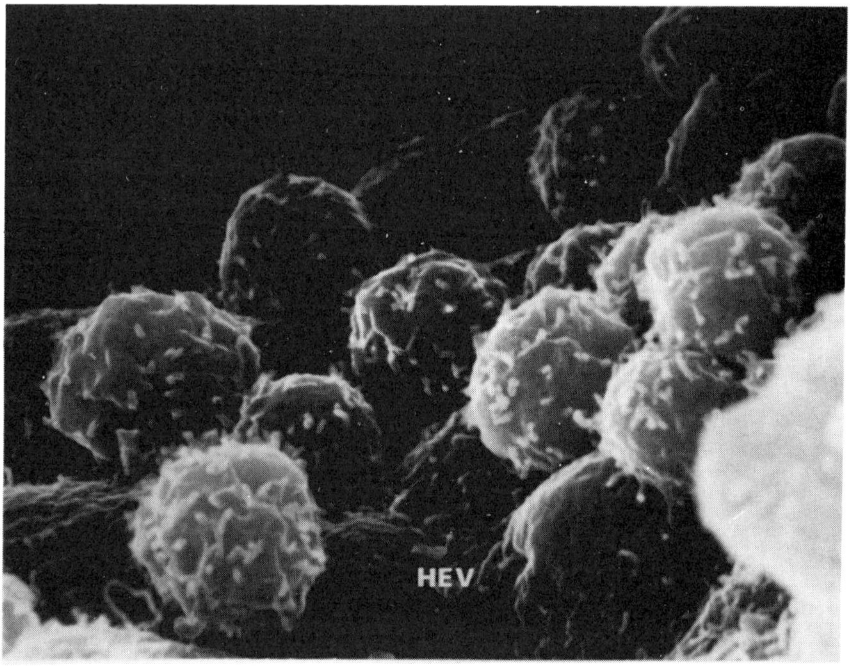

FIG. 24 Circulating lymphocytes adhere to luminal surfaces of HEV prior to emigrating into the lymph node parenchyma.

In addition, studies of lymphocyte binding to frozen sections of lymph node HEV (Butcher *et al.*, 1979) have indicated that the phylogenetic nearness of the source of adhering cells to the species of the substratum (HEV), determines the affinity of binding. That is, human lymphocytes bind better to mouse HEV *in vitro* than do chicken or lizard lymphoid cells.

Transvascular migration in normal lymph nodes is not entirely restricted to lymphocytes, since monocytes, basophils and cells resembling novel dendritic cells are infrequently found among the lymphoid cells crossing HEV walls. Lymphocytes and monocytes attach to luminal surfaces of HEV, squeeze between the endothelial cells, and enter the perivascular sheath composed of multiple laminations of reticular cell processes (Fig. 25). After gaining access to the paracortical interstitium, these cells may either crawl along reticular

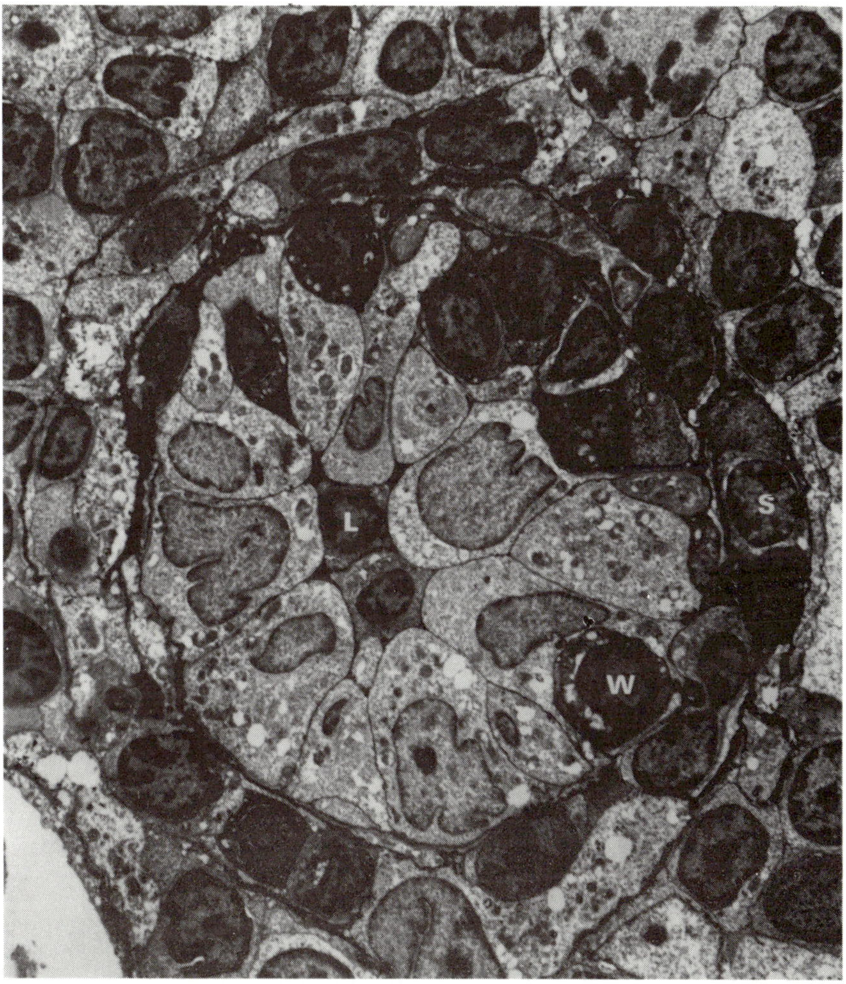

FIG. 25 Migrating lymphocytes can be seen in the lumen (L), wall (W) and sheath (S) of HEV.

fibers toward reactive foci in T or B cell areas or they may cross lymphatic endothelium and enter intermediate sinuses which ultimately delivers them into the efferent lymph. Sprent (1973) and Ford (1975) showed that the mean transit time for migration of normal lymphocytes across lymph nodes was 18 to 20 h for T cells and 28 to 30 h for B cells. The observation that B cells transit lymph nodes more slowly than T cells probably is related to the motile behavior of the respective cells. B cells locomote less frequently and more slowly than T cells. T cells appear to be attracted by short-range factors secreted by B cells, since T cells turn and migrate toward B cells whenever they pass within a 30 to 40 μm radius (Anderson and Warren, 1980). This may obviate the need for equal locomotory activity by B cells in establishing T-B interactions within lymphatic tissues, since T cells can overtake B cells during their journey from blood to lymph.

Controversy about whether lymphocytes passed through or between HEV endothelial cells (Marchesi and Gowans, 1964) has been resolved to some extent by numerous recent studies using extracellular tracers, serial sections and SEM which showed that lymphocytes enter and cross HEV by migrating between the endothelial cells (Schoefl, 1972; Wenk *et al.*, 1974; Van Ewijk *et al.*, 1976; Anderson and Anderson, 1976). The controversy had some basis, since lymphocytes deeply indent the endothelial cells as they cross HEV without breaking the macular interendothelial junctions. In acute inflammation, these endothelial junctions separate so that all varieties of blood leukocytes may pass through.

Special permeability characteristics of the HEV wall permit limited intravasation of macromolecules from within the lymph node parenchyma without allowing significant extravasation, even in the presence of transmigrating lymphocytes. This unidirectional permeability derives from the "flap-guarded valve" structure of the HEV wall composed of overlapping endothelial and reticular cells. Diffusion of materials from the lymphatic tissue into the interendothelial spaces may provide a mechanism by which chemotactic gradients are generated. This is especially true under circumstances of antigen stimulation where there is altered blood flow and increased tissue fluid pressures.

2. *The spleen*

The spleen acts as a large discriminatory filter set across the blood stream. The spleen is largely a meshwork of reticular cells and their fibers containing entrapped macrophages which can remove and destroy foreign pathogens in the blood and also provide for the selective monitoring and removal of aged and damaged erythrocytes, leukocytes and platelets passing through its interstices.

In immune reactions, the spleen provides for the same processes of antigen trapping, cellular collaboration, lymphocyte proliferation and antibody production seen in peripheral lymph nodes. As a rule, the immune responses to antigens and pathogens invading the blood stream are concentrated within the spleen. In addition, some of the antigen administered locally at distant tissue sites can pass through the regional node and be sequestered within the spleen. The immature lymphocytes mobilized into efferent lymph during immune responses in peripheral lymph nodes pass through the blood and frequently establish secondary residence in splenic cords and sinuses, where the B cells mature into antibody-secreting plasma cells.

a. *Structure*

The spleen is composed of a dense fibrous capsule with trabeculae extending inward which subdivides the organ into lobules and merges with the reticular meshwork supporting the splenic pulp. The spleen has no cortex and medulla, but its interior is grossly divisible into white pulp, which forms cylindrical collections of lymphocytes about the arteries, and red pulp, which contains erythrocyte-rich blood. The red pulp contains the splenic cords which are continuous partitions of tissue criss-crossed by reticulum lying between the splenic sinuses. The cords contain erythrocytes, lymphocytes, macrophages, granulocytes and numerous antibody-secreting plasma cells. The splenic sinuses are vascular channels between the cords which are lined by endothelial (stave) cells and hoop-like arrangements of basement membrane. The erythrocytes liberated into the splenic cords must squeeze through slits between these endothelial cells to enter the sinuses. The spleen monitors for abnormal erythrocytes by this mechanical sieving and cells which have lost their plasticity are destroyed as they pass from pulp to sinus (Chen and Weiss, 1973).

The spleen is supplied by the splenic artery which passes through the hilus and branches to pass through trabeculae into medium-sized arteries surrounded by a sheath of lymphatic tissue (periarteriolar lymphatic sheath). These vessels terminate in small arterioles which empty into the pulp cords, pulp sinuses or the white pulp and its surrounding marginal zone, which is rich in macrophages. Blood leaves the spleen through a sinusoidal system which connects by gradual transition to pulp veins, trabecular veins and finally the splenic veins. The spleen has no afferent lymphatic vessels, but

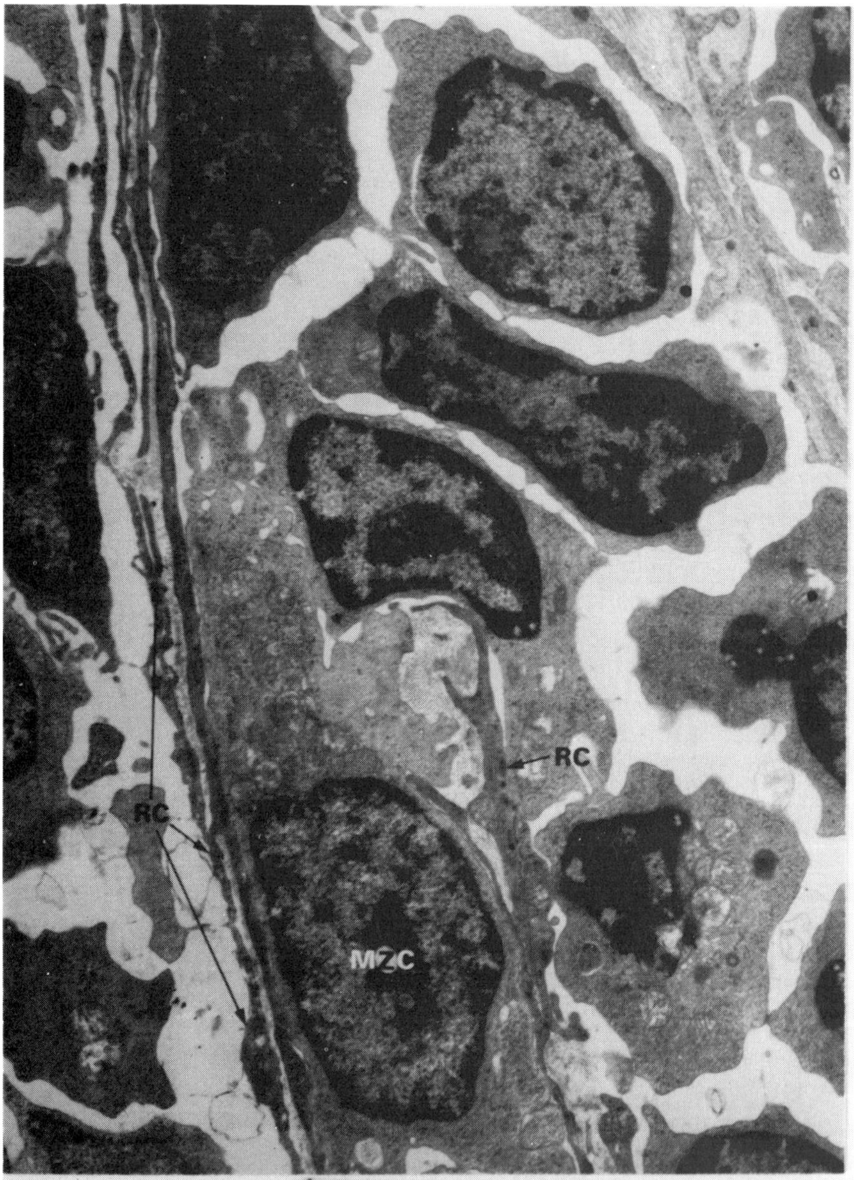
RC
RC
MZC
PALS
MZ

does possess efferent lymphatics which arise within the white pulp, pass through trabeculae and exit at the hilus.

b. *Lymphocyte emigration into the spleen*

Lymphocyte traffic through the splenic red and white pulp is not regulated by the same surface recognition mechanisms which determine selective lymphocyte homing into lymph nodes. Many of the lymphocytes entering the spleen in the arterial blood bypass the white pulp and flow along with other blood elements into the reticulum of the red pulp cords and sinuses to exit via the splenic vein. These cells would be returned to the blood within 2 to 3 h after entering the spleen. However, some small arterioles terminate in sinuses adjacent to the white pulp and others empty directly into the marginal zone. Lymphocytes arriving at these sites move across an antigen-binding interface provided macrophages in the marginal zone (Fig. 26) and enter the PALS. Cells entering here may remain within the spleen for up to 12 h. There is no clear-cut segregation of T and B cells into discrete zones within the splenic white pulp, but follicles and their mantels contain B cells; recirculating T and B cells are found in the PALS. After variable periods of residence here, some recirculating cells exit through the efferent lymphatics, while others appear to move back out via bridging zones into the red pulp sinuses (Mitchell, 1973). The magnitude of lymphocyte recirculation via splenic efferent lymph or venous return remains to be determined. However, if these immunocompetent cells encounter an appropriate antigenic stimulus, they proliferate in the same manner as that seen in peripheral nodes; the B cells can form large germinal centers in this process. A few antibody-secreting cells can be found within the periarteriolar lymphatic sheath, but most of the mature plasma cells appear within the splenic cords in the red pulp following B cell migration through the blood or their direct movement out from the white pulp.

3. *The mucosal immune system*

The mucosal immune system consists of nonencapsulated lymphoid nodules and diffuse lymphocytic infiltrates which are closely associated with the epithelium lining the intestinal and respiratory tracts. These

FIG. 26 The marginal zone of the spleen is composed of concentric "onion skin" laminations of reticular cell (RC) processes. Esterase-positive macrophage-like marginal zone cells (MZC) display antigens to lymphocytes which traverse the marginal zone *en route* to the PALS.

structures provide for the local synthesis and selective transport of secretory IgA antibodies into external secretions promoting local immunity to pathogens and foreign proteins which invade the body through mucosal surfaces. This modified immunoglobulin consists of two IgA molecules linked together by a J chain (MW 15 000) and contains a molecule of secretory component coiled about the Fc portions of the joined immunoglobulin molecules. This structure stabilizes secretory IgA against proteolysis and facilitates its transport across the mucosal epithelium.

Secretory IgA plays an important role in host resistance against many viral diseases by impairing colonization of the mucous membranes and preventing reinfection by the same virus. The efficacy of this process has been well established by the use of oral immunization with live, attenuated viruses, such as the Sabin poliovaccine, which prevents both reinfection and the establishment of the carrier state. Absence of adequate mucosal immunity can result in severe local hypersensitivity reactions when the pulmonary or intestinal epithelium is reinfected by the same viral agent, despite evidence of potent systemic immunity (i.e. the hypersensitivity pneumonitis seen in children immunized parenterally with killed measles vaccine and subsequently infected with live virus). Although secretory IgA probably does not promote direct lysis or phagocytosis of bacteria, it does interfere with bacterial adherence to mucous membranes. When this effect is combined with the normal cleansing actions provided by mucous secretion, cilial beating, cellular desquamation, intestinal motility, etc., secretory IgA can contribute in preventing bacterial colonization within the lung and gut. In addition, there is evidence that secretory IgA can combine with toxins and macromolecules within the gut lumen inhibiting their binding and absorption by intestinal epithelium.

a. *Structure*

The organized lymphatic tissue components of the mucosal immune system consist of nodular collections of lymphocytes within a reticular meshwork, which are located in the lamina propria and submucosa of the small intestine, appendix, colon, bronchi, tear ducts, salivary glands and mammary glands. Their structure differs from that seen in lymph nodes, because they lack a well-developed capsule, afferent lymphatic connections and a discrete medulla containing cords of plasma cells (Parrott, 1976).

The correlation between structure and function of these organs is best established in the Peyer's patches (Fig. 27). These patches are discrete, subepithelial collections of lymphoid tissue found along the antimesenteric wall of the intestines. Individual patches are found from the duodenum to the ileum, but are more numerous and larger in

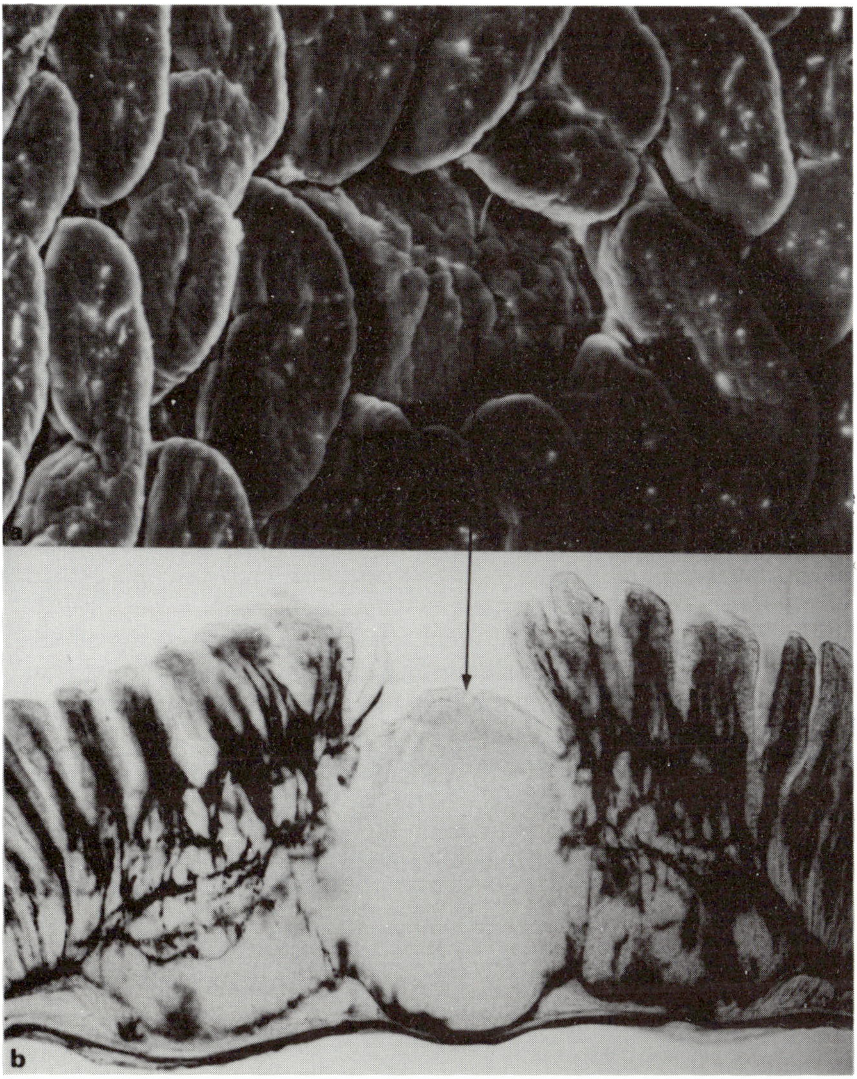

FIG. 27 In Peyer's patches, the epithelium overlying follicles (arrows) is devoid of microvilli but is capable of endocytosis. Lymphocytes often peer out between these microfold cells and are exposed to intact antigens in the gut lumen.

the distal intestinal tract. Each patch contains multiple individual follicles containing dendritic cells, macrophages and proliferating B cells and is surrounded by a mantel of small B cells. The interfollicular spaces are diffusely infiltrated with small and medium sized lymphocytes, usually of T cell origin. The patches contain specialized HEV and efferent lymphatics which provide for lymphocyte entry and egress. Although Peyer's patches lack true afferent lymphatics, about 30% of the efferent intestinal lymph from the lamina propria lymphatic plexus diffuses through them before emptying into lymphatic trunks which originate beneath the follicles and drain into mesenteric lymphatics. Regardless of how many follicles a patch contains, each is only one follicle thick, providing an intimate association between the follicle and the overlying epithelium. The specialized intestinal epithelium covering each follicle is heavily infiltrated by lymphocytes. These epithelial cells called microfold or M cells are stretched by their burden of interepithelial lymphocytes and lack prominent microvilli; their cytoplasm contains numerous transport vesicles which appear to be specifically adapted to sample intestinal contents (Owen, 1977). These cells endocytose and transport small quantitites of antigens across their cytoplasm in vesicles and deposit them among the lymphoid cells which lie above germinal follicles. The direct transport of intact antigens into the patch probably explains how these structures provide immune surveillance in the absence of afferent lymphatics (Bockman and Cooper, 1973). Recent studies have demonstrated remarkably similar transcellular transport of antigen and structural organization in the bronchial associated lymphatic tissues, so these features may be common to all components of the mucosal immune system (Rácz *et al.*, 1977).

Peyer's patches are heavily populated with B lymphocytes, but virtually no IgA secretion occurs in them, despite evidence that many of the B cells in the patch are precommitted for IgA synthesis (Cebra *et al.*, 1977). When antigen is delivered into the patch, these cells, with the help of macrophages and T lymphocytes undergo a clonal burst of proliferation. However, maturation to antibody-secreting cells does not occur in the patch. The immature cells leave through efferent lymphatics, move through the mesenteric nodes and thoracic duct back into the bloodstream. After completing various differentiation steps in the mesenteric node or the spleen, these cells preferentially establish residence at submucosal sites, such as the lamina propria of the intestine (Cebra *et al.*, 1977; Husband and Gowans, 1978). Although still unproven, this distinctive lymphocyte traffic pattern has been variously attributed to the presence of environmental antigens within intestines or the appearance of IgA dimers on the B cell surface, causing them to localize beneath epithelial cells synthesizing and releasing the secretory component of IgA. Once they have reached these submucosal sites, the B cells mature into plasma cells.

b. *Migration cycles of lymphocytes associated with mucosal immunity*

^{3}H-Uridine-labeled TDL emigrate into peripheral lymph nodes and accumulate to a peak over an 18-22-h period (Fig. 28). These same lymphocytes enter the thymic-derived area of Peyer's patches via HEV

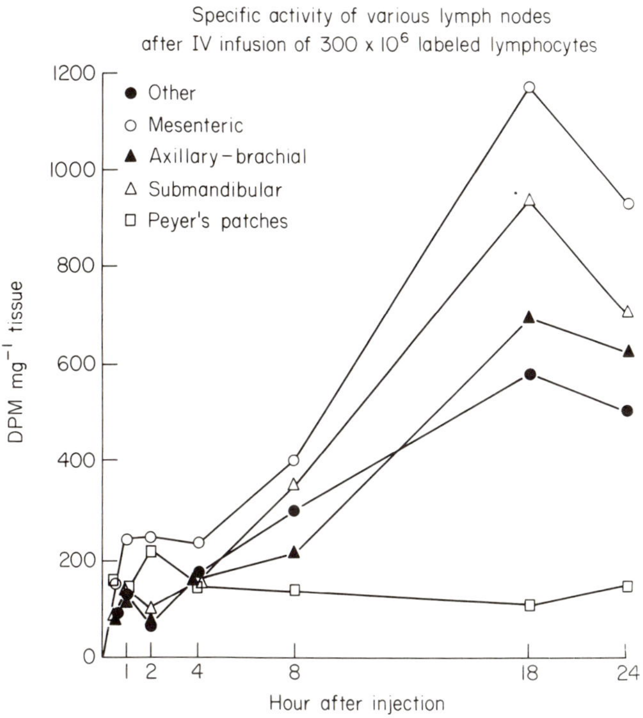

FIG. 28 The accumulation of trafficking lymphocytes in lymph nodes increases gradually over an 18-hour period. The rate of this accumulation is presumably proportional to the degree of immunological activity of the node. However, traffic to the Peyer's patch does not seem to be regulated by the same mechanisms as it is in lymph nodes. Labeled lymphocytes entering Peyer's patches peak by 2 hours and then they must leave, presumably to the mesenteric lymph node via lymphatics.

and rapidly exit via efferent lymphatics which cross the muscularis propria at the bases of germinal follicles. These cells appear in the subcapsular sinuses of mesenteric lymph nodes within 1-1/2 h and significantly contribute to the rate of accumulation of labeled lymphocytes in these nodes. Since mesenteric lymph nodes also receive lymphocytes via paracortical HEV, the steady state of lymphocyte entry into these nodes is normally two to three times that of peripheral lymph nodes. At these same time periods none of the primary or secondary chains of peripheral lymph nodes contain radiolabeled cells in their lymph sinusoidal systems. This observation is consistent with the segregation of antigen-triggering and subsequent maturation of IgA precursors which are said to occur in the Peyer's patches and mesenteric lymph node, respectively. Since long-lived recirculating T cells do not remain in the Peyer's patches long enough to participate in the maturation steps of IgM-bearing IgA precursor cells, it is possible that the T cells, exposed to identical antigens as the B cells by passage through the Peyer's patches, catch up with the IgA precursors in the lymph sinuses of the mesenteric node. Passage of these appropriately "helped" B lymphoblasts through the lymph to the blood and ultimately the gut completes the cycle of migration, since the "secondary" B cells lose their motility and lodge as antibody-secreting cells in the lamina propria.

The frequency and potential of IgA "memory" cells in TDL has not yet been well studied. However, Husband and Gowans (1978) found a subpopulation of presumably recirculating cells in TDL of rats 3 to 4 days after secondary intraluminal challenge which, when transferred to rats bearing an isolated intestinal loop containing antigen, localized in the loop, divided there and expressed IgA antibody. Thus, one aspect of the secretory antibody response may be the release of long-lived IgA precursors by Peyer's patches, which circulate through and/or lodge in mucosal tissue. Local reapplication or persistence of the antigen may then initiate their division and maturation to IgA cells at the site, presenting the aspect of a "true local secondary response".

Either the mucosal follicles can selectively accumulate IgA precursors, which differentiate elsewhere, or these cells are generated in the special milieu of the mucosal follicles. Cebra *et al.* (1977) proposed that the special feature of mucosal follicles that promotes the generation of IgA-only clonal precursors in an environment that allows antigen-driven division without maturation to plasma cells. The feature of the Peyer's patches environment that might promote this situation could include inaccessibility of T "helper" cells, excessive presence of T "suppressor" cells or humoral factors (Faulk *et al.*, 1971;

Waksman *et al.*, 1973; Kamin *et al.*, 1974; Ngan and Kind, 1978). This process might operate on the B cell which generates clones expressing both IgM and IgA.

Virtually all the IgA found in external body secretions is produced by local synthesis within plasma cells. After the IgA molecules are synthesized and assembled, the J piece is added during secretion and release of the dimers into submucosal tissue. These dimers diffuse across the basement membrane where they are coupled to secretory components which are synthesized and bound to the surface of epithelial cells. The resulting complex is endocytosed and transported through the epithelial cell cytoplasm to be secreted into the intestinal or bronchial lumens. In the lumens, it can bind with the appropriate antigen or be lost from the body during normal passage of the intestinal contents and mucous to the exterior. In addition, some IgA may be reabsorbed into the blood, removed by the liver and secreted back into the intestine with the bile, providing a form of enterohepatic circulation which may greatly augment intestinal immunity (Orlans *et al.*, 1978).

4. *Peripheral sites of chronic inflammation*

Antigens presented in a form not easily removed by cells of the mononuclear phagocyte system, e.g. emulsified in a non-degradable oily base, result in the formation of chronic inflammatory foci. These lesions possess follicular and diffuse lymphocytic infiltrates in addition to collections of foam, epithelioid and giant cells and other monocyte components of granulomata (Spector and Willoughby, 1963). Similar collections of diffuse lymphoid tissue may be seen: in lesions resulting from infections by facultative intracellular organisms of viral, bacterial and parasitic origin; in tissues exposed chronically to microbes present in the fluids which bathe them, such as the bladder or renal pelves of patients with chronic bacilluria due to pyelonephritis; in organs which are undergoing chronic rejection following transplantation; and in organs attacked by autoallergic phenomena, such as Hashimoto's thyroiditis, allergic orchitis and allergic encephalomyelitis.

All of the above chronic inflammatory lesions contain structural elements which are similar to those of non-encapsulated lymphatic tissue. The inflammatory infiltrate which succeeds neutrophils in these sites is composed predominantly of monocytes, macrophages and lymphoid cells. While monocytes and lymphocytes usually arrive at the site simultaneously, large-scale lymphoid cell emigration occurs only after additional microenvironmental structures are generated. Chronic inflammation typically develops in connective tissue sites which are well supplied by lymphatic channels. The inductive stimulus, which is possibly provided by a number of factors released by monocytes and lymphoblastic cells, results in proliferation of fibroblasts and lymphatic and blood vascular endothelium (Fig. 29). Specialized vascular segments develop by mitotic division, which morphologically, histochemically and functionally resemble HEV of lymph nodes (Astrom *et al.*, 1968; Smith *et al.*, 1970; Graham and Shannon, 1972). Such new vessels lined by plump, esterase-positive endothelial cells arise in chronic inflammatory foci prior to the appearance of dense aggregates of small lymphocytes. Circulating lymphocytes home to these vessels, emigrate from the blood and accumulate temporarily in the lesion before passing into afferent lymphatics and regional lymph nodes. Lymphoblastic cells also enter the lesion at such sites and differentiate into plasma cells or participate in the formation of germinal follicles. The antibody specificities of these cells are frequently unrelated to the antigens present at the site.

This large-scale lymphoid cell traffic through sites of chronic inflammation has been documented in studies where the outputs of cannulated afferent lymphatics draining adjuvant-induced granulomata were measured (Smith *et al.*, 1970) or where the distributions of transfused ^{3}H-uridine-labeled lymphocytes were traced in tissues by autoradiography (Anderson and Reynolds, 1979). In the former studies, the afferent lymph output in sheep inoculated with Freund's adjuvant reached $3{\cdot}1 \times 10^{7}$ lymphocytes per hour, which is nearly equal to the output of a normal lymph node, and is at least ten times that of normal afferent lymph. Increased lymphocyte traffic via the granuloma site persisted through the 70 days of the study and probably would have continued as long as the lesion was present. In the latter study the lymphocytes present in the afferent lymph were identified as predominantly B cells. This augmentation of B cell traffic to the regional lymph node via the granuloma site correlated with the pronounced increase in antibody production and with the altered ratios of T and B lymphocytes found in these nodes. The enriched B cell populations present in the afferent lymph may have been recruited from the circulation, but their formation in germinal follicles is also possible.

Macrophages in the lesion, which are unable to completely remove the antigen-containing material, become activated and secrete mediators which affect the local microenvironment and that of the regional lymph nodes by stimulating lymphocyte division, chemotaxis of monocytes and lymphocytes, vascular permeability, blood flow and cell proliferation (Unanue *et al.*, 1976). These peripheral sites of chronic inflammation resolve when all the antigen is neutralized and eliminated by phagocytes; they may, therefore, serve a beneficial

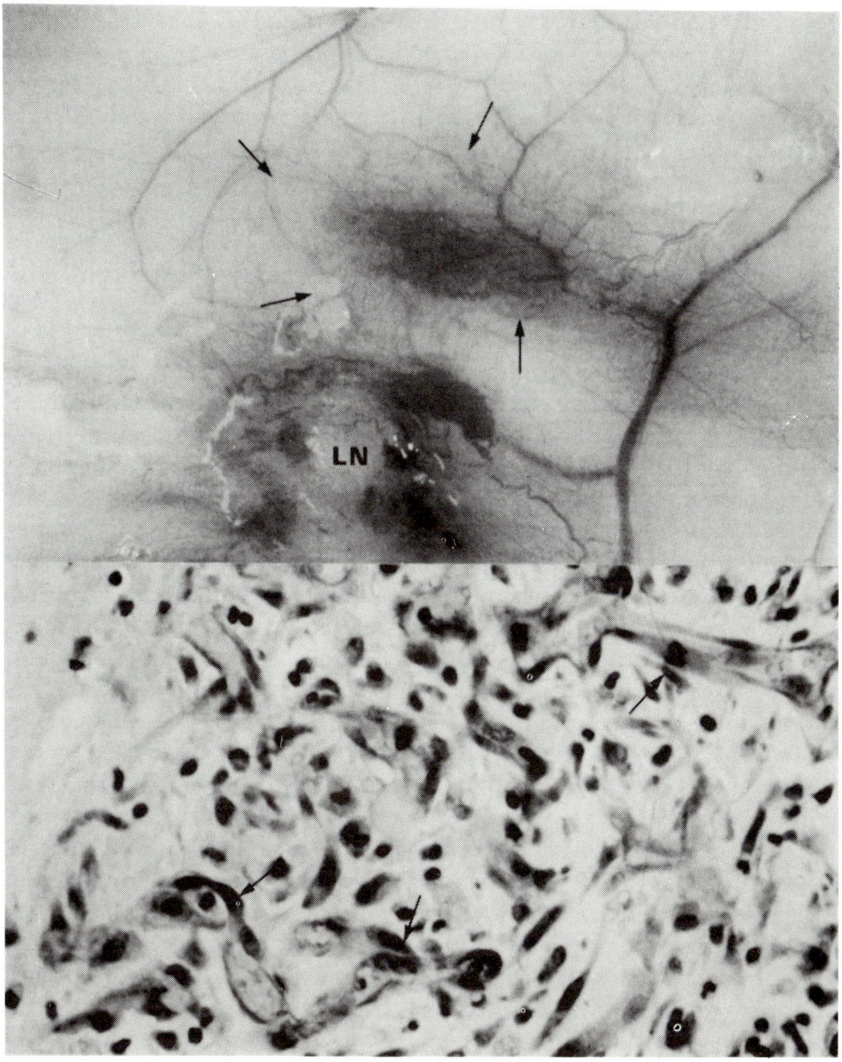

FIG. 29 Chronic inflammation is associated with hyperemia and vascular proliferation. This is illustrated here by undersurface of rat skin, which shows these vascular changes overlying the site of injection (arrows) of a water-soluble adjuvant. The regional lymph (LN) is located nearby and also has hyperemic vessels along the afferent lymphatics.

purpose by establishing new reticular microenvironments which serve the same antigen- and cell-sorting functions as peripheral lymphatic tissues. However, these foci also cause discomfort and disease when the antigen is (a) a normal constituent of the host, (b) not degradable or neutralizable or (c) capable of changing its antigenic determinants in response to immunological pressure. In addition, hydrolytic enzymes which may be released in the course of phagocytosis may damage other neighboring structures, such as the articular surfaces of joints in rheumatoid arthritis and the arthritis associated with autoallergic diseases.

VI. Circulation of lymphocytes during an immune response

Successful initiation of a specific immune response requires that the lymphocytes must engage and bind the appropriate antigen with its surface receptor. Studies in non-immune animals have shown that only a tiny minority of the lymphocytes present within a single lymph node are capable of reacting with a given antigenic determinant. If these cells were static or their movements were randomly sorted throughout the body, the likelihood of chance collisions between reactive lymphocytes and the appropriate antigen displayed on an accessory cell would be very remote. However, this is clearly not the case *in vivo*, where immunocompetent T and B cells continually recirculate between blood and lymphatic tissues (Sprent, 1973). Long-lived lymphocytes flowing in the blood show a unique "homing instinct" for lymph node HEV. These cells cross HEV and emigrate into the reticular meshwork, where they crawl along reticular cell surfaces, collide with macrophages and other lymphocytes and either stay to initiate proliferation or leave.

Lymphocytes recirculate through other lymph nodes and mucosal lymphatic tissues via HEV, providing a constant form of surveillance by immunocompetent lymphocytes that move through antigen-binding meshworks. This phenomenon probably enables a small depot of antigen to recruit a large number of antigen-specific cells from the body's lymphocyte pool.

When an individual lymphocyte encounters an appropriate antigenic stimulus within the node, it binds the antigen, interacts with other cell types and is trapped in the node, where it gives rise to a clonal burst of proliferation and differentiation of lymphocytes which mediate immune responses. Many of the immature lymphocyte progeny leave the stimulated node 48-100 h after antigen exposure and disseminate to distant nodes, the spleen and other tissues, where they can mature into specific effector cells. The B cells activated in this response move into the medullary cords of regional and distant nodes, where they mature into antibody-secreting plasma cells (Frost *et al.*, 1976).

Although T and B lymphocytes emigrate from the same segments of HEV, they are sorted by unknown mechanisms within the nodal parenchyma. The T lymphocytes establish residence in the deep cortex for relatively short time intervals before moving out into the efferent sinuses. B cells emigrate into the superficial cortex and probably remain there for longer periods before exiting via the sinusoidal pathways. This migration pattern appears to permit the T and B cells to interact with antigen-binding macrophages and engage in cellular collaboration before they redistribute into their respective zones within the nodal cortex.

Other factors also influence lymphocyte traffic patterns in the body. The ability of T cell subpopulations to recirculate appears to depend upon their state of maturation (i.e. at least some effector T cells leave the circulation at random to enter sites of inflammation). B lymphocytes display similar variations in their emigration patterns. The immature B cells appearing shortly after antigenic challenge may leave the node, but they frequently lodge in the spleen and do not recirculate through the thoracic duct. However, "memory B cells" arising at the late stages of an immune response do recirculate in a typical manner between blood and lymph (Ponzio *et al.*, 1977). The B cell precursors of IgA secretion also possess distinct and quite different migration pathways. This circuit include generation of precursor progeny in Peyer's patch follicles, which complete various maturational steps in the mesenteric node and spleen before finally lodging in the lamina propria of the gut as IgA-secreting plasma cells.

In non-stimulated animals, lymphocyte recirculation is characterized by a balanced flux of cellular traffic across afferent and efferent terminals of lymphatic tissues (Fig. 30). This kinetic equilibrium is rapidly distorted in the regional nodes draining sites of inflammation, infection or antigenic challenge (Hall and Morris, 1965; Cahill *et al.*, 1976). This is accompanied by a rapid increase in lymphocyte accumulation within the lymph node cortex, which is not associated with cellular replication. Such nodal enlargement probably reflects the combined result of increased lymphocyte traffic into the node and decreased egress, or markedly increased entry with normal rates of exiting. These early changes are believed to be produced, in part, by changes in blood flow and by release of secretory factors and lysosomal enzymes from activated macrophages, which alter lymphocyte surface

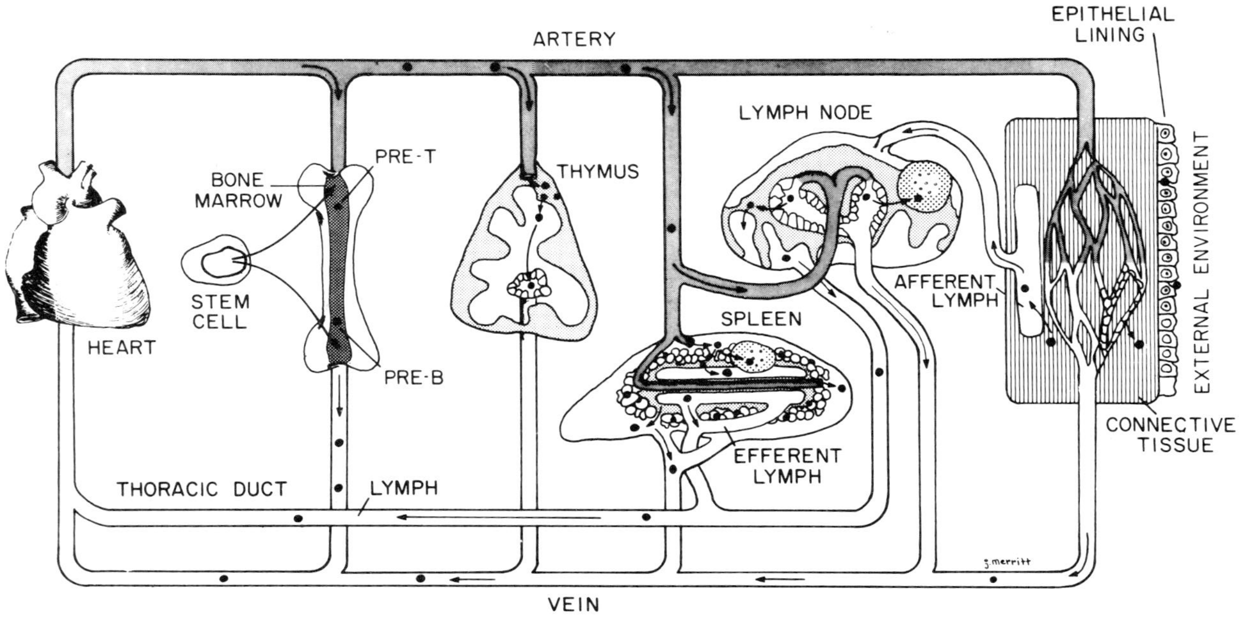

FIG. 30 This diagram depicts the circuits of lymphocyte traffic explained in the text.

adhesiveness and transit times within the node (Unanue *et al.*, 1976). As this early sequestration of recirculating lymphocytes within the stimulated node subsides, blast cell transformation and mitotic activity appear in the T and B cell zones of the cortex, reflecting the antigen-dependent cellular proliferation.

The specificities of the lymphocytes entering lymphatic tissues in the immediate 6- to 48-h period following stimulation are largely unrelated to the antigen which initiated the response. In fact, similarly non-specific lymphocytic accumulations can be induced by adjuvants which themselves are poorly immunogenic. However, as the sequestered lymphocytes are released into the efferent lymph, they are depleted of cells specifically reactive to the priming antigen (Rowley *et al.*, 1977). The retention of antigen-specific lymphocytes in regional lymph nodes has been termed "specific recruitment", and was documented using double-label techniques. Specific memory cells generated *in vivo* in the presence of ^{14}C-thymidine were mixed with equal numbers of ^{3}H-thymidine-labeled control memory cells and subsequently transfused to immunized syngeneic recipients. The relative accumulation of specific versus non-specific cells was measured in regional and contralateral nodes by scintillation spectroscopy of extracted DNA. These kinds of studies clearly demonstrated increased traffic of specifically reactive cells in antigen-draining nodes which withstood reciprocal specificity controls (Sprent *et al.*, 1971; Thursh and Emeson, 1972, Parrott and Ferguson, 1974). The numbers of labeled immunospecific cells available to lodge selectively were small enough to tax the resolving power of the assays, but studies of efferent lymph indicated that specific cell traffic remained elevated throughout the immune response. Specifically reactive lymphocytes enter the efferent lymph in maximal numbers between 72 and 100 h. Peak accumulations of antigen-reactive lymphocytes correlated chronologically with early formation of reactive centers in the cortex and proliferation of new segments of HEV (Anderson *et al.*, 1975), suggesting that these vascular structures may have some function in selective recruitment, but lymphocyte chemotactic factors or modified antigens secreted by macrophages may also facor the emigration of specific cells to HEV.

The increased migration of lymphocytes into antigen-stimulated lymphatic tissues is not restricted to long-lived recirculating lymphocytes. Lymphocytes in the cortex of the thymus undergo enhanced proliferation within the first three days following peripheral antigen inoculation. The systemic stimulus which causes thymocyte proliferation is presently unknown, but these newly formed cells leave the thymus and accumulate in the marginal zone of the spleen, Peyer's patches and some lymph nodes (Durkin *et al.*, 1978). These cells comprised predominantly of $Ly^{(1+,2+,3+)}$ cells may be precursors of antigen-specific suppressor cells which require T cell help in order ot complete their differentiation. Adult thymectomy, which removes the short-lived, cortical thymocytes but not the long-lived recirculating cells, prevents the formation of Freund's adjuvant-induced T-suppressor cell populations, further supporting the suggestion that the cortical thymocytes which lodge in the spleen are precursors of suppressor cells. As early as 6 days after immunization, the numbers of antigen-specific suppressor cells begin to increase until the immune response is terminated.

These changes in lymphocyte traffic combined with local proliferation of immunoreactive cells are responsible for the biphasic 2- to 6-fold enlargement of regional lymph nodes draining sites of antigen inoculation or infection. In the absence of additional free antigen, the suppressive effects of anti-idiotypic antibodies and/or suppressor cells eventually result in gradual reduction in traffic and proliferation. It may take a month or more for the regional lymph node to return to its normal size and physiologic activity. Following secondary exposure to antigen, the kinetics of lymphocyte traffic and immunocyte proliferation in the regional and distant lymph nodes are greatly accelerated, possibly because of the dissemination of foci of immunological memory to nearly all the lymphatic tissues of the body.

References

ANDERSON, A. O. and ANDERSON, N. D. (1975). *Am. J. Path.* **80**, 387-418.

ANDERSON, A. O. and ANDERSON, N. D. (1976). *Immunology,* **31**, 731-748.

ANDERSON, A. O. and REYNOLDS, J. A. (1979). *J. Reticuloendothel. Soc.* **26**, 667-680.

ANDERSON, A. O. and WARREN, J. T. (1979). *Fedn Proc. Fedn Am. Socs exp. Biol.* **38**, 1429 (abstr.).

ANDERSON, A. O. and WARREN, J. T. (1980). *Fedn Proc. Fedn Am. Socs exp. Biol.* **39**, 698 (abstr.).

ANDERSON, A. O., ANDERSON, N. D., HOFFMAN, R. D. and WHITE, J. D. (1978a). *Fedn Proc. Fedn Am. Socs exp. Biol.* **37**, 591 (abstr.).

ANDERSON, A. O., ANDERSON, N. D. and WHITE, J. D. (1979). *In* "Function and Structure of the Immune System" (Eds W. Müller-Ruchholtz and H. K. Müller-Hermelink), pp. 77-83. Plenum Press, New York.

ANDERSON, N. D., ANDERSON, A. O., HOFFMAN, R. D. and WHITE, J. D. (1978b). *Fedn Proc. Fedn Am. Socs exp. Biol.* **37**, 591 (abstr.).

ANDERSON, N. D., ANDERSON, A. O. and WYLLIE, R. G. (1975). *Am. J. Path.* **81**, 131-160.

ANDERSON, N. D., ANDERSON, A. O. and WYLLIE, R. G. (1976). *Immunology*, **31**, 455-473.

ASTROM, K. E., WEBSTER, H. deF. and ARNSON, B. G. (1968). *J. exp. Med.* **128**, 469-495.

ATHERTON, A. and BORN, G. V. R. (1972). *J. Physio.* **222**, 447-474.

BAILEY, R. P. and WEISS, L. (1975a). *Am. J. Anat.* **142**, 15-27.

BAILEY, R. P. and WEISS, L. (1975b). *Am. J. Anat.* **142**, 43-58.

BANGHAM, A. D. (1964). *Ann. N.Y. Acad. Sci.* **116**, 945-949.

BAUMEL, J. J., O'DORISIO, T. M. and WURTH, A. R. (1970). *Microvasc. Res.* **2**, 500-503.

BELLER, D. I. and UNANUE, R. R. (1978). *J. Immun.* **121**, 1861-1864.

BINZ, H. and WIGZELL, H. (1975a). *J. exp. Med.* **142**, 197-211.

BINZ, H. and WIGZELL, H. (1975b). *Scand. J. Immun.* **4**, 591-600.

BINZ, H. and WIGZELL, H. (1976). *Scand. J. Immun.* **5**, 559-571.

BINZ, H., FRISCHKNECHT, H., MERCOLLI, C., DUNST, S., and WIGZELL, H. (1979). *J. exp. Med.* **150**, 1084-1097.

BLUMENSTOCK, F. A., SABA, T. M., WEBER, P. and LAFFIN, R. (1978). *J. biol. Chem.* **253**, 4287-4291.

BOCKMAN, D. E. and COOPER, M. D. (1973). *Am. J. Anat.* **136**, 455-477.

BOLLMAN, J. L., CAIN, J. C. and GRINDLAY, J. H. (1948). *J. Lab. clin. Med.* **33**, 1348-1352.

BURNET, F. M. (1959). "The Clonal Selection Theory of Acquired Immunity". Vanderbilt University Press, Nashville, Tennessee.

BUTCHER, E., SCOLLAY, R. and WEISSMAN, I. (1979). *In* "Function and Structure of the Immune System" (Eds W. Müller-Ruchholtz and H. K. Müller-Hermelink), pp. 65-72. Plenum Press, New York.

CAHILL, R. N. P., FROST, H. and TRNKA, Z. (1976). *J. exp. Med.* **143**, 870-888.

CALVERT, W. J. (1897). *Anat. Anz.* **13**, 174-180.

CANTOR, H. and BOYCE, E. A. (1977). *Contemp. Top. Immun.* **7**, 47-67.

CEBRA, J. J., GEARHART, P. J., KAMAT, R., ROBERTSON, S. M. and TSENG, J. (1977). *Cold Spring Harb. Symp. quant. Biol.* **XLI**, 201-215.

CHAPMAN, A. L. and BOPP, W. J. (1970). *Am. J. vet. Res.* **31**, 1255-1268.

CHEN, L.-T. and WEISS, L. (1973). *Blood*, **41**, 529-537.

CLAMAN, H. N. and CHAPERON, E. A. (1969). *Transplant. Rev.* **1**, 92-113.

COOPER, M. D., KEIGHTLEY, R. G., WU, L.-Y. and LAWTON, A. R. (1973). *Transplant. Rev.* **16**, 51-84.

COTRAN, R. S., KARNOVSKY, M. J. and GOTH, A. (1968). *J. Histochem. Cytochem.* **16**, 382-383.

CURTIS, A. S. G. and de SOUSA, M. (1973). *Nature New Biol.* **244**, 45-47.

DABELOW, A. (1939). *Verh. anat. Ges., Jena,* **46**, 179-224.

DAVIDSON, J. W., HOBBS, B. B. and FLETCH, A. L. (1973). *Biblphie Anat.* **11**, 423-427.

DE BONO, D. (1976). *Cell. Immun.* **26**, 78-88.

DEGOS, L., PLA, M. and COLOMBANI, J. M. (1979). *Eur. J. Immun.* **9**, 808-814.
DE SOUSA, M., FREITAS, A., HUBER, B., CANTOR, B. and BOYSE, E. A. (1979). *In* "Function and Structure of the Immune System" (Eds Müller-Ruchholtz and H. K. Müller-Hermelink), pp. 51-54. Plenum Press, New York.
DUKOR, P., BIANCO, C. and NUSSENZWEIG, V. (1970). *Proc. natn. Acad. Sci. U.S.A.* **67**, 991-997.
DURKIN, H. G., CARBONI, J. M. and WAKSMAN, B. H. (1978). *J. Immun.* **121**, 1075-1081.
FAULK, W. P., McCORMICK, J. N., GOODMAN, J. R., YOFFEY, J. M. and FUDENBERG, H. H. (1971). *Cell. Immun.* **1**, 500-520.
FELDMANN, M. (1973). *Transplant. Proc.* **5**, 43-48.
FORD, W. L. (1969). *Cell. Tissue Kinet.* **2**, 171-191.
FORD, W. L. (1975). *Prog. Allergy,* **19**, 1-59.
FORD, W. L. and SIMMONDS, S. J. (1972). *Cell. Tissue Kinet.* **5**, 175-189.
FORD, W. L., SMITH, M. E. and ANDREWS, P. (1978). *Symp. Soc. exp. Biol.* **XXXII**, 359-392.
FREITAS, A. A. and BOGNACKI, J. (1979). *Immunology,* **36**, 247-255.
FROST, H. D., CAHILL, R. N. P. and TRNKA, Z. (1975). *Eur. J. Immun.* **5**, 839-843.
FROST, H., BROWN, D. G., POSKITT, D., CAHILL, R. N. P. and TRNKA, Z. (1976). *J. exp. Med.* **143**, 707-711.
GERY, I., NOAVAK, T. and STUPP, Y. (1977). *Immunology,* **33**, 727-731.
GESNER, B. M. and GINSBURG, V. (1964). *Proc. Natn. Acad. Sci. U.S.A.* **52**, 750-755.
GLICK, B., CHANG, T. S. and JAAP, R. G. (1956). *Poultry Sci.* **35**, 224-225.
GOLDSCHNEIDER, I. and McGREGOR, D. D. (1967). *J. exp. Med.* **127**, 155-168.
GOWANS, J. L. (1957). *Br. J. exp. Path.* **38**, 67-78.
GOWANS, J. L. (1959). *J. Physiol.* **146**, 54-69.
GOWANS, J. L. and KNIGHT, E. J. (1964). *Proc. R. Soc. London Ser. B,* **159**, 257-282.
GRAHAM, R. C., Jr. and SHANNON, S. L. (1972). *Am. J. Path.* **69**, 7-24.
HALL, J. G. and MORRIS, B. (1965). *Br. J. exp. Path.* **46**, 450-454.
HANNA, M. G., Jr. and SZAKAL, A. K. (1968). *J. Immun.* **101**, 949-962.
HARRIS, H. (1954). *Physiol. Rev.* **34**, 529-562.
HAY, J. B. and HOBBS, B. B. (1977). *J. exp. Med.* **45**, 31-44.
HERMAN, P. G., OHBA, S. and MELLINS, H. Z. (1969). *Radiology,* 92, 1073-1080.
HERMAN, P. G., YAMAMOTO, I. and MELLINS, H. Z. (1972). *J. exp. Med.* **136**, 697-714.
HERMAN, P. G., UTSUNOMIYA, R. and HESSLE, S. J. (1979). *Immunology,* **36**, 793-797.
HERZENBERG, L. A., CHEN, E. L., RAVITCH, M. M., RIBLET, R. J. and HERZENBERG, L. A. (1973). *J. exp. Med.* **137**, 1311-1324.
HESLOP, B. F. and HARDY, B. E. (1971). *Transplantation,* **11**, 128-134.
HORIUCHI, A. and WAKSMAN, B. H. (1968). *J. Immun.* **101**, 1322-1332.
HOWARD, J. C. and WILSON, D. B. (1974). *J. exp. Med.* **140**, 660-672.

HOWARD, J. C., HUNT, S. V. and GOWANS, J. L. (1972). *J. exp. Med.* **135**, 200-219.

HUMPHREY, J. H. (1976). *In* "Immune Reactivities of Lymphocytes. Development, Expression and Control" (Eds M. Feldmann and A. Globerson), pp. 711-723. Plenum Press, New York.

HUSBAND, A. J. and GOWANS, J. L. (1978). *J. exp. Med.* **148**, 1146-1160.

JACOBSON, E. B. and HERZENBERG, L. A. (1972). *J. exp. Med.* **135**, 1151-1162.

KAMIN, R. M., HENRY, C. and FUDENBERG, H. H. (1974). *J. Immun.* **113**, 1151-1161.

KATZ, D. H. (ed.) (1977). "Lymphocyte Differentiation, Recognition and Regulation." Academic Press, New York and London.

KELLY, R. H., WOLSTENCROFT, R. A., DUMONDE, D. C. and BALFOUR, B. M. (1972). *Clin. exp. Immun.* **10**, 49-65.

KISHIMOTO, T. and ISHIZAKA, K. (1973). *J. Immun.* **111**, 1-9.

LANDSTEINER, K. and CHASE, M. W. (1942). *Proc. Soc. exp. Biol. Med.* **49**, 688-690.

LEAK, L. V. and BURKE, J. F. (1968). *J. Cell. Biol.* **36**, 129-149.

LEWIS, W. H. (1931). *Bull. Johns Hopkins Hosp.* **49**, 29-36.

LIPSKY, P. E. and ROSENTHAL, A. S. (1973). *J. exp. Med.* **138**, 900-924.

LUNDGREN, O. and WALLENTIN, I. (1964). *Angiolica (Basel),* **1**, 284-296.

MARCHESI, V. T. and GOWANS, J. L. (1964). *Proc. R. Soc. London Ser. B,* **159**, 283-290.

MARSHALL, A. H. E. and WHITE, R. G. (1961). *Br. J. exp. Path.* **42**, 374-385.

MCCUTCHEON, M. (1946). *Physiol. Rev.* **26**, 319-336.

MCNEILAGE, L. J. and HESLOP, B. F. (1980). *Cell. Immun.* **50**, 58-70.

MICHALSKI, J. P., MCCOMBS, C. C. and WALTER, H. (1980). *Fedn Proc. Fedn Am. Socs exp. Biol.* **39**, 909 (abstr.).

MILLER, J. F. A. P. (1962a). *Ann. N.Y. Acad. Sci.* **99**, 340-354.

MILLER, J. F. A. P. (1962b). *Proc. R. Soc. London Ser. B,* **156**, 415-428.

MILLER, J. F. A. P. (1975). *Ann. N.Y. Acad. Sci.* **249**, 9-26.

MITCHELL, G. F. and MILLER, J. F. A. P. (1968). *Proc. Natnl Acad. Sci. U.S.A.* **59**, 296-303.

MITCHELL, J. (1973). *Immunology,* **24**, 93-107.

MITCHIESON, N. A. (1971). *Eur. J. Immun.* **1**, 68-75.

MOSHER, D. F. (1975). *J. Biol. Chem.* **250**, 6614-6621.

NGAN, J. and KIND, L. S. (1978). *J. Immun.* **120**, 861-865.

NOSSAL, G. J. V. (1979). *In* "Function and Structure of the Immune System" (Eds W. Müller-Ruchholtz and H. K. Müller-Hermelink), pp. 253-258. Plenum Press, New York.

NOSSAL, G. J. V. and ADA, G. L. (1971). "Antigens, Lymphoid Cells and the Immune Response". Academic Press, New York and London.

NOSSAL, G. J. V., ABBOTT, A., MITCHELL, J. and LUMMUS, Z. (1968a). *J. exp. Med.* **127**, 277-290.

NOSSAL, G. J. V., CUNNINGHAM, A., MITCHELL, G. F. and MILLER, J. F. A. P. (1968b). *J. exp. Med.* **128**, 839-853.

OLÁH, I., RÖHLICH, P. and TÖRÖ, I. (1975). "Ultrastructure of Lymphoid Organs: An Electron-Microscopic Atlas". J. B. Lippincott, Philadelphia.
O'NEILL, G. J. and PARROTT, D. M. V. (1977). *Cell. Immun.* **33**, 257-267.
OPPENHEIM, J. J. (1981). *In* "Cellular Functions in Immunity and Inflammation" (Eds J. J. Oppenheim, D. A. Rosenstreich and M. Potter), pp. 259–279. Elsevier/North Holland, Amsterdam.
ORLANS, E., PEPPARD, J., REYNOLDS, J. and HALL, J. (1978). *J. exp. Med.* **147**, 588-592.
OSOBA, D. and MILLER, J. F. A. P. (1964). *J. exp. Med.* **119**, 177-194.
OTTAWAY, C. A. and PARROTT, D. M. V. (1979). *J. exp. Med.* **150**, 218-230.
OWEN, R. L. (1977). *Gastroenterology,* **72**, 440-451.
PARROTT, D. M. V. (1976). *Clin. Gastroenterol.* **5**, 211-228.
PARROTT, D. M. V. and FERGUSON, A. (1974). *Immunology,* **26**, 571-588.
PARROTT, D. M. V., DE SOUSA, M. A. B. and EAST, J. (1966). *J. exp. Med.* **123**, 191-203.
PONZIO, N. M., CHAPMAN-ALEXANDER, J. M. and THORBECKE, G. I., (1977). *Cell Immun.* **34**, 79-92.
PRYJMA, J. and HUMPHREY, J. H (1975). *Immunology,* **28**, 569-576.
RÁCZ, P., TENNER-RÁCZ, K., MYRVIK, Q. N. and FAINTER, L. K. (1977). *J. Reticuloendothel. Soc.* **22**, 59-83.
RAVIOLA, E. and KARNOVSKY, M. J. (1972). *J. exp. Med.* **136**, 466-498.
ROUSE, R. V., VAN EWIJK, W., JONES, P. P. and WEISSMAN, I. L. (1979). *J. Immun.* **122**, 2508-2515.
ROWLEY, D. A., GOWANS, J. L., ATKINS, R. C., FORD, W. L. and SMITH, M. E. (1972). *J. exp. Med.* **136**, 499-513.
RUSSELL, R. J., WILKINSON, P. C., SLESS, F. and PARROTT, D. M. V. (1975). *Nature,* **256**, 646-648.
SAINTE-MARIE, G. and SIN, Y. M. (1970). *in* "Regulation of Hematopoiesis" (Ed. A. S. Gordon), pp. 1339-1382. Appleton-Century-Crofts, New York.
SCHOEFL, G. I. (1972). *J. exp. Med.* **136**, 568-588.
SCHREINER, G. F. and UNANUE, E. R. (1976). *Adv. Immun.* **24**, 37-165.
SCHULZE, W. (1925). *Z. Anat. Entwicklungsgesch.* **76**, 421-462.
SHEVACH, E. M. (1981). *In* "Cellular Functions in Immunity and Inflammation" (Eds J. J. Oppenheim, D. A. Rosenstreich and M. Potter), pp.161–183. Elsevier/North Holland, Amsterdam.
SILBERBERG-SINAKIN, I., THORBECKE, G. J., BAER, R. L., ROSENTHAL, S. A. and BEREZOWSKY, V. (1976). *Cell. Immun.* **25**, 137-151.
SMITH, J. B., MCINTOSH, G. H. and MORRIS, B. (1970). *J. Path.* **100**, 21-29.
SMITH, M. E. and FORD, W. L. (1979). *In* "Function and Structure of the Immune System" (Eds W. Müller-Ruchholtz and H. K. Müller-Hermelink), pp. 85-91. Plenum Press, New York.
SORDAT, B., HESS, M. W. and COTTIER, H. (1971). *Immunology,* **20**, 115-118.
SPECTOR, W. G. and WILLOUGHBY, D. A. (1963). *Bact. Rev.* **27**, 117-154.
SPRENT, J. (1973). *Cell. Immun.* **7**, 10-39.
SPRENT, J. (1977). *In* "B and T Cells in Immune Recognition" (Eds F. Loor and G. E. Roelants,), pp. 59-82. John Wiley, New York.

SPRENT, J. and BASTEN, A. (1973). *Cell. Immun.* **7**, 40-59.

SPRENT, J. and MILLER, J. F. A. P. (1976). *J. exp. Med.* **143**, 585-600.

SPRENT, J., MILLER, J. F. A. P. and MITCHELL, G. F. (1971). *Cell. Immun.* **2**, 171-181.

STAMPER, H. B., Jr. and WOODRUFF, J. J. (1976). *J. exp. Med.* **144**, 828-833.

STEINMAN, R. M. and WITMER, M. D. (1978). *Proc. Natnl. Acad. Sci. U.S.A.* **75**, 5132-5136.

STEINMAN, R. M., ADAMS, J. C. and COHN, Z. A. (1975). *J. exp. Med.* **141**, 804-820.

STENMAN, S. and VAHERI, A. (1978). *J. exp. Med.* **147**, 1054-1064.

STINGL, G., KATZ, S. I., SHEVACH, E. M., WOLFF-SCHREINER, E. W. and GREEN, I. (1978). *J. Immun.* **120**, 570-578.

THURSH, D. R. and EMESON, E. E. (1972). *J. exp. Med.* **135**, 754-763.

UNANUE, E. R., BELLER, D. I., CALDERON, J., KIELY, J. M. and STADECKER, M. J. (1976). *Am. J. Path.* **85**, 465-478.

VAHERI, A., RUOSLAHTI, L. E., WARTIOVAARA, J., KESKI-OJA, J., KUUSELA, P., and SAKSELA, O. (1976). *J. Supramol. Struct.* **4**, 63-70.

VAN DEURS, B., RÖPKE, C. and WESTERGAARD, E. (1976). *Cell. Tissue Res.* **168**, 507-525.

VAN EWIJK, W., BRONS, N. H. C. and ROZING, J. (1975). *Cell. Immun.* **19**, 245-261.

VIKLICKÝ, V., PEKNICOVÁ, J. and POLÁCKOVÄ, M. (1976). *Folia Biol. (Praha),* **12**, 159-168.

VIKLICKÝ, V. and MICKOVÁ, M. (1979). *J. Immunogenet.* **6**, 245-252.

WAKSMAN, B. H., ONZER, H. and BLYTHMAN, H. E. (1973). *Lab. Invest.* **28**, 614-626.

WARD, P. A., OFFEN, C. D. and MONTGOMERY, J. R. (1971). *Fedn Proc. Fedn Am. Socs exp. Biol.* **30**, 1721-1724.

WARD, P. A., UNANUE, E. R., SCHREINER, S. J. and GORALNICK, S. J. (1977). *J. Immun.* **119**, 416-421.

WEISS, L. (1972). "The Cells and Tissues of the Immune System. Structure, Functions, and Interactions". Prentice-Hall, Englewood Cliffs, N.J.

WEISSMAN, I. L. (1975). *Transplant. Rev.* **24**, 159-176.

WEKERLE, H., KETELSEN, U.-P. and ERNST, M. (1980). *J. exp. Med.* **151**, 925-944.

WENK, E. J., ORLIC, D., REITH, E. J. and RHODIN, J. A. G. (1974). *J. Ultrastruct. Res.* **47**, 214-241.

WILKINSON, P. C., PARROTT, D. M. V., RUSSELL, R. J. and SLESS, F. (1977). *J. exp. Med.* **145**, 1158-1168.

WILSON, D. B., MARSHAK, A. and HOWARD, J. C. (1976). *J. Immun.* **116**, 1030-1040.

WOODRUFF, J. and GESNER, B. M. (1968). *Science,* **161**, 176-178.

WOODRUFF, J. J. (1974). *Cell. Immun.* **13**, 378-384.

YOFFEY, J. and COURTICE, F. (1956). "Lymphatics, Lymph and Lymphoid Tissue". Harvard University Press, Cambridge, Massachusetts.

ZIMMERMAN, K. W. (1923). *Z. Anat. Entwicklungsgesch.* **68**, 29-110.

ZINKERNAGEL, R. M. and DOHERTY, P. C. (1975). *J. exp. Med.* **141**, 1427-1436.

3 *Lymphocyte Migration Patterns in Sheep*

J. B. HAY and R. N. P. CAHILL

I. Introduction

Just as the enigma of the migratory habits of different species of birds continues to capture the imagination of biologists, so too has lymphocyte migration caused cell experimentalists (albeit a small number of them) to marvel at the variety, complexity, dynamics and beauty of the patterns of living cell migration streams. Most cells which are classed as blood cells do not normally display the "desire" to leave the blood compartment that lymphocytes do. Furthermore, lymphocytes have preferred exit routes. It is also evident – to us at least – that certain populations of small lymphocytes preferentially migrate through different sites. Several of these emerging patterns have only been described in sheep and while it would be wrong to generalize to other species without evidence, it seems likely to us that these patterns are probably general ones. For example, the non-random migratory patterns of surface Ig-positive cells in afferent compared with efferent lymph have now been demonstrated in man as well as in sheep (Miller and Adams, 1977; Godal and Engeset, 1978). It is our contention that most of the lymphocytes in the body are recirculating cells, and while we sometimes refer to "fixed lymphoid tissue", there may be no such thing as a fixed small lymphocyte. "The recirculating lymphocyte pool" may be a misnomer because it implies that only some lymphocytes have this property. Excluding blast cells and plasma cells, we adopt the working hypothesis that all small lymphocytes migrate from blood to secondary lymphoid tissue. Indeed, a lymphocyte, by its very name, implies a free-floating cell from lymph and not a fixed cell. Cell interactions are obviously fundamental to the functional integrity of all multicellular organisms and are not only the prerogative of the immunologist. Can the large animals provide sufficient numbers of homogeneous interacting cells to enable the eventual identification of cellular recognition mechanisms which may be common to or analogous with the recognition mechanisms of embryologic and morphogenetic systems as well as to the immune system?

II. Blood lymphocytes

When lymphocytes from efferent (leaving a lymph node) lymph are labelled with a radioisotope and injected intravenously (their normal site of entry to the blood via the major lymph ducts), they rapidly disappear from the blood. For cells which are generally considered to be long-lived, they have disappearance curves more like the short-lived polymorphonuclear leukocyte (PMN). Most lymphocytes seem to have a blood half-life of about two hours, compared with monocytes — around 40 hours (Issekutz *et al.*, 1981), PMNs four hours (Issekutz and Movat, 1980), red cells — several days. Unfortunately, there is no stringent comparison of these disappearance curves using the same species and the same labelling procedure, and therefore this interpretation must be qualified. A further complication is the probability that some alteration is induced in leukocytes by the blood cell separation methods. From a first glance at Fig. 1 it would seem that most blood lymphocytes might enter lymph nodes (preferred traffic sites) in the first five hours and then reappear in lymph. However, the relationships between the disappearance from the blood, the accumulation in lymph nodes and the output of labelled cells in the lymph are not clear. Fig. 1 is a schematic, composite representation of these curves. At the time when the disappearance from the blood is the most rapid, lymphocytes are not collecting at the greatest rate in the lymph nodes. Based on data from rodents (Smith *et al.*, 1980) and sheep (Cahill *et al.*, 1976), the lymphocytes are not simply in either the spleen, liver or lungs but in all of these and other organs for varying periods of time. Spleenectomy, for example, does not substantially alter these patterns nor does intra-arterial (to by-pass the lungs) versus intravenous injection. The lung appears to temporarily and probably physiologically retard the passage of lymphocytes and maybe all leukocytes through it and studies on leukocyte margination should be referred to (Thakur *et al.*, 1977). Experiments by Cybulsky and Movat (to be published) using rabbit neutrophils clearly demonstrate this retention.

This phenomenon needs to be examined further with some consideration given to cells associated with diffuse lymphoid tissue within the walls of the larger airways compared with cells within the alveolar microcirculatory bed. Cahill and Trnka, for example, have observed differences in the accumulation of lymphocytes in the fetal lung versus that of young or adult sheep (Cahill and Trnka, 1980).

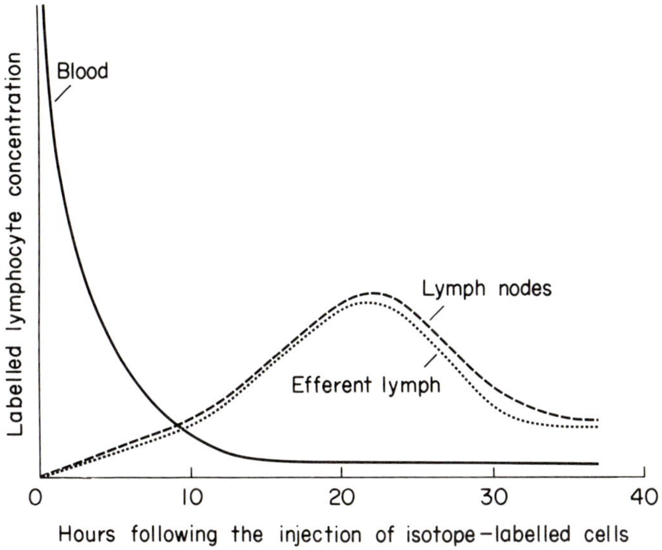

FIG. 1 A schematic interpretation of data from Cahill *et al.* (1976) and Smith *et al.* (1980) showing the disappearance of isotope-labelled lymphocytes from the blood and the subsequent accumulation of labelled cells in lymph nodes and efferent lymph.

There is a similar kinetic pattern of the appearance of labelled lymphocytes in lymph following their injection into the blood, regardless of whether the cells must traverse lymph nodes of a few milligrams in mice or a few grams in sheep. The highest concentration of cells in the lymph invariably appears near one day. The data to date has led some investigators to conclude that the blood to lymph transit time through a node is about four hours (Hall *et al.*, 1976), since some of the first intravenously labelled cells appear then. In contrast, others, including ourselves (Frost *et al.*, 1975; Issekutz *et al.*, 1980a), have referred to modal transit times of 18-22 hours (time when the highest concentration of labelled cells appear in lymph), thinking that most lymphocytes take this long. Neither analysis is satisfying in view of the rather complicated distribution in the compartments, shown in Fig. 1.

Are all the lymphocytes in the blood recirculating cells, or are there some lymphocytes which continually circulate in the blood but which never cross the blood vascular endothelium? There is no evidence for the latter and at present we prefer the hypothesis that lymphocytes in the blood are all "in transit". In later sections of this discussion, variations in the lymphocyte populations from different lymph sources are considered. The nature of this composite picture which is characteristic of the blood is important when it is realized that nearly all lymphocyte biology in man and in several animal species has been deduced by an analysis of the easily accessible blood lymphocytes. Furthermore, although blood lymphocytes seem easily accessible, it is not nearly so easy to obtain them free from contaminating monocytes and platelets. Monocytes in particular modulate most lymphocyte reactions *in vitro* (Unanue and Rosenthal, 1979).

Although lymphocytes are unique amongst the blood leukocytes in their capacity to recirculate, the monocyte also has the capability of normally migrating out of the blood, through connective tissue spaces and into afferent lymph, where some take on the morphological appearance of macrophages. These cells do not recirculate as do lymphocytes, and are absent from efferent lymph.

III. Thoracic duct lymphocytes

Most of the lymphocytes in the thoracic duct of sheep and other species are derived from efferent intestinal lymph from the small bowel and from efferent hepatic lymph (Yoffey and Courtice, 1980). Efferent lymph from subcutaneous lymph nodes contributes less than these two vital organs. In sheep, as in other species, approximately 75% of the lymphocytes in efferent lymph are surface immunoglobulin negative (Beh and Lascelles, 1974; Miller and Adams, 1977). These are probably T cells for the most part, since thymectomy (performed in utero in fetal lambs) depletes efferent lymphocytes by at least 75% (Cole and Morris, 1973). Efferent lymph contains approximately 25% surface Ig-positive cells (B cells) in most species and also in sheep (Morris and Courtice, 1977; Sprent, 1977). However, the surface Ig-positive cells in intestinal lymph have a much higher proportion of IgM-positive cells than other efferent lymph sources (Fahy *et al.*, 1980). Therefore, for B cells, the proportions will differ in intestinal vessels and thoracic duct, and both will differ from the blood. The right lymph duct is the other main lymphatic vessel which might contribute significant numbers of lymphocytes to the blood, but cervical lymph from the head and neck should also be considered. The output of lymphocytes in cervical lymph from sheep can be 2×10^8 h-1, or approximately one-tenth that of the thoracic duct output. The nature of the surface immunoglobulin on B cells from these sources is not known. However, the cervical duct drains the naso-pharynx and buccal mucosa and this lymph may have some similarties to intestinal lymph. The right lymph duct drains the thoracic and peritoneal cavity and some lung tissue (Yoffey and Courtice, 1980). One might guess that the proportion of cells with IgM or IgA on their surface may be higher than is seen on lymphocytes from other non-intestinal sites.

Differences in the nature and distribution of the B cells from these regions should be recalled in a later section dealing with differences in T cell migration through different sites.

IV. Changes in the output of lymphocytes from antigenically challenged popliteal lymph nodes

The popliteal lymph nodes of sheep are easily accessible and, under general anaesthetic, plastic catheters (usually 1·5 mm outside diameter) can be inserted into the efferent lymphatic and tied in place. Lymph can thereafter be collected in a quantitative manner into a plastic bottle attached to the flank of the sheep. As originally described by Lascelles and Morris (1961) and Hall and Morris (1962), lymph can be collected for various periods from hours to months. Fibrin formation in the catheter (collection bottles contain heparin) is the most common antagonizing factor which limits the life of the preparation, although in many situations replacement of a clotted catheter is feasible.

By perfusing the resting popliteal lymph node with ^{3}H-thymidine via an indwelling afferent lymphatic catheter (usually 0·6 mm outside diameter), Hall and Morris (1965) showed that only about 2-4% of the cells in efferent lymph were recently formed within the node. Invariably these were basophilic, blast-like forms and not small lymphocytes. Furthermore, based upon physiological collections of normal afferent lymph which has a much lower cell content, they concluded that about 90% of efferent cells were derived from the blood within the lymph node. Local irradiation of single nodes did not obliterate the cell output and this also supported a blood origin for the efferent lymph cells (Hall and Morris, 1964).

Morris and colleagues compared the cell output of a variety of nodes (Hall and Morris, 1962; Morris, 1972). An average one gram popliteal lymph node has an output of approximately 30 million lymphocytes per hour via the efferent lymph, and this value has been found in several laboratories (Cahill *et al.*, 1974; Hay and Hobbs, 1977). These lymph nodes contain an estimated $1{\cdot}2 \times 10^9$ lymphocytes and therefore an equivalent to the entire complement of lymphocytes in a node at any given time leaves the node every two or three days. From measurements of blood flow (lymphocyte delivery) to lymph nodes, it was calculated that the resting popliteal node extracts 25% of all blood-borne lymphocytes which enter it (Hay and Hobbs, 1977). The popliteal lymph node drains the tissue near the lower leg such as the foot in man, footpad of rodents and tissues near the hoof and hock of sheep. These regions and the nearby skin provide a convenient area to introduce antigens by subcutaneous injection. When bacterial and heterologous mammalian cellular antigens were introduced in this manner, Hall *et al.* (1967) found that several cellular changes were induced in the efferent popliteal lymph. Since the original description of these events a wide variety of materials ranging from saline to viral, protein, bacterial and cellular antigens have been injected (Smith and Morris, 1970; Cole and Morris, 1971; Murphy *et al.*, 1972; Hay *et al.*, 1973; English *et al.*, 1976; Frost *et al.*, 1976; Poskitt *et al.*, 1977).

A generalized summary of the cellular events which, for the most part are characteristic of all antigens, would include the stages discussed in sections A-D below.

A. PERIOD OF ACUTE INFLAMMATION AND LYMPHOCYTE SHUTDOWN

In the intact animal many cellular events associated with the reaction of the tissues to injury (inflammation) are seemingly inseparable from the early cellular events of the immune response, particularly so in natural infections or even following subcutaneous administration of bacteria or viruses. However, insofar as acquired immunity has to do with the production of antibody or the "sensitization" of T cells, the inflammatory reaction is probably a modulating rather than an obligatory influence. Specific antibody responses can be generated *in vitro*, for example, seemingly in the complete absence of the redness, swelling, heat and pain of inflammation. However, the significance of the cellular events of inflammation is absolutely vital to the maintenance of homeostasis and natural immunity cannot be ignored simply because it lacks the specificity of antibody and sensitized cells. The neutrophil deficient animal rapidly becomes the dead animal when challenged with pathogenic microorganisms in spite of lymphocytes and antibodies (Movat, 1980).

Two cellular events characterize this stage of the response of a lymph node. The output of lymphocytes begins to fall, often within the first hour (Hall and Morris, 1965). The most dramatic example of this lymphocyte shutdown is seen following the injection of influenza virus (Smith and Morris, 1970), where the efferent lymph may remain virtually acellular for 12 hours or more. The bacteriophage ϕX174 is also effective (Tao and Dresser, 1972; Cahill *et al.*, 1976). It has been shown that this deficiency is an effect of the antigen on lymphocytes which were within the node already and that the entry of lymphocytes from the blood is not compromised during this time. In fact, there is an increased entry of cells from the blood to the node at a time when the exit in the efferent lymph is reduced (Cahill *et al.*, 1976; Cahill and Trnka, 1980). It is our contention that this shutdown phenomenon has no direct bearing on the subsequent magnitude of the specific immune response. Allogeneic or even heterologous lymphocytes give rise to substantial cellular responses in efferent lymph (recruitment and blast responses) but are not very effective at producing the shutdown phenomenon. The possible mechanism of this shutdown is considered in a subsequent section.

The second early cellular change often observed in the efferent lymph is the appearance of PMNs (Hall *et al.*, 1967; Johnston *et al.*, 1979a). Normally these cells are not present in efferent lymph. The numbers of PMNs vary but bacterial antigens are usually good stimuli (Smith *et al.*, 1970d; Hay, 1979). The immune status of the animal may influence the PMN response, presumably via the generation of $C5_a$, since zymosan activated plasma induces a substantial PMN response in the draining lymph (A. Issekutz and Burrowes, unpublished observations). An antigen preparation from the protoscolices contained within hydatid cysts (*Echinococcus granulosis*) initiated an outpouring of nearly 10^9 PMNs per hour from a popliteal lymph node. The rate of lymph flow increased from 3 ml h^{-1} to 59 ml h^{-1} during this inflammatory episode (Hay, 1979). Purified protein derivative (PPD) of the tubercle bacillus, when injected into BCG-sensitized sheep does not usually invoke a PMN response in efferent lymph, although it triggers lymphocyte shutdown, recruitment and transformation (Hay *et al.*, 1973). The magnitude of the PMN response does not seem to relate to the magnitude of the lymphocyte response.

Although PMNs do not appear in the efferent lymph, they invariably appear at the site of antigen injection and, subsequently, at the site of antigen localization within the node (Frost *et al.*, 1975; Johnston *et al.*, 1979a). PMNs can be recruited into afferent lymph following the mild trauma of a 0·9% NaCl injection, for example. Although the

PMNs may constitute a substantial proportion of the afferent cell population, they may be of insufficient numbers to be conspicuous in efferent lymph, due to their short life span and phagocytic removal by the lymph node.

This early phase of cellular changes in efferent lymph is usually complete within 24 hours.

B. RECRUITMENT OF LYMPHOCYTES FROM THE BLOOD

A consequence of the stimulation of a single lymph node with antigen which is indicative of an antigen-specific immune response is the increase in output of lymphocytes seen in the efferent lymph. The timing of this increased output varies with the nature and dose of the antigen and the previous antigenic experience of the animal. However, approximately 24-48 hours after challenge is a common period for this phase of lymphocyte recruitment. Freund's complete adjuvant may give rise to a clearly delineated and protracted peak of increased lymphocyte output (Hay *et al.*, 1977; Hay *et al.*, 1973). During the response to other antigens and during secondary immune responses, the recruitment phase may be represented as the ascending portion of a single peak in cell output (Cahill *et al.*, 1976). The lymph node is increasing in size during this time and this is due both to edema and to an infiltration of the node with lymphocytes from the blood. Proliferation of cells is not a major factor during this phase.

The increase in cell output is due to small lymphocytes. The small percentage of blasts normally seen in efferent lymph are in fact diluted to an even smaller proportion during this period (Hay *et al.*, 1972; Hay *et al.*, 1973). While it is likely that the output of both T and B small lymphocytes is increased, there is some indication that T cells are enriched more than B cells (Frost, 1978). Based on studies using intravenously injected ^{51}Cr-labelled lymphocytes it seems likely that these cells were recruited from the blood into the node some hours before they appeared as a wave in efferent lymph (Cahill *et al.*, 1976). It is clear that these cells do not arise from afferent lymph since the pattern is similar when the antigenic stimulus is delivered to the node via an indwelling, afferent lymphatic catheter (Cahill and Trnka, 1980).

It has been shown that antigen promotes an increase in blood flow to lymph nodes within the first day of the immune response. The magnitude of the enhanced blood flow and enhanced lymphocyte recruitment (output in efferent lymph) were of a comparable order of magnitude and it was postulated that the hyperemia caused the increase in the lymphocyte traffic (Hay and Hobbs, 1977; Hay *et al.*,

1980). Stimuli such as allogeneic lymphocytes caused the most pronounced hyperemia and also the most pronounced recruitment phenomenon (Hay *et al.*, 1978; Hay *et al.*, 1980). Some of the possible vaso-active mediators which are implicated are discussed in section VII.

Although recruitment is a hallmark of the immune response of a single lymph node, it is probably not an obligatory step in the induction of a specific immune response. For example, a suspension of lymph node cells can give rise to an immune response *in vitro*, without the recruitment of cells from blood. Secondly, when small doses of antigen are injected, the more flamboyant changes in cell numbers in lymph cannot be detected, but subsequent evidence of a specific immune response, such as the appearance of sensitized cells, can be detected (Cahill *et al.*, 1979).

It has been suggested that this recruitment of lymphocytes provides an effective way to maximize the number of lymphocytes which may interact with a given antigen (Bell, 1978).

The second feature of this second (recruitment) phase of the immune response is the functional disappearance of specific antigen-reactive cells from the efferent lymph (Hay *et al.*, 1973). A similar phenomenon has been described in the thoracic duct of rats and mice following antigen stimulation of the spleen (Sprent *et al.*, 1971). It is our hypothesis that the lymphocytes which were capable of responding to the antigen were selectively removed within the lymph node during this period and that these cells later appear in the lymph as antigen-stimulated blast cells (Hay *et al.*, 1973). There is no proof of this hypothesis however, and the possibility that tolerant cells are responsible for the observation continues to be debated (Cahill *et al.*, 1974; McCullagh, 1980).

C. APPEARANCE OF BLAST CELLS, SPECIFIC ANTIBODY-FORMING CELLS AND NON-SPECIFIC ANTIBODY-FORMING CELLS IN LYMPH

Lymphocyte proliferation usually starts to increase significantly towards the end of the second day of the immune response in a lymph node. In the efferent lymph there is an increase in the output of lymphoblasts, most of which will incorporate radioactive thymidine *in vitro*, are large and have basophilic cytoplasm (Hall *et al.*, 1967; Hay *et al.*, 1972). The proportion of these antigen-stimulated cells which have been shown to contain or secrete specific antibody varies with different antigens and assay systems used. Cunningham *et al.* (1966) demonstrated that individual plaque-forming cells (PFCs) producing antibody to Salmonella lipopolysaccharide had the ultrastructural appearance of blast cells. Analysis of the density and size of PFCs in efferent lymph and lymph nodes suggested that most of the antibody-forming cells in lymph were large blast-forms but that an additional population of more dense, plasma cells remained in the lymph node. These cells were about three times as concentrated in the medulla compared with the cortex. At the peak of an immune response, concentrations as high as 50 000 PFC $\times$ 10^{-6} lymph cells were observed (Yamashita *et al.*, 1970). The concentration of PFCs was enriched to 120 000 $\times$ 10^{-6} *in vivo* using anti-lymphocyte serum as is described subsequently (Hay *et al.*, 1974). To our knowledge this concentration of specific plaque-forming cells is the highest seen in any *in vivo* or *in vitro* system. In experiments using horseradish peroxidase (HRP) as an antigen, as many as 50% of lymph blasts were shown to contain specific antibody with the light microscope and when examined with the electron microscope, as many as 70% of the lymph blasts contained specific antibody. In secondary immune responses, where 40% of the cells in the lymph were blasts, this meant that one in three lymph cells were making antibody to HRP. When the blast response in the lymph had waned mature, classical plasma cells were still present in the node. However, at this stage of an immune response, the most vigorous period of antibody synthesis was past and it is our conclusion that the blast cell contribution to antibody production is greater than that of plasma cells (Hay *et al.*, 1972). English *et al.* (1976) have shown that only about 5% of the newly synthesized immunoglobulin in a Salmonella response is actually specific antibody. Non-specific PFCs have been described in lymph by Poskitt *et al.* (1977).

When other antigens are used to stimulate lymph nodes, the proportion of blasts synthesizing specific antibody is quite different. Following the injection of allogeneic lymphocytes, a vigorous blast cell response follows. When these cells are stained with fluorescent anti-sheep immunoglobulin, there are very few positive cells compared with, say, a Salmonella blast response (unpublished observations). Presumably, many of these cells are T blasts, as has been shown in the thoracic duct of mice undergoing graft versus host responses (Sprent and Miller, 1971). High titres of allo-antibody do, however, appear in efferent lymph during these allogeneic responses (Hay, 1979).

Non-specific PFCs have been described during the blast cell response to several antigens (Poskitt *et al.*, 1977). Lymphocytes which bind antigen and, in the case of chicken erythrocytes give rise to rosettes, also increase in number during this blast cell phase. It was found that a low level of antigen-binding cells (about 1 in 8000) was seen in lymph prior to antigenic challenge and, that after challenge, most PFCs would also form rosettes. Rosetting cells remained at elevated levels in the efferent lymph after the PFC response had fallen to undetectable levels (Heron *et al.*, 1978).

Important questions can be asked regarding the fate of lymph blast cells. Some of these features have been examined such as their role in the propagation and dissemination of antibody production and immunological memory (Smith *et al.*, 1970a), their effect on subsequent (lumbar) lymph nodes (Trevella and Morris, 1980), and their migration to the gastro-intestinal tract (Hall, 1980). These aspects are discussed in a later section.

The blast response in efferent lymph merges with the final phase. In primary responses, the peak of blast cell output and PFC output is usually near day four. This is invariably earlier in the secondary response.

D. THE APPEARANCE OF SENSITIZED CELLS IN EFFERENT LYMPH

As the blast cell output from a primary immune response declines, sensitized cells appear in the efferent lymph. There are three documented examples of this in the sheep system involving tuberculin-sensitive cells, allo-reactive cells and the antigen-binding cells (rosettes) already referred to. These sensitized cells are a consequence of an antigen-induced proliferative response and can be considered the memory cells of predominantly T lymphocyte reactions.

When normal efferent lymphocytes are cultured with the purified protein derivative (PPD) of the tubercle bacillus there is no detectable induction of a proliferative response. However, when sheep are first injected with Bacillus Calmette Guerin (BCG) or with Freund's complete adjuvant (FCA) containing tubercle bacillus, PPD-sensitive cells subsequently appear. The kinetics of the output of these cells in efferent lymph has been described for FCA (Hay *et al.*, 1972) and BCG (Hay and Morris, 1975). Fig. 2 shows such a response to BCG and the appearance of PPD-sensitive cells. The timing of the appearance of sensitive or "sensitized" cells in this example is much more rapid than has been observed on other occasions where several weeks passed before sensitized lymphocytes could be detected (Hay and Morris, 1975). The reasons for this are not known, although the strain of bacilus may cross-react with other natural bacilli previously seen by the animal. Although PPD-sensitive cells first appear during the blast response, they are more difficult to assay at this time, due to the high background of cell replication in cultures made in the absence of PPD.

As the blast cell response declines, a greater difference between cultures set up in the presence versus the absence of PPD becomes evident. The ratio of stimulation may range from about 2-100-fold, and the reasons for this variation are not known. Furthermore, in several animals, daily or near-daily collections of efferent lymph cells over periods of several weeks have been cultured with and without PPD. A rise and fall in the magnitude of the response often (but not always) displays a periodicity of about four days and it is not known how these changes related to the general physiological status of the animal or to the growth of this facultative intracellular parasite within the macrophages of the sheep (Hay and Morris, 1975).

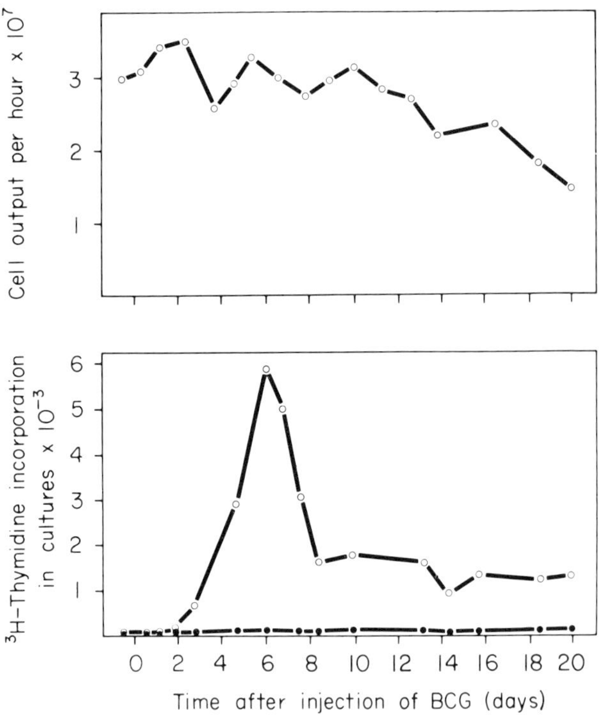

FIG. 2 The appearance of PPD-sensitive cells in efferent lymph following the subcutaneous injection of BCG into the drainage area of the cannulated lymph node. Top panel: output of lymph cells. Bottom panel: the uptake of ^{3}H-thymidine into 3-day lymph cell cultures done in the presence (o) and absence (•) of PPD.

It seems clear to us that the regional node is instrumental in the generation of these sensitized cells and that the efferent lymph is fundamental to the dissemination of sensitized cells throughout the body, where they become part of the recirculating lymphocyte pool. Furthermore, the presence of sensitized lymphocytes in afferent lymph (see section VIII) is fundamental to the initiation and development of the tuberculin reaction in the skin and may be analogous to other related pathological phenomena in a variety of tissues (Hay *et al.*, 1980).

Lymphocytes responsive to PPD are undetectable in normal sheep but are presumably present at a very low frequency. The expansion of this population of cells is the very essence of the generation of delayed hypersensitivity (Hay, 1980). The practicality of the situation with allo-reactive cells detected in mixed lymphocyte reactions (MLR) *in vitro* is substantially different, since the MLR cells can be assayed prior to immunization with allogeneic lymphocytes. Nevertheless, sensitized MLR cells are generated in stimulated lymph nodes and these sensitized cells emigrate into efferent lymph (Cahill *et al.*, 1979). They are T cells, small lymphocytes, which respond more rapidly *in vitro* than unprimed cells and become part of the recirculating pool of lymphocytes (Cahill *et al.*, 1979; Cahill and Trnka, 1980). The sensitized MLR cells appear to leave the node in maximum numbers two to three days after the peak output of blast cells. Most of these cells are probably generated in the node, although the normal lymphocyte transfer lesion induced at the injection site may contribute a significant number of cells to the regional node via the afferent lymph. Afferent cell outputs have been recorded at about 30 times greater than normal at the peak of such lesions (Hay, 1979) (see section IX, B on afferent lymph).

It is presumed that these sensitized small lymphocytes are descendants of the blast cells. Based upon the capacity of these cells to respond in a more rapid manner than in the usual MLR, it might be concluded that they are qualitatively different from unprimed cells (Fig. 3). The quantitative expansion of antigen-reactive cells is the most significant feature of this sensitization process.

There are insufficient studies on the dissemination and recirculation of these sensitized cells in the sheep. They should be further studied in the various lymph pools and in afferent lymph. Do these cells recirculate as effectively, or maybe more effectively, than normal lymphocytes? What is the significance and the mechanism of the systemic fluctuations of MLR and PPD sensitive cells (Hay *et al.*, 1973; Hay and Morris, 1975)? If these cells are the consequence of a proliferative response in the regional lymph node, can they be purified by using anti-lymphocyte serum in a manner which has proved to be particularly effective for PFCs? (Hay *et al.*, 1974). Is there a polyclonal, non-specific generation of other sensitized cells analogous to the non-specific PFC response in lymph?

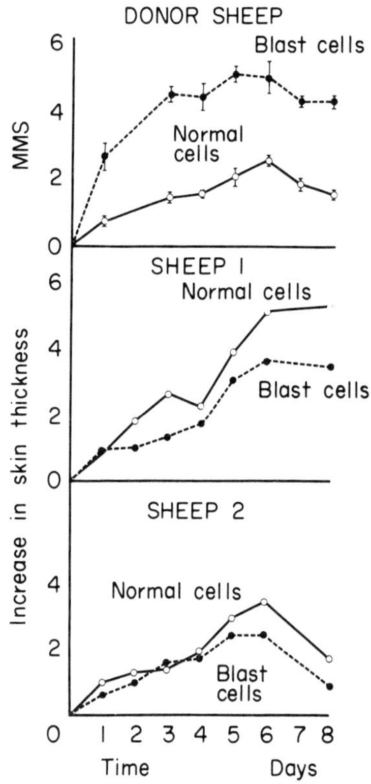

FIG. 3 Lymphocyte transfer reactions produced by the intra-dermal injection of efferent lymph cells obtained 5 days following the subcutaneous injection of normal lymphocytes from a donor sheep. The sensitized cells were more reactive when injected back into the donor than they were in two unrelated sheep. Data from PhD thesis (J. B. Hay) Australian National University, 1971.

V. Effects of local and systemic anti-lymphocyte antibody on the cellular migration from popliteal lymph nodes

A polyclonal antibody produced in rabbits by the injection of efferent lymph cells from sheep has been used to modulate the immune response as it is observed in efferent lymph (Hay *et al.*, 1974). It was found that the subcutaneous injection of 1 ml of a 1:100 dilution of such an ALS could produce a rapid fall in the output of cells from the popliteal node. The lymph remained nearly acellular for about twelve hours, and this was followed by a recruitment and blast cell response. The ALS in fact was a potent *in vitro* lymphocyte mitogen in the absence of complement. In a series of primary and secondary immune responses to Salmonella, ALS was administered locally or systemically in an attempt to suppress the number of PFCs which emigrated from stimulated popliteal nodes. Local administration included the continuous infusion of ALS into the node via an indwelling afferent lymphatic catheter. ALS was given before, with or after the Salmonella. No suppression of the PFC response was detectable. The out put of small lymphocytes could be eliminated but the cells formed in the node (blasts and PFC) entered the lymph in the usual numbers. However, instead of the blasts comprising, say, 30% of the total lymph cells at the peak of the response, the blast cells comprised over 96% of the cells in efferent lymph. Direct PFC assays as high as 120 000/10^6 cells were found. Furthermore, ALS administration proved to be an effective method to obtain large numbers of pure eosinophils or PMNs if an appropriate stimulus for these cells was given. This type of manipulation should be re-examined in an attempt to purify sensitized T cells. What effect would ALS have on the lymphocyte traffic through NLTs and granulomas (see section IX,B)? Could afferent lymph macrophages be purified in this manner? Can more subtle antisera be raised against lymphocyte sub-populations and be used to manipulate and analyze the cellular responses seen in lymph? Hybridoma methodology may be helpful in this respect. Cahill and Heron (unpublished data) have produced monoclonal antibody against a sub-population of sheep T cells and the further development of markers for sheep lymphocytes may be a potent tool for the analysis of lymph cells.

VI. Changes in the lymph plasma from antigenically challenged popliteal lymph nodes

There are many changes in the lymph plasma following antigenic stimulation of a lymph node. Some of these have been described in relation to inflammatory events rather than immunological events (Hay, 1979; Johnston *et al.*, 1979a). However, the distinction between inflammatory and immunological is often vague, particularly in the case of chronic inflammation. Since the cells of the immune response are continuously bathed in lymph plasma, any changes in the constitution of this plasma could modulate the reactive potential or the fate of the cells. There is strong evidence to support this contention.

Recent experiments by Morris and colleagues have focussed on the immune respone of lymph nodes which receive the whole lymph from a node which has been directly stimulated with antigen (Trevella and Morris, 1980). In sheep, lumbar lymph nodes receive lymph from the popliteal nodes. Earlier experiments by Hall *et al.* (1967) suggested that there was an amplification of the immune response by the second lymph node in a chain. Evidence was presented that the antigens used were quantitatively removed by the first (popliteal) node. This suggested to them that the lymph cells were responsible for the amplification in the lumbar nodes. These types of experiments have been repeated in greater detail and a role for "factors" in the lymph as well as the cells themselves have been implicated (Trevella and Morris, 1980). Infusion of popliteal lymph collected from 0-24 hours after challenge with chicken erythrocytes produced a shutdown in the cell output in the lumbar lymph. There was no subsequent recruitment, blast response or antibody production in this lumbar node. Lymph collected from the popliteal node 0-48 hours after challenge also transmitted a signal for recruitment by the lumbar node, but still did not induce a blast or PFC response. Later collections of popliteal lymph however were capable of propagating an immune response and the cells continued to demonstrate a limited proliferative capacity.

Before describing further the changes in lymph plasma from stimulated nodes and the different effects that this plasma can have on cells, it is relevant to take into account some more general physiological properties of lymph plasma.

VII. Lymph plasma proteins

Lymph formation is a consequence of a cardiovascular system which delivers the blood under pressure. There is a leakage of plasma. An examination of an immuno-electrophoresis slide made with lymph plasma shows that virtually all of the blood plasma proteins are present (Smeaton *et al.*, 1969). Efferent popliteal lymph has approximately 60% the protein concentration of blood plasma, and afferent popliteal lymph approximately 40-50% of the blood value. It has been shown that the protein concentration of efferent lymph falls if lymphocyte traffic in the node is decreased by inducing a lymphopenia (Quin and Shannon, 1977). This suggests that some protein escapes with the emigrating cells. All the constituents necessary for the polymerization of fibrin are present in lymph and without the use of anticoagulants in collecting bottles, both afferent and efferent lymph readily clot. There is some molecular sieving involved in the formation of lymph and the albumin-to-globulin ratio is higher in lymph plasma than in blood plasma. This preferential exclusion may be particularly significant with respect to very large molecules. IgM concentrations in afferent lymph are very low (Ey, 1973) and natural inhibitors of proteolytic enzymes such as alpha$_2$ macroglobulin are probably also dilute. During the first day of the immune response there is often an increase in vascular permeability associated with the inflammatory episode (Hay, 1979). This is reflected in an increase in the protein content of the lymph as well as in the flow rate.

A. IMMUNOGLOBULINS

Returning the discussion to more specific changes in lymph which may affect the cells of the immune response, the first class of molecules which are probably significant are the immunoglobulins. Specific antibody has been titrated in the efferent lymph following a variety of antigenic challenges (Hay, 1979). In many cases an IgM phase precedes the appearance of IgG. The levels and kinetics of these two change during the secondary response of a single lymph node. The antibody response in lymph can be quantitated more easily than it can be in blood. In the latter compartment the titre is the net concentration and is dependent on synthesis, accumulation as well as catabolism. In the lymph model the antibody does not accumulate since the lymph is quantitatively removed in the collection bottles. The actual antibody output of a node can be measured (antibody concentration × lymph flow rate). English *et al.* (1976) quantitated the amount of protein and immunoglobulin synthesized by a single lymph node by perfusing the node with labelled amino acids during the immune response to Salmonella lipopolysaccharide. Antigen-binding immunoglobulin as well as non-specific immunoglobulin and immunoglobulin-like protein was measured. Comparisons have been made between the protein synthesizing capacity of efferent blast cells and the blast cells in the lymph from rejecting renal allografts (Pedersen *et al.*, 1975). Frost *et al.* (1976) have shown that a popliteal node can produce and secrete into lymph 800 mg h^{-1} of specific antibody against a variant of streptococcal vaccine.

The concentration of IgA in efferent intestinal lymph is much higher than in other efferent lymph and is even higher than in the blood (Lascelles and McDowell, 1974; Beh, 1977). The gut-associated lymphoid tissue is the major source of this Ig and nearly all of the blood IgA is delivered via the lymph. It seems likely that the immunoglobulin synthesized by a lymph node exits exclusively via the efferent lymph. Two types of experiment support this view. There is evidence that immune responses can be confined to single lymph nodes, giving rise to high titres of antibody in the efferent lymph and no detectable antibody in the blood (Smith *et al.*, 1970a). Secondly, when radiolabelled proteins are infused into nodes via an afferent lymphatic vessel, virtually 100% of the protein can be recovered in the efferent lymph (Trevella and Morris, 1980).

B. SOLUBLE FACTORS IN LYMPH WHICH MODULATE LYMPHOCYTE AND MACROPHAGE FUNCTIONS

Lymph plasma obtained during the early stage of an immune response to tuberculin and to Concanavalin A was found to contain substances which stimulated DNA synthesis in normal lymphocyte cultures (Hay, 1973; Hay *et al.*, 1973). Lymph plasma has been shown to either enhance or suppress the synthesis and secretion of antibody-forming cells (English *et al.*, 1977). The background level of immunoglobulin synthesis by resting lymph nodes can be reduced to very low levels by a lymph plasma constituent obtained early in an immune response (English *et al.*, 1976). A substance which inhibited the migration of guinea pig macrophages *in vitro* has been found in lymph plasma following stimulation with tuberculin or Concanavalin A (Hay, 1973; Hay *et al.*, 1973). It would be of interest to know the identity of any substance that appears in lymph plasma which can induce shutdown or recruitment.

At present there are several potential molecular candidates for these biologically active factors although conclusive data is lacking.

C. PHOSPHOLIPASE AND ARACHIDONIC ACID METABOLITES

The stimulus for lymphocyte recruitment has been of particular interest to us. Our hypothesis is that this phenomenon is a direct consequence of an increase in the delivery rate of lymphocytes to the node via an antigen-stimulated increase in blood flow. The most potent vasoactive mediators which have been identified are the prostaglandins. In this context PGE_1, PGE_2 and PGI_2 have been the most potent in the skin of rabbits (Vadas, 1980) and sheep (Johnston, 1979). Johnston has measured the levels of PGE and PGF in afferent and efferent lymph following stimulation with a variety of immune and inflammatory agents (Johnston *et al.*, 1979a). High levels of PG appeared in the early phase of such responses. However, very little PG could be attributed to the lymph cells themselves. The possibility that a phospholipase A_2 was released by the lymph cells and that a variety of surrounding cell membranes might then provide the cyclooxygenase machinery seemed a possibility to Johnston and others (Johnston, 1979; Johnston *et al.*, 1979b). More recently, Vadas and Hay (1980) have described a vasoactive factor which induces hyperemia in rabbit skin. This material was produced by macrophage-containing cell cultures of sheep and rabbit. It did not appear to be histamine, bradykinin or prostaglandin, although the data was compatible with the elaboration of an indomethacin-sensitive step in the final vasoactive phenomenon (Vadas, 1980; Vadas and Hay, 1980). Phospholipase A_2 was assayed in these cell culture fluids and the data suggests that stimulation of macrophages (possibly via lymphocyte products) results in the release of phospholipase which, in turn, can liberate cell membrane arachidonic acid for PG synthesis (Vadas, 1980). Although hyperemia may be the cause of recruitment phenomenon seen in efferent lymph such vascular mechanisms do not further our understanding of resting lymphocyte traffic in lymphoid tissues. Nevertheless, hyperemia may modulate other aspects of immune and inflammatory phenomena as has been suggested for enhanced vascular permeability (Johnston *et al.*, 1979b; Johnston *et al.*, 1976).

Prostaglandins may modulate the functions of lymph cells via cyclic nucleotide interference or by some other mechanism as has been described in the mouse (Johnston *et al.*, 1979b). It is possible that these compounds were responsible for the modulating influence of lymph plasma described by English *et al.* (1977).

D. COAGULATION AND FIBRINOLYSIS

When studying the lymph plasma for macrophage inhibition factor (MIF) it was observed that active lymph was particularly prone to clotting and it was mentioned that the clotting system might interfere with the assay of MIF (Hay *et al.*, 1973). This was investigated further by Meade *et al.* (1976). Although it was assumed that this lymph MIF was a lymphokine, it was difficult to demonstrate MIF production with pure efferent lymph cells and PPD *in vitro*. It would have been interesting to also consider macrophage-containing afferent lymph as a source. This is particularly so since Burrowes (personal communication) has shown that stimulated afferent cells can release a thromboplastin-like material. Furthermore, during immune and inflammatory responses, the clotting time of the draining lymph is considerably shortened, most likely via activation of the extrinsic (thromboplastin) pathway of fibrin formation (Burrowes, personal communication).

Although fibrin deposition is relevant to the inflammatory process, the possibility that it can modulate lymphocyte migration should also be considered. Delayed hypersensitivity reactions can be inhibited with systemic heparin administration (Nelson, 1965). Does fibrin deposition simply lead to induration by promoting imbibition of water, or is the degree of lymphocyte infiltration (traffic) also less? The capacity of stimulated macrophages from afferent lymph to synthesize and secrete plasminogen activator may also play a role in these phenomena (Vadas *et al.*, 1979). Finally, high levels of interferon have been found in efferent lymph following challenge of the node with influenza virus (Heron *et al.*, 1980).

The modulation of the immune response as it occurs *in vivo* is a microvascular as well as a lymphoid cell phenomenon, and is much more complex than the interaction of cells in the *in vitro* systems would suggest. It seems reasonable that the immune response ultimately could be better controlled by further delineating these interacting systems and molecules.

VIII. Cells from normal afferent lymph

Afferent lymph contains some of the most interesting and functionally diverse types of cells found in any of the lymphoid tissues. Since afferent lymph flows into the subcapsular sinus of lymph nodes, it follows that lymph nodes contain all of the cell types present in afferent lymph. While this is correct, it is also apparent that any cell suspension of a lymph node contains only a diluted representation of afferent lymph, since the cell concentration of this lymph is low (about 1×10^6 ml^{-1} in sheep). Afferent lymphatics begin as blind-ended capillaries in most connective tissues of the body (Yoffey and Courtice, 1980). As these microvascular structures come together larger, collecting vessels can be observed with the naked eye. Such afferent lymphatics have a beaded appearance due to numerous valves interspersed every few millimetres along the vessel. The only species in which such afferent vessels have been drained and systematically examined under unanaesthetized, physiological and resting conditions are the sheep (Hall and Morris, 1962), man (Engeset *et al.*, 1973) and the pig (Binns, 1980). The most extensive studies have been done on the sheep and afferent lymph from various regions of skin, liver (Smith *et al.*, 1970b), heart (Simpson-Morgan, 1970), kidney (McIntosh and Morris, 1971), thyroid (Smith *et al.*, 1970b), testes (Morris and McIntosh, 1970), ovary, uterus (Morris and Sass, 1966) and gut (Lascelles and Morris, 1961; Reynolds, 1980a) have been examined. Hepatic and intestinal afferent lymph stand out in such a comparison because the cell content is approximately ten times that of afferent lymph from other sources (Smith *et al.*, 1970). Afferent lymph drainage from pathological sites is considered in section IX.

Under resting conditions afferent lymph is free of erythrocytes and PMNs. However, a modest blow, massage or an injection of physiological saline with a small bore needle is often sufficient to provoke a detectable erythrocyte and PMN response. Most of the cells in afferent lymph are small lymphocytes. It is not definitely known whether most of the small lymphocytes in afferent lymph are T cells, null cells or some other cell, but it is clear that they lack surface Ig (Morris and Courtice, 1977). Macrophages, some with extensive and ruffled cytoplasmic processes, make up about 5-15% of afferent lymph cells. Sometimes a few lymphoblasts are present. The proportion of small lymphocytes with surface Ig is approximately 25% that of efferent lymph, or about 6% of the total cells. Intestinal afferent lymph is an exception, and the proportion of surface Ig-positive cells is about the same as in efferent lymph (data referred to in Trevella and Morris (1980) and Reynolds (1980a). Values for hepatic afferent lymph are not known. Intestinal afferent (and efferent) lymph has a higher proportion of large cells containing intracellular IgA than is seen in other afferent lymph preparations (Reynolds, 1980a). Afferent cells are probably equivalent to the cells normally found in the peritoneal and pleural cavity. These are cells which, for the most part, are derived from the blood and which migrate from the blood into connective tissue or body spaces and then into lymph. In the case of the peritoneal and pleural cavity, the lymph drainage is probably via the right lymph duct.

The macrophages of afferent lymph do not enter efferent lymph. Based upon calculations and estimates on the input and output of cells from a one-gram popliteal node, it can be estimated that about 5×10^5 macrophages enter this node per hour. A centrifuged, one-gram pellet of alveolar macrophages contains approximately 5×10^8 cells and based on this estimate, it would therefore take some 40 days to replace the equivalent mass of the popliteal node with macrophages or to double the normal weight of this node. By assuming a life span of many days for the average macrophage a balanced size of the node would be maintained. Van Furth has estimated the rate of production of macrophages in mice (Van Furth and Willemz, 1979). However, as has been described previously, mesenteric nodes and hepatic nodes seem to have a higher afferent input of cells and the fate of hepatic macrophages is more difficult to analyze. Smith *et al.* (1970b) have shown that some of the cells in afferent hepatic lymph are derived from the Kupffer cell population lining the liver sinusoids.

Any attempt to rationalize how and why lymphocytes leave the blood and recirculate should incorporate an awareness that the monocyte-macrophage displays this interrupted circulation pattern from blood to afferent lymph to lymph nodes. It is possible that a substantial number of monocytes leave the blood from the post-capillary venules within lymph nodes associated with lymphocytes. Furthermore it is interesting that in all pathological situations where the output of mononuclear cells can be increased in afferent lymph to several times normal, the increase in lymphocyte output is paralleled by an increase in macrophage output. In other words, the 5-15% proportion of macrophages remains constant. Either large-scale proliferation of macrophages occurs at these pathological sites, or the emigration of monocytes and lymphocytes from the blood are interrelated in some fashion. The proportion of monocytes to lymphocytes in the blood is not unlike the proportion of macrophages to lymphocytes in afferent lymph.

Recent interest has focussed on a subpopulation of these macrophages seen in afferent lymph and several investigators have described a population of large mononuclear (veiled cells with "Ia-like" membrane antigens) in man (Spry *et al.*, 1980). A relationship between these cells, Langerhans' cells in the skin and interdigitating cells in the paracortex of lymph nodes has been suggested. It has also been claimed that these cells lack some of the surface markers characteristic for cells of the monocyte line. An anti-Ia antibody prepared in mice (ATH anti-ATL) has been found to stain predominantly B cells (based on nylon wool separation) in sheep but some large, macrophage-like cells in afferent lymph also stain very strongly (Chin, personal communication).

Relatively few functional studies have been carried out on afferent lymph cells, simply because these cells are difficult to obtain, even in sheep. Scollay and Lafferty (1975) have shown that these cells are much less effective at producing NLTs or local graft versus host reactions in the skin of recipient sheep. They also showed that afferent lymph cells produced a very early inflammatory response in the skin of both an allogeneic recipient and also in the skin of sheep which donated the cells. It would be interesting to investigate this further, in view of the description of the vasoactive product released from afferent macrophages described by Vadas and Hay (1980). Mixed lymphocyte reaction data suggests that afferent cells are poorer responders than efferent cells but that they are good stimulators (Scollay *et al.*, 1976a). Afferent cell cultures have a high background uptake of ^{3}H-thymidine and this complicates the interpretation of data comparing the stimulation index of different populations. Table 1 shows some data obtained by Cahill and Hay which illustrates the high background incorporation in normal afferent cell cultures. It would be interesting to know whether the macrophages or some other accessory cells facilitate continued DNA synthesis in the small proportion of blast cells which are present when cultures are initiated. In efferent cell

TABLE 1

A comparison of 3-day cell cultures of afferent and efferent lymph cells from normal and BCG-primed sheep. Figures represent the cpm of the mean ± standard errors of the ^{3}H-thymidine incorporation into the cells. Five experiments were done on normal sheep. Experiment 2 shows simultaneous data from afferent and efferent lymph from the same animal. Four experiments were done on BCG-primed sheep and simultaneous afferent and efferent lymph cell cultures were done in experiments 1 and 3.

Normal sheep

	Afferent cells		Efferent cells	
Experiment	- PPD	+ PPD	- PPD	+ PPD
1	18 520 ± 3876	20 797 ± 3954	—	—
2	13 187 ± 2051	11 909 ± 1847	1483 ± 143	1655 ± 325
3	33 402 ± 1089	29 228 ± 381	—	—
4	—	—	1101 ± 214	1014 ± 233
5	—	—	1953 ± 529	1160 ± 194

BCG-primed sheep

	Afferent cells		Efferent cells	
Experiment	- PPD	+ PPD	- PPD	+ PPD
1	32 146 ± 1809	87 735 ± 9875	230 ± 37	5262 ± 215
2	42 525 ± 6051	98 659 ± 6904	—	—
3	32 031 ± 2910	90 259 ± 9278	1276 ± 229	4536 ± 424
4	—	—	305 ± 84	2421 ± 64

cultures, these cells may die off more rapidly. A more interesting possibility might involve a central role of, say, the large Ia-positive cells in presenting a mitogenic stimulus to the lymphocytes (Unanue and Rosenthal, 1979).

An interesting technique for obtaining greater numbers of afferent cells has been described in sheep and rats (MacPherson and Steer, 1979; Reynolds, 1980b). This involves lymphadenectomy followed by cannulation of the larger efferent lymphatic trunks some weeks later. Severed afferent vessels anastomose at the site of the extirpated node and the afferent vessels flow directly into the efferent vessel. This lymph then has the appearance of afferent lymph. It is incredible that this healing process takes place so effectively. Studies on the healing of several lymphatics in the rabbit ear (Bellman and Oden, 1958-59) provide a fascinating morphological description of these events. When mesenteric lymphadenectomy is performed in sheep, the cell output in the major intestinal trunks is still very high (Reynolds, 1980a). The lymphocytes coming directly from the gut wall in this lymph show a non-random migration pattern (Hall, 1980) similar to that described by Cahill *et al.*, 1977) for efferent intestinal lymph cells. (See section XI discussion of intestinal lymph.)

Although some of our colleagues have concluded that the cells in afferent lymph are of trivial significance since they are relatively few in number compared with efferent lymph, we strongly disagree and take quite the opposite view that they are of fundamental significance. Furthermore, the demonstration that afferent lymph contains antigen-reactive cells to PPD in BCG primed sheep (as is documented in Table 1) is very important. Consider as an example the tuberculin reaction in the skin. It is clear that the key to the initiation of this immune-inflammatory lesion is the sensitized T cell and its interaction with PPD (Hay, 1980). Since these cells are part of the recirculating lymphocyte population and can be found in afferent lymph (and therefore in the subcutaneous extravascular tissues), the initiation of the tuberculin reaction can be considered an extravascular phenomenon. All of the cell participants are normally present outside of the blood prior to the injection of PPD. It is not known whether some PPD enters the blood, but it seems reasonable that most of the PPD is washed towards the lymph along with the plasma proteins. Indeed the flow of afferent lymph usually increases in these reactions. In any case, it is not necessary that some antigen reaches the blood and interacts with PPD-sensitive lymphocytes passing in the blood as has been commonly assumed.

In one experiment an afferent popliteal lymphatic vessel was cannulated in one hind leg of a sheep and a prefemoral efferent lymphatic cannulated on the opposite side. BCG was injected into the drainage area of the afferent vessel. Cell cultures from both these lymphatics were set up each day with PPD, without PPD and with Con A (the latter serving as a positive control for the viability of the cells). PPD-sensitive cells appeared 1-2 days earlier in the regional afferent lymph than in the systemic efferent lymph. We interpret this data to indicate that sensitized cells can be generated at the skin site of BCG injection, that they enter afferent lymph and are, a day or two later, distributed in the larger, systemic, recirculating lymphocyte pool. In the normal course of events, the regional node would also be a focus and possibly the major site of the production of sensitized lymphocytes.

IX. Afferent lymph from pathological sites

Afferent lymph has been continuously collected and studied in sheep over periods of up to many days or weeks from a variety of pathological sites. These pathological tissues include the rejecting kidney (Pedersen and Morris, 1970) and heart (Simpson-Morgan, 1970) following allogeneic transplantation into the neck, skin grafts (Hall, 1967), normal lymphocyte transfer reactions (Hay *et al.*, 1978), tuberculin reactions (Hay *et al.*, 1973), adjuvant-induced granulomas (Smith *et al.*, 1970c; Issekutz *et al.*, 1980a), fluke infested livers (Smith *et al.*, 1970c), dermal contact-sensitivity lesions (Hall, 1980), *E. coli* lesions (Johnston *et al.*, 1980), endotoxin lesions (Burrowes, personal communication) and carrageenan lesions (Johnston *et al.*, 1979a).

Although only general observations such as cell outputs, flow rates, protein content and morphology of the cells has been studied for many of these situations, some other assays have been performed to try to better understand the functional role of these cells. Some of these responses are described here under the general category of acute and chronic reactions and allogeneic phenomena.

A. ACUTE REACTIONS

Hall and Morris (1965) observed that PMNs appeared in afferent lymph very quickly after the injection of bacterial antigens into the drainage site. Following the injection of Freund's adjuvant, Smith *et al.* (1970c) observed an outpouring of PMNs in afferent lymph which lasted about two days. This phase of the response was nevertheless very small compared with the subsequent gradual rise and fall in mononuclear cell output observed over the following 70 days. Johnston *et al.* (1979a, 1980) have measured E and F prostaglandins (PG) in afferent lymph plasma during the acute inflammatory response to *E. coli* and carrageenan. Prostaglandin concentrations increased very rapidly and reached a maximum near three hours after stimulation. There were large numbers of PMNs in the afferent lymph at this time, although the peak output of PMNs was usually slightly later than the peak output of PG. Using the same *E. coli* preparation but studying the migration of ^{51}Cr PMNs in rabbits, Issekutz and Movat (1980) have found that 90% of PMN entry occurs during the first four hours of the lesion and that entry is virtually complete by six hours. It would be interesting to know precisely how many of the PMNs which enter such a site reach the lymph compared with the number which expire in dermal tissues. Such experiments may be feasible in the sheep.

In an analysis of many lymph responses, Johnston was able to graphically plot the total output of PG in lymph versus the total output of PMNs. There was no correlation between these events. This suggested that cells other than PMNs such as macrophages were contributing PG. From *in vitro* studies, however, he concluded that these inflammatory cells probably did not directly contribute PG, but that they may have been a source of phospholipase A_2, a view supported by the recent data of Vadas (1980). Presumably the membranes of any surrounding cells could act as a substrate for the phospholipase A_2, release arachidonic acid and, in the presence of the cyclo-oxygenase system, so generate PG. Other investigators (Greenwood and Kerry, 1979) who have examined PG in the edema fluid from subcutaneous chambers in sheep also concluded that the PMNs did not generate the PG directly.

Another interesting series of observations by Johnston *et al.* (1980) was concerned with the metabolism of PG within lymph nodes. PGE was always higher in afferent lymph, whereas PGF was comparable in afferent and efferent lymph. By perfusing and injecting nodes with radioactive arachidonic acid and analyzing the metabolic products using thin layer chromatography, he was able to demonstrate a selective catabolism of PGE. The role that PG may play in the inflammatory response has been reviewed by Johnston *et al.* (1979b).

Other studies on afferent lymph following the injection of both *E. coli* and Salmonella lipopolysaccharide have demonstrated that the clotting time of the lymph plasma is shortened and the capacity of the lymph cells to promote fibrin polymerization is enhanced (Burrowes, personal communication). This transient effect appears to be due to the activation of the extrinsic clotting pathway and the release of a thromboplastin-like material. Both macrophages and PMNs may be the source of this factor. Large, mononuclear lung lavage cells are particularly potent in this respect (Burrowes *et al.*, 1980).

An output of 10^7 PMNs per hour in a single afferent lymphatic is common at the peak of these acute reactions. Often the rate of lymph flow increases from about 1 ml h^{-1} to about 8 ml h^{-1} at the peak of the response. However, when endotoxin (LPS) alone is injected the catheter often clots completely or the flow rate does not appreciably change. Presumably the more complex bacterial antigens and whole organisms give rise to enhanced vascular permeability as well as thromboplastin release, whereas endotoxin alone promotes mainly the release of thromboplastin.

B. CHRONIC REACTIONS

Some of the most severe chronic inflammatory reactions are produced in the skin by the injection of Freund's adjuvant. These lesions are familiar to most immunologists when they use adjuvant in the skin of rabbits to stimulate antibody production. The cell output in afferent lymph from such lesions rises to about 30 times normal, or 3×10^7 cells per hour at the peak of the reaction (around four weeks). Smith *et al.* (1970c) have shown that even at 70 days, the afferent cell output is still much higher than normal. It has been shown that this is truly a migration of lymphocytes from the blood rather than local proliferation (Issekutz *et al.*, 1980a) and the recovery of intravenously injected labelled cells was comparable, if not greater, than the recovery of labelled lymphocytes in efferent lymph. These lesions are, therefore, as much a traffic site as is a lymph node. As was described earlier, the macrophage output in afferent lymph also increases to about 30-fold higher than normal. When afferent cells are labelled, returned to the blood and the appearance of labelled cells is followed in afferent lymph, the recovered radioactivity is associated with small lymphocytes which lack surface Ig (Chin, Issekutz and Hay, unpublished observations). The macrophages, when returned to the blood in this somewhat artificially contrived manner, probably do not leave the blood and enter afferent lymph again (except maybe in the liver). Some differences between the recovery of cells in granuloma afferent lymph and normal afferent lymph, and particularly intestinal efferent lymph, is described in a later section.

Three separate and distinct cell products have been studied which are released from afferent granuloma cells (macrophages) *in vitro*. They are not detectable from either normal afferent lymph cells or efferent lymph cells. These cell products are an hyperemia-inducing factor (probably phospholipase A_2 (Vadas and Hay, 1980), plasminogen activator (Vadas *et al.*, 1979) and tissue thromboplastin (Burrowes *et al.*, 1980). Possibly, with appropriate assays, other macrophage products could also be detected. Nevertheless, these studies suggest that the macrophages in this chronically inflammed afferent lymph are more active than those of normal afferent lymph. Tuberculin reactions in the skin give rise to an output of mononuclear cells in the afferent lymph which can reach some 25 times normal. This cell output reaches a maximum around 48 hours (Hay *et al.*, 1973). No functional studies have yet been done on these cells. A large migration of lymphocytes into the kidney and into renal afferent lymph was seen in chronic hydronephrosis (Smith *et al.*, 1970c). It is not known how changes in the hydrodynamics of renal fluids could promote this migration.

C. ALLOGENEIC REACTIONS

Normal lymphocyte transfer (NLT) reactions have been studied in sheep by Jones and Lafferty (1969) and others. When allogeneic lymphocytes are injected intradermally, particularly in the skin in the groin of a sheep, an erythematous, indurated but rather hard lesion develops. Depending upon the number of lymphocytes injected and the degree of genetic dissimilarity between donor and host, these lesions can become necrotic in the centre by six days. The blood flow of these lesions is many times that of normal skin and it has been shown that at this increase in lymphocyte delivery is sufficient to account for the increased numbers of lymphocytes leaving such sites in the afferent lymph (Hay *et al.*, 1978). The maximum output of cells in the afferent lymph occurs near six days, the time when the skin lesion is the largest. When sensitized cells are compared with normal lymphocytes the skin lesion develops more rapidly and appears to be more severe (Fig. 3). In view of the studies on MLRs using sensitized cells (Cahill *et al.*, 1979), it would be interesting to determine whether the blast cells or the small cells are responsible for this rapid NLT. Also, the use of afferent lymph cells would be an interesting comparison to see if sensitized cells are in the afferent lymph or whether afferent cells are less effective than efferent as has been shown for the normal cells (Scollay and Lafferty, 1975). Studies by Pedersen and Morris have shown that the capacity to induce NLT lesions depends on which lymph cells are used and the time after the allogeneic stimulus (Pedersen and Morris, 1974).

The most spectacular changes in afferent lymph have been shown during the rejection of renal allografts by Pedersen and Morris (1970). During the eight days or so of the rejection process, litres of renal afferent lymph have been drained off via the lymph catheter. Several grams net weight of lymphocytes and macrophages leave the blood within the kidney, migrate through this highly structured tissue and enter the afferent lymph. These physical processes also must severely compromise the functional integrity of this organ. Although many of these cells in the afferent lymph are blasts, they do not appear to be making much antibody when compared with other blast cells from efferent lymph (Pedersen *et al.*, 1975). Presumably a large proportion of such cells are T blasts. The significance of the proteins that they are synthesizing is not known.

X. Similarities and differences between chronic inflammatory sites and lymph nodes

Most of the functional analyses of the cells in stimulated afferent lymph compare these cells with the cells from efferent lymph. How closely does a chronic inflammatory site like the adjuvant granuloma resemble a lymph node? There are several similarities. The cell output can be comparable, the traffic through them can be comparable, the blood flow can be comparable. It has been shown that NLT lesions and the adjuvant lesions have a large number of cells within them which have the ultrastructural appearance of plasma cells (Smith *et al.*, 1970c; Hay, 1979). In contrast, Frost *et al.* (1975) reported that the shutdown phase of a lymph node response to antigen did not have a counterpart in afferent lymph, although chronically stimulated lesions were not examined. The lesions do not have a capsule, afferent lymphatic input, clearly defined follicles and germinal centres. It would be interesting to test how much antibody a granuloma can produce. Some preliminary observations come to mind in this context. We have had occasion to induce a granuloma with adjuvant containing Salmonella organisms. Several days later when blasts were apparent in both the regional afferent and efferent lymph and the cell outputs were increased, specific PFCs could be detected in efferent but not afferent lymph. In another experiment granulomas produced by Freund's complete adjuvant were injected with PPD. Evan's blue was mixed with the PPD and the blue appeared in the cannulated afferent lymph. No effect on the cell output was observed (i.e. no shutdown or recruitment of cells). Qualitative changes in the capacity of the macrophages to produce plasminogen activator did, however, occur (Wasi,

Vadas and Hay, unpublished observations). More studies of this nature are required, but it seems possible that in spite of the fact that a granuloma contains the cells necessary (T, B and macrophages) for an immune response and an intact vascular system, it may be fundamentally different from a lymph node. A more complete understanding of these lymphocyte traffic sites may lead to a more rational approach to the eventual control of the immune response.

XI. Intestinal lymph

Most lymphocyte migration occurs through the gut and the gut-associated lymphoid tissue. Reynolds (1980a) has documented the magnitude of the gut-associated lymphoid tissue (GALT) in the lamb before and after birth. The increase in mass of the mesenteric nodes and of Peyer's patches is remarkable. A variety of mesenteric lymph nodes has been cannulated in sheep. The efferent lymphatics of mesenteric nodes which drain the jejunum and maybe some of the duodenum are usually white with chyle. This is not apparent in lymph from the lower ileum and ileo-caecal junction. By far the largest mass of mesenteric lymph nodes in sheep is associated with the small bowel, compared with the caecum and large bowel. This seems to be in contrast to the microbial load within the bowel. One interpretation of this distribution might be that the mesenteric nodes are concerned more with the food antigens of the gut than with the microbial antigens. The gut contains a large mass of lymphoid tissue within its walls. In addition to the organized tissues of Peyer's patches there are many lymphocytes in the lamina propria and in the epithelial mucosa. The small bowel and Peyer's patches in particular are probably the source of most of the Ig-bearing small lymphocytes in the sheep (based upon data referred to by Fahy *et al.*, (1980) and Reynolds (1980a)). Reynolds concluded that Peyer's patches can be considered primary lymphoid tissue since much of the lymphopoeisis takes place *in utero* in the absence of antigen. In addition, antigen can modify the development of the GALT after birth and, therefore, such tissue also responds as secondary lymphoid tissue.

There is some difficulty in analyzing the intestinal lymph as a reflection of immune reactions in the gut for several reasons. The level of "background" stimulation is high because of constant antigenic bombardment and the delivery of lymph and cells from the lymphoid tissue of the gut wall. Therefore, the cellular changes may be masked. Furthermore, it is difficult to stimulate a single mesenteric node in a meaningful fashion, i.e. via the intestinal lumen. Beh (1977) found that the immune response of mesenteric nodes following intraluminal administration of antigen was meagre compared with the response of other lymph nodes. More recently Beh (1979) has used DEAE-dextran as an adjuvant and specific immune responses have been recorded in the efferent lymph of an ileal lymph node. The antibody-containing cells which entered the lymph included an early output of IgM-specific cells, followed by IgG-specific cells. Beh *et al.* (1979) found that these two classes of antibody-containing cells entered the intestinal efferent lymph following the administration of antigen directly into the node. Therefore, it may be significant that the more recent studies with adjuvant also showed an increased output of IgA-containing cells in the efferent lymph. A contribution of IgA precursors by Peyer's patches is suggested by such studies and it will be interesting to see further developments in this area. The contribution of IgA precursor cells by Peyer's patches in rabbits had been conclusively shown (see Chapter 5).

There is another advantage of intestinal lymph cannulation from single mesenteric nodes that could be exploited in the future. The blood vascular compartment of the node and the GALT is technically approachable. For example, a small indwelling arterial catheter can be positioned via the superior mesenteric artery in such a manner as to not occlude the blood flow but to permit the the intra-arterial perfusion of a region of gut and mesenteric node. When this is done and dye is introduced intra-arterially, a well-defined area can be visualized. We have perfused such a region with prostaglandin, for example (unpublished observation), and hope to study the formation and changes in lymph following such procedures. In Basel, Cahill and colleagues have used such an approach to perfuse a defined region of fetal bowel with radioactive thymidine.

The migration of lymphoblasts from the GALT lymphatics back to the GALT in mice, rats and sheep further distinguishes this lymphoid tissue from the subcutaneous lymphoid tissue (Hall, 1980). The role that these cells and their products play in the maintenance of the secretory immune system is discussed in Chapter 5. Differential migration patterns of small lymphocytes between the GALT and other lymphoid tissues has been described in sheep and this topic warrants a more detailed discussion.

XII. Differences in lymphocyte migration patterns in lymph draining subcutaneous lymph nodes, mesenteric lymph nodes and chronic inflammatory sites

The experiments to be described here have been performed only in sheep and are concerned with the collection and labelling of lymph cells and their subsequent migration back to lymph following intravenous injection. There are quantitative differences in the recovery of different lymphocytes in different lymph compartments and it is our hypothesis that the differences are due to different subpopulations of lymphocytes. Both Chromium-51 and Indium III have been used for these studies and Issekutz *et al.* have compared the use of these two isotopes in the sheep (Issekutz *et al.*, 1980b).

Cahill *et al.* (1977) labelled lymphocytes from a main intestinal trunk of sheep and monitored the blood-to-lymph migration of such cells through subcutaneous nodes and mesenteric nodes. Lymphocytes of intestinal origin always reappeared in higher concentrations in intestinal lymph than in subcutaneous lymph. The reverse was observed when subcutaneous lymph was the source of the cells for labelling. These patterns were also found by Scollay *et al.* (1976b). In addition, Cahill *et al.* (1977) showed that such migration was a property of lymphocytes which lacked surface Ig and were presumably T cells. Experiments of a similar nature were performed by Chin and Hay (1980) and evidence was presented to document that popliteal and prefemoral node patterns were indistinguishable from one another, that groups of mesenteric nodes were similar to one another but that the mesenteric patterns differed from the subcutaneous patterns as shown by Cahill *et al.* Chin *et al.* demonstrated that small lymphocytes and not lymphoblasts were responsible for these patterns. It seems likely that the lymphocyte responsible for this preferential intestinal migration are present in both afferent and efferent intestinal lymph based upon labelling experiments combined with mesenteric lymphodenectomy as performed by Hall (1980).

In other experiments, the recovery of Indium III-labelled lymphocytes in normal efferent lymph differed from the recovery in afferent lymph-draining granulomas (Issekutz *et al.*, 1980a). When afferent granuloma lymphocytes are labelled, the recovery is always higher in such afferent lymph than in normal efferent lymph. The efferent lymph of the regional node has a pattern which is intermediate between the other two regions (Issekutz *et al.*, 1980). Based upon recovery data it can also be added that the extent of migration of lymphocytes from blood to lymph in a granuloma is equal to the traffic through a lymph node. In the experiments of Chin and Hay (1980) a most dramatic difference in labelled lymphocytes was observed when afferent granuloma cells were recovered in the lymph of origin at concentrations seventy-fold higher than in the intestinal lymph. When intestinal lymph cells were labelled and injected intravenously higher concentrations of labelled cells were always recovered in the intestinal lymph than in the lymph from subcutaneous lymph nodes or from skin granulomas (see Fig. 4).

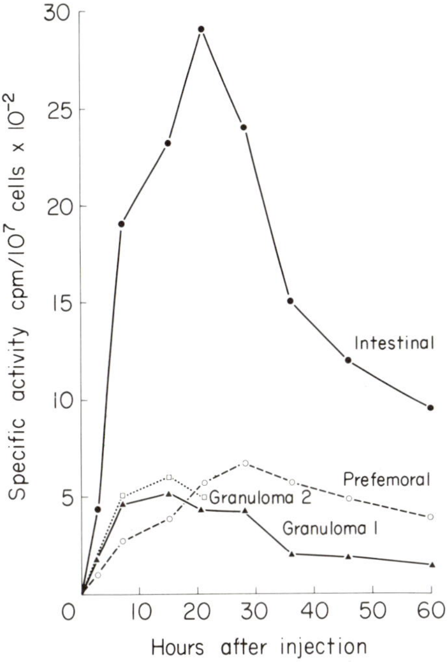

FIG. 4 Profiles of cell-specific activities in efferent intestinal lymph, efferent prefemoral lymph and afferent lymph draining a granuloma in the right hind leg and the left hind leg following the intravenous injection of $4{\cdot}0 \times 10^8$ efferent intestinal lymphocytes labelled with $31{\cdot}59 \times 10^6$ cpm of ^{111}Indium (with permission of W. Chin and American Gastroenterological Association).

From recent unpublished data (Chin, Issekutz and Hay), it can be added that these afferent lymph patterns are due to small, surface Ig-negative lymphocytes. Such patterns are probably not a consequence of the chronic inflammation. Normal afferent lymphocytes give rise to the same patterns. From Hall's studies, it would seem that intestinal afferent cells are quite different from granuloma afferent cells. Chin (unpublished observations) has observed that chronic inflammatory lesions induced in the caecum conform to intestinal lymphocyte migration patterns rather than subcutaneous granuloma patterns.

The significance of these different migration patterns is not known but may have some bearing on systemic versus local mucosal immunity. However, cervical efferent lymph cells conform to the pattern of subcutaneous nodes even though this node drains the naso-pharyngeal tissues (Chin, Cahill and Hay, unpublished observations). It would be interesting to examine the cells leaving the lung and the liver using this approach. It is important to determine whether these patterns exist only in sheep or whether they are more universal. Since such protocols are impossible in small animals, perhaps data can be collected from other large animals or eventually from man. Studies by Butcher *et al.* (1980) provide evidence that there is an organ specificity of lymphocyte binding to vascular endothelium in the mouse. Using thymic lymphoma cells almost exclusive specificity was shown between venules from Peyer's patches compared with lymph nodes.

XIII. Lymphocyte migration in the fetal lamb

It is not easy to claim that antigen stimulation produces these patterns since Cahill *et al.* (1980) have tested this proposition to some degree in subcutaneous nodes and found comparable concentrations of labelled lymphocytes in the lymph from normal and stimulated nodes. Nevertheless the intestinal versus subcutaneous lymph differences are not apparent in the fetal lamb, implying that post-natal stimulation of the GALT induces these differences (Butcher *et al.*, 1980). If the differences are due to differences in cell populations, are more universal and occur in most species, then further experimental analysis of these patterns should be informative and rewarding.

References

Beh, K. (1977). *Aust. J. exp. Biol. med. Sci.* 55, 263-274.

Beh, K. J. (1979). *Immunology*, **37**, 279-286.

Beh, K. J., Husband, A. J. and Lascelles, A. K. (1979). *Immunology*, 37, 385-388.

Beh, K. J. and Lascelles, A. K. (1974). *Aust. J. exp. Biol. med. Sci.* 52, 505-514.

BELL, G. I. (1978). *In* "Theoretical Immunology" (Eds G. I. Bell, A. S. Perelson, and G. H. Pimbley), pp. 341-378. Dekker.
BELLMAN, S. and ODEN, B. (1958-59). *Acta. chir. scand.* **116**, 99-117.
BINNS, R. M. (1980) *Monographs Alergy* **16**, 19-37.
BURROWES, C., WASI, S., CHIN, W. Z., HAY, J. B. and MOVAT, H. Z. (1980). Submitted for publication.
BUTCHER, E. C., SCOLLAY, R. G. and WEISSMAN, I-L. (1980). *Eur. J. Immun.* **10**, 556-561.
CAHILL, R. N. P., HAY, J. B., FROST, H. and TRNKA, Z. (1974). *Haematologia,* **8**, 321-334.
CAHILL, R. N. P., FROST, H. and TRNKA, Z. (1976). *J. exp. Med.* **143**, 870-888.
CAHILL, R. N. P., POSKITT, D. C., FROST, H. and TRNKA, Z. (1977). *J. exp. Med.* **145**, 420-428.
CAHILL, R. N. P., FROST, H., HAY, J. B., LAFLEUR, L. and TRNKA, Z. (1979). *Transplantation,* **27**, 102-106.
CAHILL, R. N. P., POSKITT, D. C., HAY, J. B., HERON, I. and TRNKA, Z. (1980). *Eur. J. Immun.* **9**, 251-253.
CAHILL, R. N. P. and TRNKA, Z. (1980). *Monographs Allergy,* **16**, 38-49.
CHIN, W. G. and HAY, J. B (1980). *Gastroenterology,* **79**, 1231-1242.
COLE, G. J. and MORRIS, B. (1971). *Aust. J. exp. Biol. med. Sci.* **49**, 75-88.
COLE, G. J. and MORRIS, B. (1973). *Adv. vet. Sci. comp. Med.* **17**, 225-263.
CUNNINGHAM, A. J., SMITH, J. B. and MERCER, E. H. (1966). *J. exp. Med.* **124**, 701-704.
ENGESET, A., HAGER, B., NESHEIM, A. and KOLBENSTVEDT, A. (1973). *Lymphology,* **6**, 1-5.
ENGLISH, L. S., ADAMS, E. P., and MORRIS, B. (1976). *J. exp. Med.* **144**, 586-603.
ENGLISH, L., MORRIS, B. and ADAMS, E. (1977). *Cell. Immun.* **28**, 90-100.
EY, P. L. (1973). *Eur. J. Immun.* **3**, 37-43.
FAHY, V. A., GERBER, H. A., MORRIS, B., TREVELLA, W. and ZUKOSKI, C. F. (1980). *Prog. Allergy,* **16**, 82-99.
FROST, H. (1978). *Cell. Immun.* **37**, 390-396.
FROST, H., CAHILL, R. N. P. and TRNKA, Z. (1975). *Eur. J. Immun.* 839-843.
FROST, H., BRAUN, D. G., POSKITT, D. C., CAHILL, R. N. P. and TRNKA, Z. (1976). *J. exp. Med.* **143**, 707-711.
GODAL, T. and ENGESET, A. (1978). *Lymphology,* **11**, 208-210.
GREENWOOD, B. and KERRY, P. J. (1979). *J. Physiol.* **288**, 379-391.
HALL, J. G. (1967). *J. exp. Med.* **125**, 737-754.
HALL, J. G. (1980). *Monographs Allergy,* **16**, 100-111.
HALL, J. G. (1980). *In* "Blood Cells and Vessel Walls". Cibe Foundation Symposium 77, pp. 197-204. Ebeviur/North Holland.
HALL, J. G. and MORRIS, B. (1962). *Q. Jl. exp. Physiol.* **47**, 360-368.
HALL, J. G. and MORRIS, B. (1964). *Lancet,* **i**, 1077-1080.
HALL, J. G. and MORRIS, B. (1965). *Brit. J. exp. Path.* **46**, 450-454.
HALL, J. G. and MORRIS, B. (1965). *J. exp. Med.* **121**, 901-910.

HALL, J. G., MORRIS, B., MORENO, G. D. and BESSIS, M. G. (1967). *J. exp. Med.* **125**, 91-110.
HALL, J. G., SCOLLAY, R. G. and SMITH, M. F. (1976). *Eur. J. Immun.* **6**, 117-120.
HAY, J. B. (1973). *Int. Archs Allergy appl. Immun.* **44**, 569-584.
HAY, J. B. (1979). *Curr. Topics Path.* **68**, 89-109.
HAY, J. B. (1980). *In* "Inflammation, Immunity and Hypersensitivity" (Ed. H. Z. Movat), 2nd edition, pp. 271-318. Harper & Row, Baltimore.
HAY, J. B. and HOBBS, B. B. (1977). *J. exp. Med.* **145**, 31-44.
HAY, J. B. and MORRIS, B. (1975). *Br. med. Bull.* **32**, 135-140.
HAY, J. B., LACHMANN, P. J. and TRNKA, Z. (1972). *In* "Proceedings of the Seventh Leukocyte Culture Conference" (Ed. F. Dagillard), pp. 341-350. Academic Press, New York and London.
HAY, J. B., MURPHY, M. J., MORRIS, B. and BESSIS, M. C. (1972). *Am. J. Path.* **66**, 1-24.
HAY, J. B., CAHILL, R. N. P. and TRNKA, Z. (1973). *Cell. Immun.* **10**, 145-153.
HAY, J. B. LACHMANN, P. J. and TRNKA, Z. (1973). *Eur. J. Immunol.* **3**, 127-131.
HAY, J. B., YAMASHITA, A. and MORRIS, B. (1974). *Lab. Invest.* **31**, 276-285.
HAY, J. B., HOBBS, B. B., JOHNSTON, M. G. and MOVAT, H. Z. (1978). *Int. Archs. Allergy appl. Immun.* **55**, 324-331.
HAY, J. B., CHIN, W. Z. and ISSEKUTZ, T. B., J. (1980). *In* "Immunological Aspects of Rheumatic Diseases" (Ed. W. C. Dick). MTP Press, Lancaster, U.K.
HAY, J. B., JOHNSTON, M. G., VADAS, P., CHIN, W., ISSEKUTZ, T. and MOVAT, H. Z. (1980). *Monographs Allergy,* **16**, 112-125.
HERON, I., POSKITT, D. C., CAHILL, R. N. P. and TRNKA, Z. (1978). *Cell. Immun.* **41**, 178-187.
HERON, I., TRNKA, Z. and CAHILL, R. N. P. (1980). Unpublished observations.
ISSEKUTZ, A. C. and MOVAT, H. Z. (1980). *Lab. Invest.* **42**, 310-317.
ISSEKUTZ, T. B., CHIN, W. and HAY, J. B. (1980a). *Cell. Immun.* **54**, 79-86.
ISSEKUTZ, T. B., CHIN, W. G. and HAY, J. B. (1980b). *Clin. exp. Immunol.* **39**, 215-221.
ISSEKUTZ, T. B. and ISSEKUTZ, A. C. and MOVAT, H. Z. (1981). *Am. J. Path.* **102**, 47–52.
JOHNSTON, M. G. (1979). Ph.D. thesis, University of Toronto.
JOHNSTON, M. G., HAY, J. B. and MOVAT, H. Z. (1976). *Agents Actions,* **6**, 705-711.
JOHNSTON, M. G., HAY, J. B. and MOVAT, H. Z. (1979a). *Am. J. Path.* **95**, 225-238.
JOHNSTON, M. G., HAY, J. B. and MOVAT, H. Z. (1979b). *Curr. Topics Path.* **68**, 259-287.
JOHNSTON, M. G., HAY, J. B. and MOVAT, H. Z. (1980). *Am. J. Path.* **99**, 695-714.

Jones, M. A. S. and Lafferty, K. J. (1969). *Aust. J. exp. Biol. med. Sci.* **47**, 159-169.
Lascelles, A. K. and Morris, B. (1961). *Q.Jl exp. Physiol.* **46**, 199-205.
Lascelles, A. K. and McDowell, G. H. (1974). *Transplant. Rev.* **19**, 170-208.
McCullagh, P. (1980). *Monographs Allergy,* **16**, 143-156.
McIntosh, G. H. and Morris, B. (1971). *J. Physiol.* **214**, 365-376.
Meade, C. J., Lachmann, P. J. and Binns, R. M. (1976). *Scand. J. Immun.* **5**, 529-539.
Miller, H. R. P. and Adams, E. P. (1977). *Am. J. Path.* **87**, 59-80.
Morris, B. (1972). *In* "Handbuch der allgemeinen Pathologie", vol. 3, part 6, pp. 405-456. Springer-Verlag, Berlin.
Morris, B. and Courtice, F. C. (1977). *Lymphology,* **10**, 62.
Morris, B. and McIntosh, G. H. (1970). *In* "Progress in Lymphology II", pp. 173-175. Springer-Verlag, Berlin.
Morris, B. and Sass, M. B. (1966). *Proc. R. Soc. B.* **164**, 577-591.
Movat, H. Z. (1980). *In* "Inflammation, Immunity and Hypersensitivity: Molecular and Cellular Mechanisms", pp. 1-162. Harper and Row, Baltimore.
Murphy, M. J., Hay, J. B., Morris, B. and Bessis, M. C. (1972). *Am. J. Path.* **6**, 25-42.
Nelson, D. S. (1965). *Immunology,* **9**, 219-234.
Pedersen, N. C. and Morris, B. (1970). *J. exp. Med.* **131**, 936-969.
Pedersen, N. C. and Morris, B. (1974). *Transplantation,* **17**, 48-58.
Pedersen, N. C., Adams, E. P. and Morris, B. (1975). *Transplantation,* **19**, 400-409.
Poskitt, D. C., Frost, H., Cahill, R. N. P. and Trnka, Z. (1977). *Immunology,* **33**, 81-89.
Quin, J. W. and Shannon, A. D. (1977). *J. Physiol.* **264**, 307-321.
Reynolds, J. (1980a). *Allergy,* **16**, 187-202.
Reynolds, J. (1980b). Personal communication.
Scollay, R. and Lafferty, K. J. (1975). *Transplantation,* **19**, 170-176.
Scollay, R. G., Hopkins, J. and Hall, J. G. (1976a). *Nature, Lond.* **260**, 528-531.
Scollay, R. G., Hall, J. G. and Orlans, E. (1976a). *Eur. J. Immunol.* **6**, 121-125.
Simpson-Morgan, M. (1970). Personal communication.
Smeaton, T. C., Cole, G. J., Simpson-Morgan, M. W. and Morris, B. (1969). *Aust. J. exp. Biol. med. Sci.* **47**, 565-572.
Smith, J. B. and Morris, B. (1970). *Aust. J. exp. Biol. med. Sci.* **48**, 33-46.
Smith, J. B., Cunningham, A. J., Lafferty, K. J. and Morris, B. (1970a). *Aust. J. exp. Biol. med. Sci.* **48**, 57-70.
Smith, J. B., McIntosh, G. H. and Morris, B. (1970b). *J. Anat., Lond.* **107**, 87-100.
Smith, J. B., McIntosh, G. H. and Morris, B. (1970). *J. Path. Bact.* **100**, 21-29.

SMITH, J. B., PEDERSEN, N. C. and MORRIS, B. (1970d). *Series Haemat. III,* **2**, 17-61.
SMITH, M. E., MARTIN, A. F. and FORD, W. L. (1980). *Monographs Allergy,* **16**, 203-232.
SPRENT, J. (1977). *In* "The Lymphocytes: Structure and Function" (Ed. J. Marchalonis) Dekker, New York.
SPRENT, J. and MILLER, J. F. A. P. (1971). *Nature new Biol.* **234**, 195-198.
SPRENT, J., MILLER, J. F. A. P. and MITCHELL, G. F. (1971). *Cell. Immun.* **2**, 171-181.
SPRY, C. J. F., PFLUG, A. J., JANOSSY, G. and HUMPHREY, J. H. (1980). *Clin. exp. Immunol.* **39**, 750-755.
TAO, T-W and DRESSER, D. W. (1972). *Eur. J. Immun.* **2**, 262-265.
THAKUR, M. L., COLEMAN, R. E. and WELCH, M. J. (1977). *J. Lab. clin. Med.* **89**, 217-228.
TREVELLA, W. and MORRIS, B. (1980). *In* "Blood Cells and Vessel Walls: Functional Interactions". Ciba Foundation Symposium No. 71, Excerpta Medica, Amsterdam.
UNANUE, E. R. and ROSENTHAL, A. S. (Eds) (1979). *In* "Macrophage Regulation of Immunity". Academic Press, New York, London, Toronto, Sydney, San Francisco.
VADAS, P. (1980). Ph.D. thesis, University of Toronto.
VADAS, P. and HAY, J. B. (1980). *Int. Archs Allergy appl. Immun.* **62**, 142-151.
VADAS, P., WASI, S., MOVAT, H. Z. and HAY, J. B. (1979). *Proc. Soc. exp. Biol. Med.* **161**, 82-85.
VAN FURTH, R. and WILLEMZE, R. (1979). *Curr. Topics Path.* **68**, 179-212.
YAMASHITA, A., HAY, J. B. and LAFFERTY, K. J. (1970). *Aust. J. exp. Biol. Med. Sci.* **48**, 619-630.
YOFFEY, J. M. and COURTICE, F. C. (Eds) (1980). *In* "Lymphatics, Lymph and the Lymphomyeloid Complex". Academic Press, London, New York, Toronto, Sydney, San Francisco.

4 *Ontogeny of the Immune Response: Studies with Mutant Mice*

R. AUERBACH

I. Introduction

The use of mutations as probes for the study of mammalian development has been a major factor in helping to characterize a wide spectrum of developmental interactions, to delineate specific control points in the development of various organs and organ systems, and to provide variants for determining sensitivity to teratogenic agents. A prime reason for this is that the mammalian embryo is refractory to many of the standard techniques of the experimental embryologist because of its protected environment within the mother. Mutants can provide the "experiments of nature" that at least in part can replace these techniques.

Because inbred lines of mice were established beginning some seventy years ago, the mouse now occupies a unique position with respect to genetic analysis and the generation and availability of mutant animals. Given the long history of inbreeding and the relatively short gestation and maturation period it has been possible to isolate many animals bearing genetic markers and developmental deviations. When variants are observed most investigators routinely carry out simple breeding tests: many defects are due to simple Mendelian gene alterations and are thus readily identified; reporting of mutants has been simplified and encouraged through the informal channel of the *Mouse News Letter*; and several laboratories have considered the maintenance of mutant lines to be their obligation to the scientific community.

From a developmental standpoint the most "interesting" mutants have frequently been lethals, first identified because of a classical 2:1 ratio of an F2 generation of matings between two variant offspring of a test cross, i.e. a recessive lethal usually associated with a dominant, viable, visibly distinguishable phenotype. Frequently, the identifying characteristic of the dominantly expressed phenotype has been "trivial": a white belly spot against a black background, shortened tail, pigmentation changes, hind leg paralysis. The reason for this is a practical one relating to animal husbandry. An animal caretaker (or investigator or graduate student!) will notice a lame mouse or a peculiar pigment pattern; a defect in a liver enzyme or in cell shape is not likely to arouse the same initial attention; and a more serious defect would probably not survive to birth and hence be lost. Then, too, a dominant effect not associated with viability permits ready selection in test crosses. At the same time a minor dominant effect may well be a sign of a more serious recessive one: a belly spot may represent a primary defect in cell migration during ontogeny which in homozygous condition prevents germ cell, neural crest or blood cell migration (cf. Russell, 1955); a defective tail may represent a defect in the axial skeleton in animals which in homozygous condition show defects in primary inductive events underlying trunk development (Gluecksohn-Waelsch and Erickson, 1970a); a defect in limb extension in heterozygous condition may involve major mesenchymal deviations in homozygotes (Searle, 1964). For a comprehensive coverage of mouse mutants the reader is referred to the "Biology of the Laboratory Mouse", a volume prepared by the staff of the Jackson Laboratory, (Green, 1966) as well as to the *Mouse News Letter*, which was mentioned earlier.

In analyzing the ontogeny of the immune response the need to study prenatal development of mammals is particularly important. Some immunological functions have already been shown to exist among yolk sac cells of the early 9-day mouse embryo, a stage equivalent to a 48-hour chick embryo or a 4-week human embryo (Hofman and Globerson, 1973, 1976; Auerbach, 1976, 1978); fetal liver cells of many mammalian species have been shown to be capable of inducing cell-mediated immune reactions such as mixed leukocyte culture responses (MLC) and graft-versus-host reactions (GVH) (Umiel, 1973; Umiel *et al.*, 1968; cf. Umiel and Auerbach, 1973, for earlier review); the expression of antigen-specific surface immunoglobulin on fetal liver cells has been documented repeatedly (Spear and Edelman, 1974; Nossal and Pike, 1955); and with the exception of some marsupials many of the immune responses are far advanced or fully developed at birth (Solomon, 1971; Auerbach, 1972; Solomon and Horton, 1977).

Postnatal changes do still occur in mammals with reasonably precocious parturition, including the mouse (cf. Klinman and Press, 1975; Goidl and Siskind, 1974) but these changes represent later expression of some specific clonotypes or of differentiation of secretory functions, superimposed on an already present though perhaps more rudimentary immunological system.

The importance of using mammalian material in the study of ontogeny of the immune response must be stressed. While many experimental manipulations would be easier in non-mammalian embryos because of the accessibility of the eggs and the ability of the embryos to survive outside of the maternal environment, there are many features of the immune response unique to mammals: the role of the placenta as a barrier and selective membrane; the problems relating to survival of the fetus in spite of its allogeneic properties (e.g. expression of paternal antigens and the consequent immune response by maternal lymphocytes); the adoptive functions of circulating serum factors such as tolerogens, blocking factors, isoantigens and viruses or viral products; and the continuing administration through the maternal circulation of new antigens, processed antigens, antibodies or other chemical mediators of potential importance to the elaboration of immune recognition systems, establishment of immunological tolerance, or modulation of expressed clonotypes.

This chapter will, of necessity, not include a detailed discussion of all the murine mutants that have been described that could be of interest to immunologists. Many mutants have not been analyzed extensively and the possible impact of various physiological changes on immunological development is quite large, so a more systematic screening of available mutants might well prove most productive. In addition to single locus mutants, moreover, there are significant differences in ontogeny of immune responsiveness between different strains of mice. Although such differences must have an underlying genetic basis, the precise genetic controls involved may range from a primary difference in one gene region (especially that involving the major histocompatibility complex) to a multifactorial one encompassing genetic factors on several chromosomes. Here, too, a systematic screening would be useful, for most of the work on ontogeny of the immune system has been carried out in a few restricted mouse strains. Strain differences, such as those dealing with mitogen responsiveness, ease of induction of autoimmune reactions or rate of maturation of specific antigen receptors probably represent only a small fraction of the available strain variability in immunological maturation.

Finally, there can be little doubt that the major histocompatibility region (H-2) occupies a unique place in the study of immunological reactions, permitting the analysis of immune response genes and factors influencing serological detection and lymphocyte recognition. Surprisingly, however, relatively little has been done with regard to questions of ontogeny that have involved the use of the congenic lines that have been so useful in dissecting out the fine structure genetic map of this chromosomal region. Coverage of the H-2 system in this chapter will be limited to those aspects in which specific ontogenic information has become available. It should be clear, however, that the potential information that can be obtained through the use of the recombinant strains on a congenic background is vast, and there is now a rapid increase in information coming from studies involving these strains of mice.

II. Mouse mutations

A. THE nu/nu ATHYMIC MOUSE

The nude mouse, first described over a decade ago as an athymic mutant (cf. Pantelouris, 1968; 1973; Pantelouris and Hair, 1970) has become probably the most widely used developmental variant in immunology. Virtually void of functional T cells the nude mouse is currently being employed as a host animal for growth of immunologically disparate tissues including, for example, human tumor lines, as a source of "pure" B cells for numerous *in vitro* and cell transfer studies as well as for the development of anti-B cell antibodies, as a test organism for the study of T-independent immune responses, and as a host animal in studies directed at determining the role of T cell immune responses in protection against tumors or in the enhancement of tumor growth and metastasis (Wortis, 1971; Rygaard, 1973; Rygaard and Poulsen, 1973; Wodarska and Wodarski, 1976; cf. Milich and Gershwin, 1977, for references). Discussion in this chapter, however, will be restricted to studies directed at our understanding of the ontogeny of immunocompetent cells.

Although the thymus is absent or virtually absent at the time of birth a thymus rudiment can be seen in nude mice at day 12-13 of development (Wortis *et al.*, 1971), but while at this time the rudiment may appear reasonably normal (cf. discussion below) it fails to develop further, migration to the thoracic cavity does not occur, and by day 15 only a small epithelial remnant of the organ remains. Whether the rudiment does in fact become populated with stem cells during the 2-3 day period before it degenerates is a matter of some disagreement. In our laboratory we have shown that rudiments from nu/nu embryos, grown in tissue culture, become lymphoid, and moreover that the lymphocytes formed *in vitro* are immunocompetent as measured by their ability to induce a graft-versus-host reaction (Chakravarty *et al.*, 1975). John Owen and his colleagues (Jordan *et al.*, 1977) on the other hand, find no evidence for lymphopoiesis in explanted nu/nu thymus rudiments and argue that our published results are in error, due to faulty identification of homozygous embryos. Weissman (Weissman and Auerbach, 1977) suggests that an explanation for the discrepancy between these two reports may be that while Owen's group used homozygous nude mothers, our experiments were carried out with embryos developing in heterozygous mothers, permitting the transplacental passage of thymic humoral factors during ontogeny, an argument which is supported by a variety of experimental studies in which the immune capabilities of nude mice born to heterozygous versus homozygous mothers have been reported (Hale *et al.*, 1976). Indeed numerous discrepancies between different nude mice have been reported, and in addition to the question of heterozygous versus homozygous mothers, differences between nude mice based on genetic background can also not be ignored (cf. Salomon and Lynch, 1977).

Recently, however, we have repeated the experiments involving the explantation of rudiments from nu/nu embryos, using inbred BALB/c homozygous nude mothers to permit a more direct comparison between our earlier work and the studies reported by Owen and his collaborators. BALB/c homozygous nude embryos clearly are more abnormal in terms of thymus development than are the nude embryos obtained on an outcrossed background. In the BALB/c nude embryos the thymus rudiment is already quite degenerate by the end of the 13th day. Nevertheless, lymphoid development can be seen in many of the nu/nu explants, so that we must conclude that the failure of thymus rudiments to develop lymphoid cells under some conditions of tissue culture is not a mandatory accompaniment of the nu/nu genotype.

It is not surprising that stem cells may enter the thymus rudiment of the nude mouse embryos, since stem cells have been clearly demonstrated to exist in nu/nu mice (Pritchard and Micklem, 1973; Kindred and Loor, 1974; Loor and Roelants, 1975; Sato *et al.*, 1976; cf. Milich and Gershwin, 1977, for more detailed discussion). Thus, when thymus grafts are made from Thy-1·1 donors into Thy-1·2 nude recipients these grafts become populated with lymphocytes carrying the host (Thy-1·2) T cell antigenic marker. Moreover, bone marrow cells obtained from nude mice are rich in T cell precursors as shown by studies of lectin binding, assay for the presence of cell surface antigens detectable by antisera prepared against brain cells (anti-BAθ), and response to thymic humoral factors. Indeed the finding of T cell precursors must be kept in mind in interpreting studies where nude mice have been used to obtain "pure" B cells, and in studies equating the nude mouse with a mouse totally lacking in T cell responses. The latter point is especially important in the light of recent findings that T precursor cells (e.g. The Ly-1, 2, 3 lymphocyte) may be reactive in syngeneic recognition processes and the observation that even the yolk sac may already have immunological effector cells (Hofman and Globerson, 1973, 1976; Auerbach, 1976; Auerbach and Sidky, 1978).

Among the potential development problems the nude mouse may help to answer are the relation of the thymus during development to other developing systems (e.g. endocrine-thymus axis; maturation of yolk sac and liver cells; differential maturation of granulocytic and erythrocytic cells). In this connection it is interesting that restoration experiments with thymus grafts are not totally successful (Loor and Hägg, 1977). Intriguing also is the finding that nude mice may have a reduced incidence of spontaneous tumors, reflecting the possibility that immune surveillance represents activity of a stem cell rather than a definitive T cell function, if indeed the thymus is responsible for such surveillance. The prevalence of natural killer cells (NK cells) in nude mice needs to be explored further. Nude mice may also be particularly useful in studies of transplacental carcinogenesis, in analysis of dependent versus independent development of splenic lymphocytes, and in the study of immunological tolerance and recognition of "self" during embryogenesis.

A new allele of nude has been described recently, whimsically named nude streaker (nu^{str}) which in homozygous condition also is athymic but appears to be viable for a considerable time even under conventional conditions of animal husbandry (Eicher, 1976; Shultz *et al.*, 1978). There appears to be a severe reduction in the percentage of Thy-1 bearing lymphocytes in lymph node and spleen as well as a general depletion of lymphocytes in the thymus-dependent areas of these organs. The immunological properties of streaker mice are similar to those of nude mice: $nu^{str}-nu^{str}$ animals have reduced T cell functions including an inability to reject H-2 histoincompatible skin allografts, poor response to PHA and Con A, and a drastic reduction in humoral response to T-dependent antigens. Interestingly, serum immunoglobulin levels of all classes are also decreased.

Since the mutation arose in the AKR/J line, the nude streaker mice are of Thy-1·1 type, in contrast to the nude mice which are routinely maintained on BALB/c, C57BL and CBA backgrounds, all of which are of Thy-1·2 type.

It may be recalled that the nude mouse was initially inviable except under germ-free conditions, and it was assumed that the early death of nude animals was due to a thymic deficiency. If, however, the T cell defect of streaker mice is similar to that of nude mice, then the question of viability needs to be reconsidered. Many laboratories, indeed, now have nude mice that survive quite well in conventional animal quarters, yet have no more thymus than did the original stocks. The possibility exists that by selection the athymic mouse lines that have survived under conventional methods of animal husbandry are those with high athymic T cell activity, and this possibility must be kept in mind in extrapolating from the athymic lines to normal thymic functions.

B. THE Dh/+ ASPLENIC MOUSE

When Searle first described the mutant dominant hemimelia in 1959, interest was focussed on the skeletal defects leading to partial paralysis of the posterior part of the animal. On autopsy it was discovered, however, that the animals lacked a spleen as well, a fact that was largely forgotten until recently when several laboratories initiated studies to determine the effects of absence of the spleen on development of other lymphoid organs. A review of these studies has been published recently (Auerbach, 1978).

Most investigators have assumed, perhaps correctly, that studies of the immunological capacity of the Dh/+ mouse are studies of the role of the spleen; it should, however, at once be apparent that the Dh mutation has pleiotropic effects (e.g. the effect on the skeleton), and that there may be other, as yet unreported, tissues that are influenced by the Dh gene. There has not, to date, been a careful examination of the development or structure of Peyer's patches, for example, and embryological studies have not included an analysis of functional development of the embryonic or fetal liver. Thus, the studies reported below should be interpreted with caution in ascribing their basis to the asplenic condition of the Dh mouse.

Most provocative of the studies with Dh mice was the report of Battisto and his co-workers (1971) that neither the bone marrow nor the thymus from Dh/+ mice was capable of cooperative interactions in the reconstitution of the immune response to SRBC in lethally irradiated mice. These results were confirmed by Wargon *et al.* (1975), but contradicted by Landahl *et al.* (1976) and Auerbach *et al.* (1976). In contrast to the earlier studies carried out in non-inbred mice, Auerbach's group used Dh mice on an inbred (BALB/c) background, and under those conditions showed that Dh bone marrow and thymus cells could execute normal functions on transfer to irradiated syngeneic host animals.

Subsequently, however, intermediate results were obtained both by Russell and Golub (1976, 1977) and by Gershwin and his co-workers (Fletcher *et al.*, 1977). Russell and Golub demonstrated that although the bone marrow cells of Dh mice were normal, there was a tendency of Dh thymus cells not to settle in the spleen following transfer into irradiated mice, and hence not to be as good as normal thymus cells in restoring the immune responsiveness (T-helper function) of irradiated mice. Fletcher *et al.* (1977) showed that the thymus defect of Dh mice was a transient one, demonstrable in juvenile animals, but no longer seen when older (5-month) animals were used. Thus the currently most reasonable view is that the Dh gene affects the *rate* of maturation of thymus cells, as judged by a delay in their capacity to settle into the spleen and to function in the response to SRBC following transfer into irradiated animals (cf. Auerbach, 1978).

The asplenic Dh mouse does not appear to have any defect in T cell effector functions as judged by the capacity of Dh/+ lymphocytes to evoke a graft-versus-host reaction, to respond in MLC, or to function in delayed hypersensitivity assays (Auerbach *et al.*, 1976; Landahl *et al.*, 1976; Fletcher *et al.*, 1977). But these studies all were carried out with adult animals. In view of the more recent studies suggesting an effect on rate of maturation of thymus cells, an ontogenically oriented set of experiments would seem to be needed to determine whether, for example, the neonatal thymus can already carry out MLC and CML reactions (cf. Wu, 1978). If so, questions of differential maturation of helper cells versus effector cells may well be answered through the use of the Dh mouse. Alternatively, the asplenic mouse may provide an ideal model for studying the development of those cell surface functions necessary to achieve selective seeding in the spleen; our understanding of the development of cell properties relevant to lymphatic circulation and differential sequestering by lymphoid organs is still quite rudimentary at the present time.

C. MUTATIONS AT THE T-LOCUS

Probably the most fascinating genetic region in the mouse is that associated with chromosome XVII. Immunologists for many years have been aware of the importance of this chromosome for immunological reactions because of the central role played by the major histocompatibility complex (H-2 region) in various aspects of the immune response. Only recently, however, has it become generally known to immunologists that closely associated with the H-2 complex is another complex genetic region which for over 30 years has been recognized as critical to the development of the early embryo. This region, studied so extensively by L. C. Dunn and by Gluecksohn-Schoenheimer (Waelsch) and their students, comprising the T-locus and adjacent portions such as Fused, has been shown to influence the many distinct events of early embryogenesis, including separation of the germ layers, the primary inductive events associated with neurulation and formation of the mesoderm, and various aspects of development of the body axis (Dunn, 1964; Gluecksohn-Waelsch and Erickson, 1970a, b; cf. also Bennett, 1975). A series of recessive t-alleles, recognized by interaction with the dominant T-(Brachyury) gene to produce a tailless mouse has been described, and over a hundred such alleles, usually lethal in homozygous condition, have now been found. Complementation analysis suggests that the t genes can be classed into five complementation groups. Their presence in wild populations of *Mus musculus* suggests a selective advantage of major proportions, given the strong negative selective pressure exerted by homozygous lethality. For an excellent and thorough review of the T-locus, reference should be made to the article by Gluecksohn-Waelsch and Erickson (1970a).

That the T-locus may be significant in terms of the immune response is just now beginning to be recognized (cf. Boyse and Bennett, 1974; Artzt and Bennett, 1975; Levinson and McDevitt, 1976; Klein and Hammerberg, 1977) although this had already been proposed on the basis of embryological considerations many years ago (Auerbach, 1969; cf. Auerbach, 1977). Serological studies suggest that each complementation group has serological distinctions which can be seen by means of sperm-associated isoantigens. The suggestion that surface antigens determined by the T-locus are similar to H-2 antigens has prompted the hypothesis that indeed the H-2 antigens represent modifications by duplication of the primitive T-associated antigens (cf. Artzt and Bennett, 1975). Initial biochemical studies supported this hypothesis by showing close similarities in the sedimentation constants of subunits of the surface-associated antigens, but later work is more suggestive of a family of molecules rather than of a repetitive sequence of homologous peptides (cf. Vitetta *et al.*, 1975).

The rationale for including the T-locus in this chapter is that it seems attractive to suggest that this complex genetic region may be a prime candidate for controlling primitive recognition. Admittedly, this is speculative at the moment, but several features are present that warrant proposing this hypothesis:

1. The *type* of surface-associated molecule determined by T is similar to that of H-2 antigens. The 44 000 and 12 000 M.W. subunits found in the F-9 antigen (presumed equivalent of one t-allele determined surface antigen) conforms to this view;
2. The t-allele series is widely distributed in spite of its selective disadvantage (see above), indicating that it must have a primary function critical for survival;
3. Most of the manifestations of the t-series indicate that cell surface recognition processes are involved. Among these are segregation disequilibrium (sperm antigen associated?), sorting out of germ layers (Holtfreter-type recognition?), alteration of cell aggregation patterns (Yanagisawa and Fujimoto, 1977) and sequential expression of t-determined and H-2 determined antigens on primitive embryonic cells (Gachelin *et al.*, 1977).

Since alleles at the T-locus suppress crossing-over over much of chromosome XVII, including H-2, it is not at all clear at this time how much of what we have assumed as H-2K associated immunological function may in fact reflect functional attributes of the T-complex. Recognition of foreignness by primitive embryonic cells such as, for example, yolk sac cells (Hofman and Globerson, 1973, 1976; Auerbach, 1978) could well fall into this category.

Finally, mention should be made of other genes of chromosome XVII, such as Fu and Fu^{Ki}, both of which have major developmental effects (duplications of trunk and nervous system) which may involve cell surface phenomena. Since these genes map between T and H-2, the arguments for their function in primitive recognition mechanisms are strong. As yet serological studies using these genetic markers have not been published.

The use of teratomas in conjunction with studies of t-allele determined surface antigens has already been mentioned in relation to the work with F9 antigen. Several laboratories are now generating a variety of teratomas derived from mutants at the T-locus (McDevitt; Jacob) and Fu^{Ki} (Dahl, Kahan and Auerbach) and these may help resolve some of the questions of ontogeny of cell surface antigens determined by chromosome XVII. For a more thorough discussion of the use of teratomas in developmental studies the reader may wish to refer to recent comprehensive reviews (e.g. Sherman and Solter, 1975; Jacob, 1977; Auerbach, 1977; Bennett *et al.*, 1977).

D. THE lpr/lpr LYMPHOPROLIFERATION MUTANT

In a series of recent reports, Murphy (cf. Murphy and Roths, 1977a, b) has described a congenic strain of mice produced by inbreeding the mutant gene lpr (lymphoproliferation) in the Murphy strain MRL, originally derived by inbreeding following interstrain crosses involving C57BL/6, C3H/Di, AKR/J and G/J. Immunologically significant strain markers include H-2k, Ly-1·2, Ly-2·1, Ly-3·1, Thy-1·2 and TL- (Murphy and Roths, 1978). Homozygotes for the lpr gene develop massive lymph node enlargement, with lymph nodes reaching 100 times normal values by the time animals are 4 months old, and at which time animals begin to die with abnormal lymph node architecture and immune complex glomerulonephritis. At this time over 90% of lymphocytes in the lymph node carry the Thy-1 antigen. Antinuclear antibody as well as anti-thymus antibodies are present, and there is a marked increase in serum IgG1 and IgG2a. Expression of the mutant phenotype is suppressed by thymectomy of juvenile animals (Murphy and Roths, 1978).

The pattern of pathogenesis suggests that lpr mutant mice may serve as a model for Systemic Lupus Erythematosis, both because of the typical histopathological pattern and because of the demonstration of thymic autoantibodies (Eisenberg *et al.*, 1978). Developmental studies directed at analysis of ontogeny of thymus rudiments, development of suppressor cell populations and pattern of T-B and T-T cell collaboration have not yet been reported.

E. THE me/me MOTHEATEN MOUSE

The me/me mutation results in short-lived mice which prior to their death before two months of age manifest a variety of immunological defects such as hyperimmunoglobulinemia and autoimmune disease (Lutzner and Hansen, 1976; Shultz and Green, 1976; Shultz *et al.*, 1978). A primary general sign of the mutant effect is seen in skin lesions which develop within the first week of life and involve accumulations of neutrophils, lymphocytes and macrophages. Subsequently, monocytes are seen as the main cell type and animals develop multiple lesions over much of the body (hence the name "motheaten"). Histopathological studies (Shultz *et al.*, 1978) indicate that by three weeks of age the me/me spleen is enlarged but void of well-defined lymphoid follicles and that by four weeks of age surviving animals show thymic atrophy as well as deficiency in the B cell associated areas of the spleen, Peyer's patches and lymph nodes.

In vivo studies of immunological function have shown that there is a reduced response to SRBC as measured by the 19S direct PFC assay, and that there is also a reduced capacity of spleen and thymus cells of motheaten mice to induce a graft-versus-host reaction. Serum immunoglobulin levels are high, however, with elevations seen in all immunoglobulin classes, and there is an excess background level of PFC to SRBC. The random activation of anti-SRBC antibody-forming cells is presumed to reflect general polyclonal activation of immunoglobulin-producing cells. It may, however, be argued that the reduced 19S PFC response to SRBC reflects feedback inhibition by antibody, rather than a primary defect in B cell or T-helper cell activity.

A more recent study of the developing B cell population of the spleen of me/me mice shows that even at 3 weeks of age the predominant B cell is an immature one (similar to what is seen in the CBA/N line described below). Me/me spleen cells fail to show presence of IgD, have the high intensity Ig fluorescence typical of neonatal B cells, lack the receptor for the third component of complement on their cell surface, and are slow to cap their surface-associated immune complexes. Although the number of T cells appears normal there is seen a depression of various T cell functional responses including reactivity to mitogens, MLC stimulation and the ability to generate cytotoxic effector cells.

A number of measurements reflect autoimmune reactivity: presence of immunoglobulin deposits, serum thymocytotoxicity and serum antibodies against single stranded DNA. Initial studies on me/me bone marrow suggest some stem cell defects as well, but detailed studies of motheaten bone marrow cells have not yet been reported.

The motheaten mouse appears to combine some of the features of both the NZB strain for autoimmunity and the CBA/N strain for B cell deficiency, making it a particularly attractive mutant for study of development of immune responsiveness and tolerance. Although the poor viability of the homozygotes forces one to use heterozygotes for matings, with the disadvantage of having to run progeny tests for presence of the mutant allele, the possibility of introducing a single gene defect into animals with other deficiencies is particularly intriguing.

F. THE PITUITARY DWARF MUTATION

The pituitary dwarf mouse (dw/dw) first described by Snell in 1929 has been studied extensively in terms of ontogeny of immune functions, and has served as a model for analysis of the role of the pituitary in the development of lymphoid tissues. Notably through the work of research groups of Pierpaoli (Pierpaoli *et al.*, 1969; Pierpaoli and Sorkin, 1973; Pierpaoli *et al.*, 1976) and Baroni (Baroni *et al.*, 1969, 1971; Baroni and Doria, 1973) it has been demonstrated that dw/dw mice are deficient in the development of lymphoid tissues, notably the thymus and circulating T lymphocytes, and that cellular immune functions are delayed in onset and deficient throughout life. Immunological deficits were shown for allograft rejection, GVH reactivity and response to T-dependent antigens and T cell mitogens (Duquesnoy *et al.*, 1970; Baroni *et al.*, 1971; Fabris *et al.*, 1971; Duquesnoy and Ahrens, 1973; Okouchi, 1976; Schneider, 1976).

More recently studies of Pelletier *et al.* (1976) have demonstrated that dw/dw mice have low serum thymic hormone activity, suggesting that the pituitary defect correlated also with a defect in thymus epithelial cell functions; alternatively, the mutant effect may be simultaneously on the developing hypophysis and thymus secretory cells. Thus the possibility exists that the primary effect of the dw/dw gene on lymphoid tissues (and hence lymphoid function) is not through the pituitary itself but rather through a genetically controlled defect in secretory functions extending to the thymus. Hormone restitution studies should be capable of resolving the question of primary defect, but studies involving pituitary hormone administration (Holder and Wallis, 1977) have not addressed themselves to restitution of lymphoid functions, and restitution experiments with thymus epithelial cells or through thymus hormone administration have not yet been reported.

Other mutants involving endocrine pathology, such as the lethargic (lh/lh) gene (Dung and Swigart, 1971; Dung and Adrian, 1978) which influences the adrenal gland, or the obese (ob/ob) gene which affects pancreatic function also influence lymphoid morphology and function. Further work with these and similar mutants may clarify the complex role of other endocrine organs in the development of lymphoid cell maturation and function.

G. DYSTROPHIC MICE

A number of studies have been carried out with mice carrying a genetic defect leading to murine muscular dystrophy. The dy gene has been reported both in C57BL/6 and 129/J (ReJ) mice, and two alleles have been identified varying in severity of the dystrophic expression and in animal viability (Stevens *et al.*, 1957; Roew and Goldspink, 1969a, b; Meier and Southard, 1970; Montgomery and Swenarchuk, 1977). Because of the known association between the thymus and a variety of neuro-muscular abnormalities such as myasthenia gravis the dystrophic mutants have been analyzed both in terms of development of thymus architecture and T cell functions (cf. Meier *et al.*, 1965).

Two independent investigations indicate that the development of the thymus is retarded prior to weaning (Karmali and Horrobin, 1977; de Kretser and Livett, 1976). Later in life, on the other hand, thymus size may increase so that the thymus weight to body weight ratio ultimately may indeed be higher than normal. Histologically the defect in thymus development is seen in part as an excess of thymic epithelial cells accompanied by a severe reduction in thymic lymphoid cells. This suggests that dystrophic mice may have an abnormal amount of thymus humoral factor production. To what extent the alteration in thymus morphology and deficiency in initial thymus lymphoid cell numbers is causally related to the development of the muscular degeneration seen at 3-4 weeks of age is, however, not clear; for example neonatal thymectomy does not appear to have a beneficial effect on the expression of the dy syndrome (Walker, 1964).

Critical information on the functional capacity of thymus cells or of thymus-derived cells of dy/dy animals is lacking at this time, and this is especially important in view of the probable association between T cell function and dystrophic symptoms in other species such as the chicken. Genetic experiments involving dy and Dh genes might also be most informative, in view of the pleiotropic effects on limb development seen with both of these mutants.

III. The major histocompatibility complex

The major histocompatibility complex, or H-2 region, of the mouse occupies a unique role in immunological functions with its central role in immune recognition, immune responsiveness, control of complement activity, and determination of specificities critical for immune reactions against cells, viruses, and tumor antigens. Moreover, as more information becomes available the H-2 region seems to assume an ever more important set of controlling functions for all aspects of the immune system. For an overview of functions of the major histocompatibility complex reference can be made to the recent books of Klein (1975), Katz (1977) and Snell *et al.* (1976)

as well as a series of paper collections published in *Transplantation Reviews (Immunological Reviews)*.

Given the importance of the H-2 complex, it is most surprising that so little relevant work has been carried out in which the H-2 system has been looked at from the standpoint of developmental immunology. The bulk of developmental information deals with the *expression* of H-2 antigens as measured by serological reagents prepared in allogeneic animals rather than in congenic resistant lines. Most of what we now know about the expression of H-2 antigens on various cells, therefore, makes no distinction between H-2K, D, 1a or J regions, or between public and private specificities, and indeed has mostly involved assessment of non-lymphoid cells. As far as antigenic expression on embryonic cells is concerned, moreover, each successive study has been able to document an earlier detection of H-2 antigens: The Möllers, in 1962, described H-2 on cells in the perinatal period; Edidin and Gooding were able to demonstrate antigens on early embryonic egg cylinder stage cells (Patthey and Edidin, 1973); and Edelman's group (Webb *et al.*, 1977) has detected H-2 antigens even on the mouse blastocyst. In contrast, H-2 determinants were not found on germ cells or on the "undifferentiated" F9 teratoma cells. Whether this failure to detect H-2 antigens on these cells is due to true absence or due to tests not sensitive enough to demonstrate their presence is not clear.

While one could argue that expression of H-2 antigens is not really a major aspect of developmental immunology, reflecting antigenic expression rather than immunological function, this argument is weakened for two reasons: (1) H-2 expression may be intimately related to the development of self-recognition mechanisms relevant to the establishment of immunological tolerance; and (2) the presence of H-2 determinants may have a direct bearing on immune responsiveness because of the various H-2 restriction-associated reactions which appear to require crosslinking of H-2 determinants with antigens controlled by minor histocompatibility genes, virally determined antigens, or certain types of haptenic determinants. A full discussion of these aspects of the H-2 complex is beyond the scope of the present chapter, however, and the reader is referred to the many papers and workshops of the 3rd International Congress of Immunology for a balanced and current review of this subject (Mandel *et al.*, 1977).

Ontogenic studies of immune responsiveness deal with the H-2 complex only indirectly for although H-2 determinants may be essential for activation of effector cells the ability to respond, although presumably related to H-2 disparity has not been shown to require H-2 differences to be actually expressed on the responding cell population itself. A few recent experiments can, however, be cited. Wu *et al.* (1975; cf. Auerbach, 1976; Wu, 1978; Auerbach and Sidky, 1978) have shown that the ability of lymphoid cells from the spleen and thymus to stimulate effector cell activity is present at least from birth, as measured in MLC. Wu has also reported that at birth the thymus and spleen can already carry out MLC responses, indicating that LD-determined responses (1a determinants, primarily) are already found at this time. The detection of CML reactivity is seen in the thymus shortly after birth but is somewhat delayed (2-3 days) in the spleen. Since congenic strains were used in this study, the conclusions clearly do reflect H-2 associated immunological functions. The findings on ontogeny of spleen cell functions have been confirmed by Pilarski (1977) and both spleen and thymus ontogenic studies of Widmer and Cooper (unpublished observations) are in accord with the observations of Wu.

Whether these studies reflect an inability of cells to recognize K or D determinants at the time of birth, i.e. whether the ability to recognize 1a determinants precedes recognition mechanisms for H-2K or D determinants, is, however, not at all clear. Absence of CML effector cells could equally as well be due to absence of differentiation of a particular T cell subset. Indeed, Cantor and Boyse have suggested that the Ly-1, 2, 3 cell is the only cell present in the spleen at the time of birth, and if, indeed, CML function depends on the presence of Ly-2, 3 cells then the observations of Wu would best not be interpreted in terms of recognition, but rather in terms of maturation of effector cell functions. Then, too, the demonstrated presence of neonatal suppressor cells (Mosier *et al.*, 1977; Globerson *et al.*, 1978) may have prevented CML activity of cells that in principle were fully competent to act as effector cells.

The absence of H-2 antigen expression on F9 teratoma cells deserves further comment. Apparently there is a correlation between the expression of the F9 antigen and the absence of H-2, for as teratomas differentiate (e.g. the PCC4 line teratoma), loss of F9 antigen is correlated with expression of H-2 antigens (Jacob, 1977; Gachelin *et al.*, 1977). Since there are numerous teratoma lines now becoming available, arrested in various stages of differentiation (cf. Sherman and Solter, 1975; Jacob, 1977; Kahan, 1978; Auerbach, 1977) there may soon be available a battery of reagents for characterizing the sequence of events leading to the expression (and function?) of specific H-2 determinants.

IV. Mouse strain variations

Mouse developmental mutants such as those described in preceding sections of this chapter involve changes in a single gene or within a relatively small chromosomal segment. However, because of the long-term isolation of a variety of strains that have been selected for such properties as resistance or sensitivity to specific virus infections, for their ability to support or resist "spontaneous" or virus-mediated tumor growth, or for their fecundity or longevity, numerous lines now exist that have marked differences in the development of their immunological repertoire.

NZB mice. One of the best known variant strains is the NZB (New Zealand Black) line which has been used extensively to study the development of autoimmune lesions which are consistently observed in these animals (Helyer and Howie, 1963; Burnet and Holmes, 1964). NZB mice are characterized by the development of Coombs-positive reactions, massive splenomegaly, autoimmune lesions of the kidney, and a variety of other manifestations of autoimmune pathology. Recent studies include experiments on immunosuppressant effects, thymectomy, splenectomy, nephrectomy, virus infection, nature of immune complexes and numerous other treatments and agents (e.g. Talal and Steinberg, 1974; Gelfand *et al.*, 1976; Cohen and Ziff, 1977; Zinkernagel and Dixon, 1977; Roubinian, Papoian and Talal, 1977; Hurd, 1977).

From a developmental standpoint it is perhaps most significant that the ability to respond to antigens such as SRBC occurs earlier in this strain than in any other (Playfair, 1968), a finding which has not yet been correlated with the possibly precocious development of T-helper cells or a selected deficiency or imbalance in a variety of other T-regulator cells. On the other hand a number of hyper-active T cell functions are seen in juvenile NZB mice, including increased proliferative responses in MLC assays (Palmer *et al.*, 1976) and excessive cross-reactivity in studies with heterologous erythrocytes (Playfair and Marshall-Clarke, 1973).

Embryological studies with NZB mice, including assessment of developmental rates in the embryonic thymus, liver and yolk sac, have not been reported. These could shed much light on the nature of the defect leading to the expression of increased T cell activity and autoimmune diseases postnatally.

C3H/He sublines. Responsiveness to polyclonal stimulators such as LPS has been taken for granted for murine B cells, but within the C3H/He line there has been a divergence of responsiveness to LPS, a difference which has been subjected to considerable study recently. The C3H/HeAn subline fails to respond to LPS in contrast to the C3H/HeJ subline (Watson and Riblet, 1974; Coutinho *et al.*, 1975). Extensive studies by Glode *et al.* (1976; Glode and Rosenstreich, 1976) have demonstrated that there is a direct effect of the genetically determined difference on B cells, since the unresponsiveness seen in C3H/HeAn mice was not influenced by C3H/HeJ macrophages or spleen cells.

In view of the extensive information available on ontogeny of responsiveness to polyclonal activators including LPS, administered to fetal liver cells, and the extensive use of LPS responsiveness of these liver cells in studies of sequential expression of specific clonotypes during ontogeny (cf. Goidl *et al.*, 1976) it would seem that developmental studies of fetal liver cells of these two sublines might prove particularly interesting. It would be most informative to determine, for example, whether the development of responsiveness of fetal liver cells to specific antigens or to allogeneic cells is different for these two C3H sublines, whether there are fundamental differences in the spacing of surface receptors on developing B cells, and whether there might be a differential susceptibility of these sublines to induction of tolerance which could be in turn related to differing requirements for epitope density on tolerogenic molecules.

SJL mice. The number of experiments carried out with the SJL strain is increasing rapidly because of the exceedingly high responsiveness of this subline to various antigens such as SRBC. Yet the same line is also sensitive to induction of amyloidosis, and is probably the best strain for inducing experimental allergic encephalomyelitis (Levine and Sowinski, 1973; Bernard, 1976; Freedman, 1978). Since these latter two properties may reflect sensitivity to tolerogens and/or relative refractiveness to induction of suppressor cells, the question asked earlier with respect to the NZB strain also applies here: Can an increased responsiveness to antigens or an ontogenically premature reactivity to such antigens be correlated with variations in the generation of self-recognition properties? Data on suppressor cells, sensitivity to suppressor molecules and balance between various T cell subpopulations are not yet adequate to explain the extraordinary responsiveness of the SJL mouse.

Ha/ICR mice. The non-inbred Ha/ICR line, developed originally through selection for high litter size (Hauschka, 1973) as now available from the ARS/Sprague Dawley Company, as well as the inbred strain (HaICR/Au) developed from this line, appears to be a low-responder strain to histocompatibility antigens as determined by responsiveness in MLC, and by the ability to induce a graft-versus-host reaction either *in vitro* or following injection into neonatal semi-allogeneic host animals (Cairns, Townsend, Kubai and Auerbach, unpublished observations). Since this unresponsiveness seems to involve a failure to recognize several unrelated H-2 haplotypes this strain may have an excessive (non-specific?) suppressor cell population, or some other imbalance in T cell subpopulations (e.g. deficient Ly-1, 2, 3- cells).

From a developmental standpoint the fact that the HaICR line has been continuously selected for high litter size, rapid maturation of young, and capacity of the mother to nurse many offspring is particularly intriguing when considered in the light of the observed low response to histocompatibility antigens. It has been postulated that there is a transient gvh-type effect of maternal lymphocytes on nursing histoincompatible offspring, leading to temporary runting and retardation of postnatal development (cf. Beer *et al.*, 1974; Head *et al.*, 1977). Since Hauschka's selection did not involve inbreeding, a corollary of the postulated gvh reaction would be that unresponsiveness of maternal lymphocytes should lead to more rapid growth and higher viability of nursing offspring. Experiments involving reciprocal hybrids between HaICR mice and high responder strains (e.g. SJL) might be most informative.

The CBA/N mouse. One of the most useful recently discovered variants is the CBA/N line. The CBA/N mouse manifests a sex-linked B cell deficiency seen by an inability of the B cell to progress in its differentiation beyond the equivalent of a neonatal mouse (Amsbaugh *et al.*, 1972; Scher *et al.*, 1975a, b). It may be recalled that during the course of B cell development precursor stem cells progress from Ig- to Ig+ + + to Ig+, i.e. the neonatal B cell has a higher density of surface-associated immunoglobulin than does the B cell of the adult animal. The CBA/N mouse B cell does not progress beyond the high-density surface-associated Ig+ + + phenotype.

Several consequences of the maturational arrest have been seen in the CBA/N animal:

1. The ontogeny of clonotypes is limited. For example, while those types of cells expressing beta-galactosidase specific antigen-binding properties, known to be fully represented at birth, are present in normal numbers, phosphocholine receptor-expressing cells are completely lacking since the PC clonotype does not normally make its appearance until more than a week after birth (Mosier *et al.*, 1977; Mond *et al.*, 1977).
2. The ability to respond to tolerogenic signals remains comparable to the neonatal mouse. This follows logically from the fact that

the density of surface-associated Ig remains high, facilitating the reading of such signals.
3. The expression of mature differentiation antigens does not occur. For example, the LyB-5 antigen, characteristic only of the definitive B cell, is lacking in CBA animals (Ahmed *et al.*, 1977; Huber *et al.*, 1977).
4. There is a defect in the ability of CBA/N mice to form colonies *in vitro* (Kincade, 1977).
5. There are major differences in the affinity of antibody produced by CBA/N mice (Scher *et al.*, 1975a, b; 1976a, b; Mosier *et al.*, 1976; Gershon and Kondo, 1976; Kincade, 1977; Mond *et al.*, 1977).

The utility of the CBA/N line for studies of immunological development cannot be overemphasized. For example, the CBA/N mouse has been used for the preparation of anti-LyB-5 antibody, providing a new marker for differentiation of antibody-forming cells (Huber *et al.*, 1977; Ahmed *et al.*, 1977). Moreover, since the CBA/N deficiency is sex-linked, congenic antisera can be prepared by permitting male CBA/N mice to respond to cells from heterozygous female CBA/N (XnX+) mice. Among other findings, the strain has already provided useful information concerning the sequential elaboration of responsiveness to mitogens and it has furnished definitive proof for the view that antibody variability is expressed in an ordered pattern during ontogeny (cf. Sherwin and Rowlands, 1975; Klinman *et al.*, 1976; Metcalf *et al.*, 1977; Klinman, 1978).

In our own laboratory we have used the CBA/N mouse to investigate the question of antibody-mediated suppression of immune responsiveness, a question which arose following our finding that tolerance induced in adult mice following the administration of soluble extracts obtained from SRBC lysates could be transferred from mothers to their offspring through the milk (Auerbach and Clark, 1975). We found that while the unresponsiveness to SRBC in the mothers was long-lasting, the tolerance of offspring was limited to the period of nursing, resulting from the transmission of milk-borne suppressive factors. Suppressor cells seemed not to be directly involved, since spleen cells taken from nursing tolerant young were fully competent when tested in a cell transfer assay (Kubai and Auerbach, unpublished observations). This raised the question of whether tolerance in the adult and the neonate had the same basis, or whether there might be a differential sensitivity of the neonatal and adult animal to suppression by passively transferred antibody. Previous comparisons of neonatal and adult animals had suffered from the fact that there are many differences between young and adult animals that are unrelated to the immune cells themselves (e.g. hormonal milieu). By use of the adult CBA/N mouse it has been possible to demonstrate that antibody-mediated suppression could be readily achieved in adult animals whose B cells were arrested at the neonatal stage (Kubai and Auerbach, unpublished). Experiments to examine the concept of clonal abortion are now in progress.

Other mouse strains. Documentation of strain differences in susceptibility to tumors, responsiveness to teratogenic stimuli, developmental rates and onset of aging processes is massive, and represents only a portion of the developmentally significant events that may be approached through the comparison of different mouse strains. To what extent immunological maturation is associated with these developmental events is not at this point clear but needs to be examined. For example, one may ask whether the high sensitivity of the C3H mouse to induction of cleft palate by cortisone (Fraser, 1976) is related to the pattern or degree of immune responsiveness of this strain, and whether, perhaps, the C3H/HeJ and C3H/HeAn sublines differ in this property. The Swiss Webster mouse is particularly sensitive to transplacental carcinogenesis induction by nitrosoamine compounds (Rice, 1973) and one wonders whether this sensitivity is correlated with a differential suppression of immune responsiveness during ontogeny of the treated offspring. The C57BL/6 strain is likely to respond to leukemogenic agents such as urethane (Shimkin and Stoner, 1975), and one may ask whether this is related to the more rapid maturation of thymus rudiments during development of this strain of mice. The 129/J line (and even more so the 129/SvTer subline) is particularly susceptible to spontaneously appearing testicular teratomas, and in view of the germ cell/T cell correlation we have postulated, one should ask whether there is some unique difference in this strain in the pattern or rate of thymus stem cell differentiation.

V. Concluding comments

The examples chosen for inclusion in this chapter represent those mutants and strains of mice which have been studied most extensively specifically for the purpose of analyzing developmental aspects of the immune response. These are but a few of the vast number of variants available for study; the potential value of utilizing these animals has just begun to be appreciated.

It is of historical interest that immunologists were among the first to recognize the potential of utilizing spontaneously occurring human disease states, so-called "experiments of nature", to help in the analysis of basic biological processes. Indeed much of our understanding of mechanisms of immuno-deficiency disease, of autoimmunity, of thymic and bursal subfunctions, and of complement-associated pathology have resulted from this recognition.

For the developmental immunologist, the mouse model may serve a similar role in that the already isolated genetic variants may represent developmental "experiments of nature" that can help in the analysis of patterns of stem cell formation and migration, of endocrine functions during ontogeny, of sequential steps in the elaboration of antibody variability, and in the many other differentiative events that occur during the development of the immune response.

Acknowledgements

The author appreciates the help of Wanda Auerbach and Barbara Houser in library reference work and preparation of the manuscript. The secretarial assistance of Allyson Jabusch is acknowledged with thanks. Original research described in this chapter has been supported by grant AI14607 from the National Institutes of Health.

References

Ahmed, A., Scher, I., Sharrow, S. O., Smith, A. H., Paul, W. E., Sachs, D. H. and Sell, K. W. (1977). *J. exp. Med.* **145, 101-110.**

Amsbaugh, D. F., Hansen, C. T., Prescott, B., Stashak, P. W., Barthold, D. R. and Baker, P. J. (1972). *J. exp. Med.* **136**, 931-949.

Artzt, K. and Bennett, D. (1975). *Nature,* **256**, 545-547.

Auerbach, R. (1969). *In* "Developmental Aspects of Antibody Formation and Structure" (Eds J. Sterzl and I. Riha), pp. 23-33. Academic Press, New York and London.

Auerbach, R. (1972). *Curr. Top. Devl. Biol.* **7**, 257-280.

Auerbach, R. (1976). *Ann. d'Immunol. (Inst. Pasteur),* **127** C, 983-992.

Auerbach, R. (1977). *In* "Cell and Tissue Interactions" (Eds J. W. Lash and M. M. Burger), pp. 47-55. Raven Press, New York.

Auerbach, R. (1978). *Devl. comp. Immun.* **2**, 219-228.

Auerbach, R. and Clark, S. (1975). *Science,* **189**, 811-813.

Auerbach, R. and Sidky, Y. A. (1978). *In* "Animal Models of Comparative and Developmental Aspects of Immunity and Disease" (Eds M. E. Gershwin and E. L. Cooper), pp. 166-174. Pergamon Press, New York.

AUERBACH, R., KUBAI, L., LANDAHL, C., CHAKRAVARTY, A., and SULMAN, M. (1976). *In* "Immuno-Aspects of the Spleen" (Eds J. R. Battisto and J. W. Streilein), pp. 3-11. Elsevier/North Holland, Amsterdam.

BARONI, C. D. and DORIA, G. (1973). *Adv. exp. med. Biol.* **29**, 655-660.

BARONI, C. D., FABRIS, N. and BERTOLI, G. (1969). *Immunology,* **17**, 303-314.

BARONI, C. D., PESANDO, P. C. and BERTOLI, G. (1971). *Immunology,* **21**, 455-461.

BATTISTO, J. R., BOREK, J. F. and BUCSI, R. A. (1971). *Cell. Immun.* **2**, 627-633.

BEER, A. E., BILLINGHAM, R. E. and HEAD, J. (1974). *J. invest. Derm.* **63**, 65-74.

BENNETT, D. (1975). *Cell,* **6**, 441-454.

BENNETT, D., ARTZT, K., MAGNUSON, T. and SPIEGELMAN, M. (1977). *In* "Cell Interactions in Differentiation" (Eds J. Karkinen-Jääskeläinen, L. Saxén, and L. Weiss), pp. 389-398. Academic Press, London, New York, San Francisco.

BERNARD, C. C. A. (1976). *J. Immunogen.* **3**, 263-274.

BOYSE, E. A. and BENNETT, D. (1974). *In* "Cellular Selection and Regulation in the Immune Response" (Ed. G. M. Edelman), pp. 155-176. Raven Press, New York.

BURNET, F. M. and HOLMES, M. C. (1964). *J. Path. Bact.* **88**, 229-241.

CANTOR, H. and BOYSE, E. A. (1975). *J. exp. Med.* **141**, 1376-1389.

CHAKRAVARTY, A., KUBAI, L., SIDKY, Y. and AUERBACH, R. (1975). *Ann. N.Y. Acad. Sci.* **294**, 34-42.

COHEN, P. L. and ZIFF, M. (1977). *J. Immun.* **119**, 1534-1537.

COUTINHO, A., GRONOWICZ, E. and SULTZER, B. M. (1975). *Scand. J. Immun.* **4**, 139-143.

DUNG, H. C. (1977). *Transplantation,* **23**, 39-43.

DUNG, H. C. and ADRIAN, E. K., Jr. (1978). *Devl. comp. Immun.* **2**, 327-338.

DUNG, H. C. and SWIGART, R. H. (1971). *Tex. Rep. Biol. Med.* **29**, 273-288.

DUNN, L. C. (1964). *Science,* **144**, 260-263.

DUQUESNOY, R. J. and AHRENS, R. C. (1973). *J. Immun.* **110**, 578-580.

DUQUESNOY, R. J., KALPAKTSOGLOU, P. K. and GOOD, R. A. (1970). *Proc. Soc. exp. Biol. Med.* **133**, 201-206.

EICHER, E. (1976). *Mouse News Letter,* **54**, 40.

EISENBERG, R. A., TAN, E. M. and DIXON, F. J. (1978). *J. exp. Med.* **147**, 582-587.

FABRIS, N., PIERPAOLI, W. and SORKIN, E. (1971a). *Clin. exp. Immun.* **9**, 209-225.

FABRIS, N., PIERPAOLI, W. and SORKIN, E. (1971b). *Clin. exp. Immun.* **9**, 227-240.

FLETCHER, M. P., IKEDA, R. M. and GERSHWIN, M. E. (1977). *J. Immun.* **119**, 110-117.

FRASER, F. C. and FAINSTAT, T. D. (1951). *Pediatrics,* **8**, 527-533.

FREEDMAN, M. (1978). Undergraduate Honors Thesis, University of Wisconsin, Madison.

GACHELIN, G., KEMLER, R., KELLY, F. and JACOB, F. (1977). *Devl Biol.* **57**, 199-209.
GELFAND, M. C., SCHUR, P. H., ASOFSKY, R. and STEINBERG, A. D. (1976). *Arthritis Rheum.* **19**, 43-48.
GERSHON, R. K. and KONDO, K. (1976). *J. Immun.* **117**, 701-702.
GLOBERSON, A., RABINOVICH, H. and UMIEL, T. (1978). *In* "Developmental Immunobiology" (Eds J. B. Solomon and J. D. Horton), pp. 331-337. Elsevier/North Holland, Amsterdam.
GLODE, L. M. and ROSENSTREICH, D. L. (1976). *J. Immun.* **117**, 2061-2066.
GLODE, L. M., SCHER, I., OSBORNE, B. and ROSENSTREICH, D. L. (1976). *J. Immun.* **116**, 454-461.
GLUECKSOHN-WAELSCH, S. and ERICKSON, R. P. (1970a). *Curr. Top. devl. Biol.* **5**, 281-316.
GLUECKSOHN-WAELSCH, S. and ERICKSON, R. P. (1970b). Proc. Symp. Immunogenetics of the H-2 System, Liblice-Prague.
GOIDL, E. A., KLASS, J. and SISKIND, G. W. (1976). *J. exp. Med.* **143**, 1503-1520.
GOIDL, E. A. and SISKIND, G. W. (1974). *J. exp. Med.* **140**, 1285-1302.
GREEN, E. L. (ed.) (Staff of the Jackson Laboratory.) (1966). "Biology of the Laboratory Mouse", 2nd edition, 706 pp. McGraw-Hill, New York, Toronto, Sydney, London.
HALE, M. L., HANNA, E. E. and HANSEN, C. T. (1976). *Nature,* **260**, 44-45.
HAUSCHKA, T. S. and MIRAND, E. A. (1973). *In* "Perspectives in Cancer Research and Treatment" (Ed. C. P. Murphy), pp. 319-331. A. R. Liss, Inc., New York.
HEAD, J. R., BEER, A. E. and BILLINGHAM, R. E. (1977). *Transplantn Proc.* **9**, 1465-1471.
HELYER, B. J. and HOWIE, J. B. (1963). *Br. J. Haemat.* **9**, 119-131.
HOFMAN, F. and GLOBERSON, A. (1973). *Eur. J. Immun.* **3**, 179-181.
HOFMAN, F. and GLOBERSON, A. (1976). *In* "Immune Reactivity of Lymphocytes. Development, Expression, and Control" (Eds M. Feldman and A. Globerson). *Adv. exp. med. Biol.* **66**, 51-58.
HOLDER, A. T. and WALLIS, M. (1977). *J. Endocr.* **74**, 223-229.
HUBER, B., GERSHON, R. K. and CANTOR, H. (1977). *J. exp. Med.* **145**, 10-20.
HURD, E. R. (1977). *J. Immun.* **119**, 1552-1555.
JACOB, F. (1977). *Immun. Rev.* **33**, 3-32.
JORDAN, R. K., OWEN, J. J. T. and RAFF, M. C. (1977). *Eur. J. Immun.* **7**, 736-743.
KAHAN, B. (1978). *In* "Genetic Mosaics and Chimeras in Mammals" (Ed. L. B. Russell), pp. 297-328. Plenum Press, New York and London.
KARMALI, R. A and HORROBIN, D. F. (1976). *Nature,* **263**, 684-685.
KATZ, D. H. (1977). "Lymphocyte Differentiation, Recognition, and Regulation", 749 pp. Academic Press, New York and London.
KINCADE, P. W. (1977). *J. exp. Med.* **145**, 249-263.
KINDRED, B. and LOOR, F. (1974). *J. exp. Med.* **139**, 1215-1227.
KLEIN, J. (1975). "Biology of the Mouse Histocompatibility-2 Complex;

Principles of immunogenetics applied to a single system", 620 pp. Springer Verlag, Berlin and New York.

KLEIN, J. and HAMMERBERG, C. (1977). *Immun. Rev.* **33**, 70-104.

KLINMAN, N. R. and PRESS, J. L. (1975). *J. exp. Med.* **141**, 1133-1146.

KLINMAN, N. R., SIGAL, N. H., METCALF, E. S., PIERCE, S. K. and GEARHART, P. J. (1976). *Cold Spring Harb. Symp. quant. Biol.* **41**, 165-174.

KLINMAN, N. R., CANCRO, M. P., PIERCE, S. K., OWEN, J. A., METCALF, E. S. and SIGAL, N. H. (1979). *In* "Developmental Immunobiology" (Eds G. W. Siskind, S. D. Litwin and M. E. Weksler), pp. 179-193. Grune Stratton, New York, San Francisco, London.

KRETSER, T. A. de and LIVETT, B. G. (1976). *Nature,* **263**, 682-684.

LANDAHL, C. A., CHAKRAVARTY, A., SULMAN, M., KUBAI, L. and AUERBACH, R. (1976). *J. Immun.* **117**, 151-154.

LEVINE, S. and SOWINSKI, R. (1973). *J. Immun.* **110**, 139-143.

LEVINSON, J. R. and MCDEVITT, H. O.(1976). *J. exp. Med.* **144**, 834-839.

LOOR, F. and HÄGG, L-B. (1977). *Cell. Immun.* **29**, 200-209.

LOOR, F. and ROELANTS, G. E. (1975). *Ann. N.Y. Acad. Sci.* **254**, 226-242.

LUTZNER, M. A. and HANSEN, C. T. (1976). *J. Immun.* **116**, 1496-1497.

MANDEL, T. E., CHEERS, C., HOSKING, C. S., MCKENZIE, I. F. C. and NOSSAL, G. J. V. (eds) (1977). *In* "Progress in Immunology III" (Proc. 3rd. Internat. Congr. Immunol.), 855 pp. Australian Academy of Science.

MEIER, H. and SOUTHARD, J. L. (1970). *Life Sci.* **9**, 137-144.

MEIER, H., WEST, W. T. and HOAG, W. G. (1965). *Archs Path.* **80**, 165-170.

METCALF, E. S., SIGAL, N. H., PICKARD, A. R. and KLINMAN, N. R. (1977). *In* "Progress in Immunology III" (Eds T. E. Mandel, C. Cheers, C. S. Hosking, I. F. C. McKenzie and G. J. V. Nossal), pp. 162-170. Australian Academy of Science.

MILICH, D. R. and GERSHWIN, M. E. (1977). *Devl comp. Immun.* **1**, 289-298.

MÖLLER, G. and MÖLLER, E. (1962). *J. cell. comp. Physiol.* **60** (Suppl. 1), 107-128.

MOND, J. J., LIEBERMAN, R., INMAN, J. K., MOSIER, D. E. and PAUL, W. E. (1977). *J. exp. Med.* **146**, 1138-1142.

MONTGOMERY, A. and SWENARCHUK, L. (1977). *Nature,* **267**, 167-168.

MOSIER, D. E., MOND, J. J. and GOLDINGS, E. A. (1977). *J. Immun.* **119**, 1874-1878.

MOSIER, D. E., SCHER, I. and PAUL, W. E. (1976). *J. Immun.* **117**, 1363-1369.

MURPHY, E. D. and ROTHS, J. B. (1977a). *In* "Topics in Hematology" (Proc. 16th Internat. Cong. of Hematol., Kyoto), (Eds S. Seno, F. Takaku and S. Irino), pp. 69-72. Exerpta Medica, Amsterdam, Oxford.

MURPHY, E. D. and ROTHS, J. B. (1977b). 48th Annual Report, The Jackson Laboratory, p. 31.

NOSSAL, G. J. V. and PIKE, B. L. (1975). *J. exp. Med.* **141**, 904-917.

OKOUCHI, E. (1976). *J. physiol. Soc. Japan,* **38**, 325-335.

PALMER, D. W., DAUPHINÉE, M. J., MURPHY, E. and TALAL, N. (1976). *Clin. exp. Immun.* **23**, 578-581.

PANTELOURIS, E. M. (1968). *Nature,* **217**, 370-371.

Pantelouris, E. M. (1973). *Differentiation,* **1**, 437-450.
Pantelouris, E. M. and Hair, J. (1970). *J. Embryol. exp. Morph.* **24**, 615-623.
Patthey, H. and Edidin, M. (1973). *Transplantation,* **15**, 211-214.
Pelletier, M., Montplaisir, S., Dardenne, M. and Bach, J. F. (1976). *Immunology,* **30**, 783-788.
Pierpaoli, W., Baroni, C., Fabris, N. and Sorkin, E. (1969). *Immunology,* **16**, 217-230.
Pierpaoli, W., Kopp, H. G. and Bianchi, E. (1976). *Clin. exp. Immun.* **24**, 501-506.
Pierpaoli, W. and Sorkin, E. (1973). *Adv. exp. biol. Med.* **29**, 651-654.
Pilarski, L. (1977). *J. exp. Med.* **146**, 887-892.
Playfair, J. H. L. (1968a). *Immunology,* **15**, 35-50.
Playfair, J. H. L. (1968b). *Immunology,* **15**, 815-826.
Playfair, J. H. L. and Marshall-Clarke, S. (1973). *Immunology,* **24**, 579-588.
Playfair, J. H. L., Marshall-Clarke, S. and Hudson, L. (1974). *Eur. J. Immun.* **4**, 54-56.
Pritchard, H. and Micklem, H. S. (1973). *Clin. exp. Immun.* **14**, 597-607.
Rice, J. M. (1973). *In* "Transplacental Carcinogenesis" (Eds L. Tomatis and U. Mohr), pp. 77-83. International Agency for Research on Cancer, Lyon.
Roubinian, J. R., Papoian, R. and Talal, N. (1977). *J. Immun.* **118**, 1524-1529.
Rowe, R. W. D. and Goldspink, G. (1969a). *J. Anat.* **104**, 519-530.
Rowe, R. W. D. and Goldspink, G. (1969b). *J. Anat.* **104**, 531-538.
Russell, E. S. (1955). *In* "Aspects of Synthesis and Order in Growth" (Ed. D. Rudnick), pp. 113-126. Princeton University Press, Princeton, New Jersey.
Russell, J. L. and Golub, E. S. (1976). *In* "Immuno-Aspects of the Spleen" (Eds J. R. Battisto and J. W. Streilein), pp. 185-192. Elsevier/North-Holland Biomedical Press, Amsterdam.
Russell, J. L. and Golub, E. S. (1977). *Eur. J. Immun.* **7**, 305-309.
Rygaard, J. (1973). "Thymus and Self, Immunobiology of the Mouse Mutant Nude," 193 pp. F.A.D.L. Copenhagen, Denmark.
Rygaard, J. and Polvsen, C. O. (eds) (1973). "Proc. 1st. Internat. Workshop on Nude Mice", 301 pp. Gustav Fischer Verlag, Stuttgard.
Salomon, J. C. and Lynch, N. (1977). *Biomedicine,* **26**, 77-78.
Sato, V. L., Waksel, S. D. and Herzenberg, L. A. (1976). *Cell. Immun.* **24**, 173-185.
Scher, I., Ahmed, A., Strong, D. M., Steinberg, A. D. and Paul, W. E. (1975a). *J. exp. Med.* **141**, 788-803.
Scher, I., Steinberg, A. D., Berning, A. K. and Paul, W. E. (1975b). *J. exp. Med.* **142**, 637-650.
Scher, I., Ahmed, A., Sharrow, S. O. and Paul, W. E. (1976a). *In* "Development and Host Defenses" (Eds M. D. Cooper and D. Dayton), pp. 55-74. Raven Press, New York.
Scher, I., Sharrow, S. O. and Paul, W. E. (1976b). *J. exp. Med.* **144**, 507-518.
Schneider, G. B. (1976). *Am. J. Anat.* **145**, 371-393.

SEARLE, A. G. (1964). *Genet. Res.* **5**, 171-197.

SHERMAN, M. I. and SOLTER, D. (eds) (1975). "Teratomas and Differentiation", 324 pp. Academic Press, New York, San Francisco, London.

SHERWIN, W. K. and ROWLANDS, D. T., JR. (1975). *J. Immun.* **115**, 1549-1554.

SHIMKIN, M. B. and STONER, G. D. (1975). *Adv. Cancer Res.* **21**, 2-58.

SCHULTZ, L. D. and GREEN, M. C. (1976). *J. Immun.* **116**, 936-943.

SCHULTZ, L. D., HEINIGER, H-J. and EICHER, E. M. (1978). *In* "Animal Models of Comparative and Developmental Aspects of Immunity and Disease" (M. E. Gershwin and E. L. Cooper, eds), pp. 211-222. Pergamon Press, New York.

SCHULTZ, L. D., SIDMAN, C. L. and UNANUE, E. R. (1978). *In* "Animal Models of Comparative and Developmental Aspects of Immunity and Disease" (Eds M. E. Gershwin and E. L. Cooper), pp. 260-269. Pergamon Press, New York.

SNELL, G. D. (1929). *Proc. Natn Acad. Sci. U.S.A.* **15**, 733-734.

SNELL, G. D., DAUSSET, J. and NATHENSON, S. (1976). "Histocompatibility", 401 pp. Academic Press, New York, San Francisco, London.

SOLOMON, J. B. (1971). "Foetal and Neonatal Immunology, Frontiers in Biology", 381 pp. Elsevier/North Holland, Amsterdam.

SOLOMON, J. B. and HORTON, J. D. (eds) (1977). "Developmental Immunobiology", 456 pp. Elsevier/North Holland, Amsterdam.

SPEAR, P. G. and EDELMAN, G. M. (1974). *J. exp. Med.* **139**, 249-263.

STEVENS, L. C., RUSSELL, E. S. and SOUTHARD, J. L. (1957). *Proc. Soc. exp. Biol. Med.* **95**, 161-164.

TALAL, N. and STEINBERG, A. D. (1974). *Curr. Top. Microbiol. Immun.* **64**, 79-103.

UMIEL, T. (1973). *Transplantation,* **11**, 531-535.

UMIEL, T. and AUERBACH, R. (1973). *Pathobiol. Annual,* **3**, 27-46.

UMIEL, T., GLOBERSON, A. and AUERBACH, R. (1968). *Proc. Soc. exp. Biol. Med.* **129**, 598-600.

VITETTA, E. S., ARTZT, K., BENNETT, D., BOYSE, E. A. and JACOB, F. (1975). *Proc. Natn. Acad. Sci.* **72**, 3215-3219.

WALKER, B. E. (1964). *Tex. Rep. Biol. Med.* **22**, 640-647.

WARGON, L. B., LOZZIO, B. B. and WUST, C. J. (1975). *Proc. Soc. exp. Biol. Med.* **148**, 925-928.

WATSON, J. and RIBLET, R. (1974). *J. exp. Med.* **140**, 1147-1161.

WEBB, C. G., GALL, W. E., and EDELMAN, G. M. (1977). *J. exp. Med.* **146**, 923-932.

WEISSMAN, I. L. and AUERBACH, R. (1977). *In* "Progress in Immunology III" (Proc. 3rd Intern. Cong. Immunol.), pp. 802-804. Australian Academy of Science.

WŁODARSKA, J. and WLODARSKI, K. (1976). *Post. Hig. I Med. DosW.* **30**, 31-48.

WORTIS, H. H. (1977). *Clin. exp. Immun.* **8**, 305-317.

WORTIS, H. H., NEHLSEN, S. and OWEN, J. J. (1971). *J. exp. Med.* **134**, 681-692.

WU, S. (1978). *Differentiation,* **11**, 169-174.

WU, S., BACH, F. and AUERBACH, R. (1975). *J. exp. Med* **142**, 1301-1305.
YANAGISAWA, K. O. and FUJIMOTO, H.(1977). *J. Embryol. exp. Morph.* **40**, 277-283.
ZINKERNAGEL, R. M. and DIXON, F. J. (1977). *Clin. exp. Immun.* **29**, 110-121.

Addendum (prepared spring, 1979)

Since the preparation of this chapter in April 1978 there have been extensive additional studies involving developmental studies with mutant mice. A rapid review of some of these studies is presented along with a supplementary bibliography, so that this chapter may be more current at the time of publication.

New Mutants

Among the most interesting newly described mutants is the *beige* (bg/bg) mutation (Roder, 1979; Roder and Duwe, 1979; Roder *et al.* 1979) which has been shown to involve a developmental effect expressed as an impairment of formation of natural killer (NK) cells. An interesting set of deficiencies is associated with impairment of bone marrow cell development, as seen in osteopetrotic (mi/mi) mice (Milhaud and Labat, 1979; Seaman *et al.*, 1979). Mast cell deficiencies have been associated both with beige mice and with mutants of the W series (Kitamura *et al.*, 1979), and the W mutation has been shown also to affect the circulation of lymphocytes involved in mediating delayed-type hypersensitivity (Marchal *et al.*, 1980). The hairless mouse (hr/hr) has been shown to be immunodeficient in terms of T cell functions, but unlike the nude mouse the hairless syndrome involves a disproportionate representation of the various Lyt-bearing splenic T cells (Reske-Kunz *et al.*, 1979a, b). Of particular interest in hairless mice is the fact that the Lyt-1, 2, 3 cell that is considered to be a precursor cell is present in excess, suggestive of a developmental block in T cell maturation analogous to the B cell block associated with CBA/N animals. A most useful source for information on mouse mutants has been published by the Federation of American Societies for Experimental Biology as volume III of the Biological Handbooks series (Part I, Mouse and Rat, 1979) and the reader is referred to this volume for more extensive bibliographical information on mouse mutants and mouse strains.

Endocrine mutants

Differences between genetically obese (ob/ob) and normal mice have been seen in terms of skin graft rejection and natural killer type functions, and it has been suggested that these differences represent secondary effects of adreno-cortical hyperfunction rather than a primary cellular defect, since adrenalectomy and *in vitro* functional activity of ob/ob cells demonstrated a fundamental capacity of ob/ob T cells to carry out immune functions

(Sheena and Meade, 1978; Meade *et al.*, 1979). An extensive update of hypopituitary dwarf (as well as of athymic nude) mice has been presented by Piantanelli and Fabris (1978). An extensive literature has developed involving the study of diabetic mice. Of special interest is the suggestion that there is a defect in lymphokine production in db/db animals (Kazura *et al.*, 1979), that there are major defects in both *in vitro* and *in vivo* tests of immune activity of T cells from db/db mice (Mandel and Mahmoud, 1978), and that, as with ob/ob mice, there are nontheless differences between *in vitro* and *in vivo* systems, indicating that host systemic factors also influence immune reactivity of these metabolically compromised mutant mice (Fernandes *et al.*, 1978).

Other mutants

Further work describing the motheaten mouse has been published by Sidman *et al.* (1978a, b). A major update on asplenic (Dh/ +) and athymic (nu/nu) mice has been presented by Gershwin and his co-workers (Gershwin *et al.*, 1978, 1979). Interesting, also, is the associated work described by Gershwin *et al.* (1979) in which the Dh gene has been introduced into NZB autoimmune mice. For an extensive updating of the literature of the H-2 region reference is made to the review by Klein (1978). Of the several papers involving the T-locus, the studies reported by Shur and Bennett (1979) indicating a specific defect of T-mutants in galactosyltransferase activity may prove to be of special significance in terms of cell surface interactions.

The CBA/N mouse

One of the most active areas of investigation has been the study of the maturation of B cells and of B cell subsets in the CBA/N mouse. The characterization of tolerance-sensitive and tolerance-insensitive B cell subsets has been shown to differ between CBA/N and normal mice (Merchant *et al.*, 1978; McKearn and Quintans, 1979; Metcalf *et al.*, 1980). The fact that the CBA/N mouse also involves T cell deficits must now be considered (Goodman and Weigle, 1979). Interesting indeed is the finding that some of the CBA/N defects may be overcome with advancing age (Fidler *et al.*, 1979; Whitlock and Watson, 1979; Rosenberg, 1979; Lindsten and Andersson, 1979), and this finding leads one to re-examine much of the earlier work with this variant strain. A new and potentially exciting use of the CBA/N mouse has been their employment as a source of spleen cells for generation of hybridomas (Schroer *et al.*, 1979), all of which to date have been of the IgM class. Reference to a good overview of studies with this line is made to the review by Paul *et al.* (1979).

The NZB mouse

Many of the studies with NZB mice have been directed at further understanding of autoimmune pathology. The present discussion is focussed primarily on those reports aimed at understanding developmental processes. It has been suggested that NZB mice fail to respond to prethymic bone marrow suppressor cells (Dauphin and Talal, 1979), and indeed a variety of regulatory functions seem to be impaired in the developing NZB mouse (cf. Theofilopoulos *et al.*, 1980) as well as in other mice with autoimmune deficiencies of genetic origin. Differences have been noted in terms of clonable B lymphocytes and myeloid precursors in NZB animals (Kincade *et al.*, 1979), and several other studies have emphasized B cell hyperactivity and alterations in specific B cell subsets of NZB mice (Nakajima *et al.*, 1979; Taurog *et al.*, 1979; Cohen *et al.*, 1978). More complex analysis of NZB mice bearing additional immune-modification genes has been carried out by Gershwin and his colleagues (Gershwin *et al.*, 1979; Ohsugi and Gershwin, 1979).

The C_3H/HeJ substrain

Further work has been carried out on the Lps gene associated with this substrain of the C_3H line. The Lps gene has now been assigned to chromosome 4 (Watson *et al.*, 1978), and the defect has been associated with differences in membrane-LPS interactions of both lymphocytes and macrophages (Peavy *et al.*, 1978). Macrophage differences between LPS-responsive and LPS-unresponsive mice have also been discussed by Vogel and Rosenstreich (1979) who have demonstrated that the genetic defect in responsiveness of macrophages can be overcome by lymphokine-induced stimulation of lymphocytes. Thus the macrophage alteration may be assumed to be secondary to the unresponsiveness of C_3H/HeJ lymphocytes. An interesting extension of the original studies with this strain is the work of O'Brien *et al.* (1979) which indicates that there is a whole series of susceptibility genes to *Salmonella typhimurium*, and that the high sensitivity of this substrain to *Salmonella* involves not only the Lps gene but both X-linked (xid) and autosomal (Ity^s) susceptibility genes as well. The biological function of the Lps gene has been discussed by Rosenstreich (1978) in a volume on the origins of inbred mice edited by H. C. Morse which can serve as an excellent introduction to the central theme of the work reviewed in the present chapter on the use of mutant mice in studies on the ontogeny of the immune response.

Bibliography

ALTMAN, P. L. and KATZ, D. D. (comp. and eds) (1979). "Inbred and Genetically Defined Strains of Laboratory Animals". Part 1, Mouse and Rat Biological Handbooks III, Federation of American Societies for Experimental Biology, Bethesda, Maryland.

COHEN, P., ZIFF, M. and VITETTA, E. S. (1978). *J. Immun.* **121**, 973-977.

CROWIE, A. J., JACOBSON, S. and MAY, M. (1978). *Immun. Commun.* **7**, 417-429.

DAUPHIN'EE, M. J. and TALAL, N. (1979). *J. Immun.* **122**, 936-941.

FERNANDES, G., HANDWERGER, B. S., YUNIS, E. J. and BROWN, D. M. (1978). *J. clin. Invest.* **61**, 243-250.

FIDLER, J. M., MORGAN, E. L. and WEIGLE, W. O. (1979). *J. Immun.* **124**, 13-19.

GERSHWIN, M. E., AHMED, A., IKEDA, R. M., SHIFRINE, M. and WILSON, F. (1978). *Immunology,* **34**, 631-642.

GERSHWIN, M. E., CASTLES, J. J., ERICKSON, K. and AHMED, A. (1979). *J. Immun.* **122**, 2020-2025.

GERSHWIN, M. E., CASTLES, J. J., IKEDA, R. M., ERICKSON, K. and MONTERO, J. (1979). *J. Immun.* **122**, 710-717.

GOODMAN, M. G. and WEIGLE, W. O. (1979). *J. Immun.* **123**, 2484-2487.

KAZURA, J. W., GANDOLA, C., RODMAN, H. R. and MAHMOUD, A. A. (1979). *J. Immun.* **123**, 2114-2117.

KINCADE, P. W., LEE, G., FERNANDES, G., MOORE, M. A., WILLIAMS, N. and GOOD, R. A. (1979). *Proc. Natn. Acad. Sci. U.S.A.* **76**, 3464-3468.

KITAMURA, Y., SHIMADA, M., GO, S., MATSUDA, H., HATANAKA, K. and SEKI, M. (1979). *J. exp. Med.* **150**, 482-490.

KLEIN, J. (1978). *Adv. Immun.* **26**, 55-146.

LINDSTEN, T. and ANDERSSON, B. (1979). *J. exp. Med.* **150**, 1285-1292.

MANDEL, M. A. and MAHMOUD, A. A. (1978). *J. Immun.* **120**, 1375-1377.

MARCHAL, G., MILON, G. and GUENET, J.-L. (1980). *Immunology,* **39**, 269.

MCKEARN, J. P. and QUINTANS, J. (1979). *J. Immun.* **124**, 77-80.

MEADE, C. J., SHEENA, J. and MERTIN, J. (1979). *Int. Archs Allergy appl. Immun.* **58**, 121-127.

MERCHANT, B., SNIPPE, H., LIZZIO, E. F. and INMAN, J. K. (1978). *J. exp. Med.* **147**, 1755-1770.

METCALF, E. S., SCHER, I. and KLINMAN, N. R. (1980). *J. exp. Med.* **151**, 486-491.

MILHAUD, G. and LABAT, M. L. (1979). *Biomedicine,* **30**, 71-75.

MORSE, H. C. III (ed.) (1978). "Origins of Inbred Mice". Academic Press, New York, London, San Francisco.

NAKAJIMA, P. B., DATTA, S. K., SCHWARTZ, R. S. and HUBER, B. T. (1979). *Proc. Natn. Acad. Sci. U.S.A.* **76**, 4613-4616.

O'BRIEN, A. D., ROSENSTREICH, D. L., SCHER, I., CAMPBELL, G. H., MACDERMOTT, R. P. and FORMAL, S. B. (1979). *J. Immun.* **124**, 20-24.

OHSUGI, Y. and GERSHWIN, M. E. (1979). *J. Immun.* **123**, 1260-1265.

PAUL, W. E., SUBBARAO, B., MOND, J. J., STIECKMANN, D. G., ZITON, I., AHMED, A., MOSIER, D. E. and SCHER, I. (1978). *In* "Cells of Immunoglobulin Synthesis" (Eds B. Pernis and H. J. Vogel), pp. 383-396. Academic Press, New York, London, San Francisco.

PEAVY, D. L., BAUGHN, R. E. and MUSHER, D. M. (1978). *Infect. Immun.* **21**, 310-319.

PIANTANELLI, L. and FABRIS, N. (1978). *Birth Defects,* **14**, 315-333.

RESKE-KUNZ, A. B., SCHEID, M. P., DE SOUSA, M. and BOYSE, E. A. (1979). *Adv. exp. Med. Biol.* **114**, 55-58.

RESKE-KUNZ, A. B., SCHEID, M. P. and BOYSE, E. A. (1979). *J. exp. Med.* **149**, 228-233.

RODER, J. C. (1979). *J. Immun.* **123**, 2168-2173.

RODER, J. and DUWE, A. (1979). *Nature,* **278**, 451-453.

RODER, J. C., LOHMANN-MATTHES, M. L., DOMZIG, W. and WIGZELL, H. (1979). *J. Immun.* **123**, 2174-2181.

ROSENBERG, Yvonne, J. (1979). *J. exp. Med.* **150**, 1561-1566.

ROSENSTREICH, D. L. (1978). *In* "Origins of Inbred Mice" (Ed. H. C. Morse III), pp. 457-460. Academic Press, New York, London, San Francisco.

SCHROER, K. R., KIM, K. J., PRESCOTT, B. and BAKER, P. J. (1979). *J. exp. Med.* **150**, 698-702.

SEAMAN, W. E., GINDHART, T. S., GREENSPAN, J. S., BLACKMAN, M. A., and TALAL, N. (1979). *J. Immun.* **122**, 2541-2547.

SHEENA, J. and MEADE, C. J. (1978). *Int. Archs. Allergy appl. Immun.* **57**, 263-268.

SHUR, B. D. and BENNETT, D. (1979). *Devl Biol.* **77**, 243-259.
SIDMAN, C. L., SHULTZ, L. D. and UNANUE, E. R. (1978a). *J. Immun.* **121**, 2393-2398.
SIDMAN, C. L., SHULTZ, L. D. and UNANUE, E. R. (1978b). *J. Immun.* **121**, 2399-2404.
TAUROG, J. D., MOUTSOPOULOS, H. M., ROSENBERG, Y. J., CHUSED, T. M. and STEINBERG, A. D. (1979). *J. exp. Med.* **150**, 31-43.
THEOFILOPOULOS, A. N., SHAWLER, D. L., EISENBERG, R. A. and DIXON, F. J. (1980). *J. exp. Med.* **151**, 446-466.
VAN SNICK, J. L. and MASSON, P. L. (1980). *J. exp. Med.* **151**, 45-55.
VOGEL, S. N. and ROSENSTREICH, D. L. (1979). *J. Immun.* **123** 2842-2850.
WATSON, J., KELLY, K., LARGEN, M. and TAYLOR, B. A. (1978). *J. Immun.* **120**, 422-424.
WHITLOCK, C. A. and WATSON, J. D. (1979). *J. exp. Med.* **150**, 1483-1497.

5 *The Mucosa-associated Immune System of the Rabbit**

A. D. BEFUS and J. BIENENSTOCK

I. Introduction

The rabbit has been extensively employed as an experimental animal in immunology, particularly since the early 1960s. At that time, the fundamental role of the avian bursa of Fabricius in the development of humoral immunity was being elucidated (Glick *et al.*, 1956; Cooper *et al.*, 1966a) as was the role of the thymus in cellular immunity (Miller, 1961; Cooper *et al.*, 1966a). It was a time of great excitement in the history of immunology as the characteristics of these two central lymphoid structures, so pivotal in the ontogeny of the immune system, were being unravelled.

These studies quickly led to a consideration of what was the mammalian equivalent of the avian bursa, as mammals lack an obvious bursa. It was highly probable that such an equivalent existed, not only because of the obvious distinction in mammals between humoral and cellular immunity as in birds, but also because "experiments in nature", as they were described by Good, demonstrated either thymic or bursal equivalent (or both) abnormalities (see Cooper *et al.*, 1966b). Given that both the thymus and bursa arise from the embryonic alimentary canal, the search for the bursal equivalent in mammals quickly centred upon gut-associated lymphoid tissue (GALT) (Archer *et al.*, 1963; Cooper *et al.*, 1966b), such as the appendix (APP) and sacculus rotundus (SR) of rabbits and the Peyer's patches (PP) which occur in all mammals that have been studied

* Supported by the Medical Research Council of Canada.

(e.g. Good and Finstad, 1967; Fichtelius *et al.*, 1968). The rabbit presented such a fine model for these studies as: (a) rabbit GALT exceeds in mass and cell yield the remaining lymphoid tissue (Waksman and Ozer, 1976); and (b) the size and location of rabbit GALT allow easy access for study and experimental manipulation. Although much has been learned of the function of GALT, including that it does not appear to be a bursal equivalent in the strictest sense (see section II, D), much remains to be uncovered.

Another exciting development in the early 1960s was the discovery of IgA (Heremans *et al.*, 1959) and its strong association with mucosal sites (Tomasi and Zigelbaum, 1963). This association enhanced the interest in GALT and potentiated the use of rabbits in its study. It is now clear, in large part through studies with rabbits but in other species as well, that GALT plays a paramount role in IgA and other immune responses at mucosal sites. Moreover, lymphoid aggregates similar to GALT occur at other mucosal sites such as the respiratory tract where they have been called BALT (bronchus-associated lymphoid tissue: Brundelet, 1965; Bienenstock *et al.*, 1973a, b; Chamberlain *et al.*, 1973; Bienenstock *et al.*, 1974; Bienenstock and Johnston, 1976; Rácz *et al.*, 1977). Presumably similar aggregates occur at other mucosal sites. There is increasing evidence that we must now consider a common mucosal immunologic system with complex interrelationships largely through cell traffic among all sites, including bowel, lung, breast, salivary and lacrimal glands, ear and urogenital tract (Parmely and Beer, 1977; Bienenstock *et al.*, 1978; Bienenstock *et al.*, 1979). The rabbit has been instrumental in the development of these concepts through studies of its GALT and BALT.

We intend to outline the role of the rabbit over the last two decades in the evolution of our thought concerning bursal equivalents, GALT, BALT and, most recently, the common mucosal immunologic system. For the sake of clarity, we will refer to studies in other species as well, especially those which have been significant in our conceptual progress. As many reviews on mucosal immunity and GALT have appeared recently, we will refer the reader to them frequently, and have not attempted to review all the available relevant literature, especially in the areas where little progress has occurred since the latest reviews. The following reviews are particularly recommended: Bienenstock (1974); Heremans (1974); Lamm (1976); Parrott (1976); Tomasi (1976); Waksman and Ozer, (1976); Porter and Knight (1977). In areas where recent developments have been significant, we have been more exhaustive in our coverage, even if contributions have been based upon models other than the rabbit.

II. Gut-associated lymphoid tissue (GALT)

A. FUNCTIONAL MORPHOLOGY

Rabbit GALT includes PP, SR, called by some the tonsil iliaca (Ackerman, 1966), and the APP (Fig. 1). Solitary lymphoid nodules (SLN) distributed throughout the small and large bowel (Dukes and Bussey, 1926; Bloom and Fawcett, 1968; Kealy, 1976; Cole, 1978; Keren *et al.*, 1978) should probably be included in GALT, although to date they have received little attention.

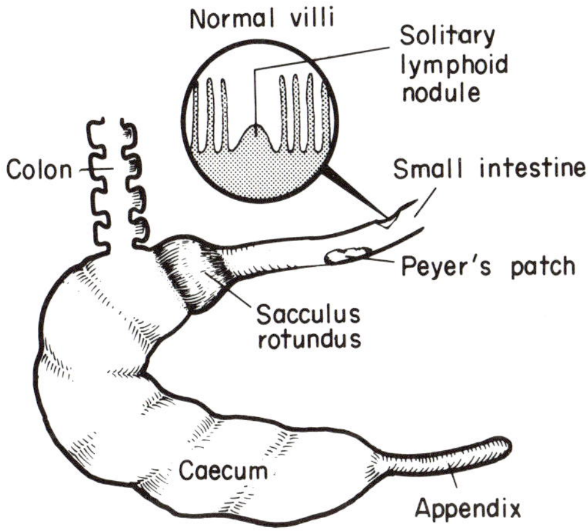

FIG. 1 Gut-associated lymphoid tissue (GALT) of the rabbit.

1. *Appendix*

The APP, which is large in the rabbit, is situated at the caudal end of the caecum like the uninflated end of an elongated balloon. In man, the APP is said to be vestigial (Waksman and Ozer, 1976) although such a description may only reflect our current knowledge. The APP is absent in rodents such as mice and rats.

The microanatomy of various GALT components is similar apart from differences in the proportions of the regions within the lymphoid aggregates (Faulk *et al.*, 1971; Waksman *et al.*, 1973; Waksman, 1973). Fig. 2 (modified from Waksman *et al.*, 1973) is a diagrammatic representation of a single follicle and overlying structures of the APP. Five regions can be recognized, namely the lymphoepithelium, dome, corona, follicle (or as called by some authors, the germinal center), and the interfollicular or thymus-dependent area (TDA). Waksman and Ozer (1976) state that the follicle, despite being a site of rapid B cell proliferation and containing tingible body macrophages, both

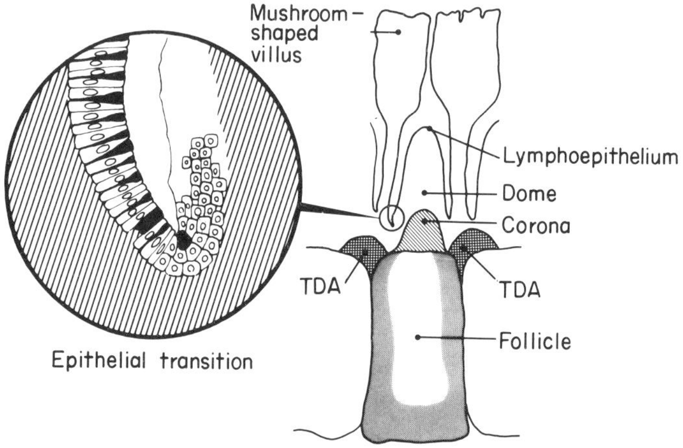

FIG. 2 Diagrammatic representation of the anatomy of a GALT component — the appendix.

characteristics of germinal centers, is nevertheless different from a classical germinal center in two ways. Firstly, the mantle zone of small lymphocytes which surrounds a germinal center is absent around GALT follicles and secondly, GALT follicles lack dendritic reticulum cells so important in antigen retention in germinal centers of lymph nodes and the spleen (Nossal and Ada, 1971). A third factor is that the major site of cell proliferation is at the periphery of the follicle (see below) rather than in the center as occurs in typical germinal centers. Between adjacent follicular complexes with their overlying lymphoepithelium, dome and corona, there are areas of normal gut mucosa, which in the APP are mushroom-shaped.

There is an abrupt transition between the typical columnar epithelium of the normal mucosa and the lymphoepithelium over the dome (Fig. 2). The lymphoepithelium consists of cuboidal epithelial cells and is heavily infiltrated by lymphocytes. Goblet cells, numerous in normal mucosal epithelium, are absent in the lymphoepithelium. This highly specialized epithelium also covers the PP, SR and SLN (Faulk *et al.*,

1971; Waksman *et al.*, 1973; Keren *et al.*, 1978). Recently, a uniquely specialized epithelial cell of the follicle-associated epithelium (Bockman and Cooper, 1973) subsequently called the microfold or M cell (Owen and Jones, 1974; Owen, 1977), has been described in the lymphoepithelium of the human and murine PP. Presumably, this cell is characteristic of all lymphoepithelia (see section III, B). M cells and lymphocytes are in intimate association and lumenal antigenic material, taken up by M cells, is quickly passed onto adjacent lymphocytes (Owen, 1977). It is clear that the lymphoepithelium, and M cells in particular, continuously sample the antigenic nature of the lumenal environment (Bockman and Cooper, 1973; Owen and Jones, 1974; Owen 1977). This movement of macromolecules is bidirectional, into the tissues, but also into the lumen as Bockman and Stevens (1977) have recently shown. As early as 1932 it was suggested by Watzka (see Nieuwenhuis, 1971, p. 88) that lymphocytes influence the differentiation of epithelial cells to maintain this lympho-epithelium. The origin and ontogeny of M cells and the nature of factors which regulate their numbers in health and disease require further investigation if we hope to understand their function and to manipulate mucosal immune mechanisms.

The transport phenomena characteristic of the specialized lympho-epithelium may not be restricted to macromolecules. It has long been suggested that lymphocytes and other leucocytes enter the intestinal lumen, although this has not been satisfactorily documented (e.g. Mitchison, 1953, Ambrus and Ambrus, 1959; Teir *et al.*, 1963; Kotani *et al.*, 1967; Nieuwenhuis, 1971; Joel *et al.*, 1972; Waksman, 1973; Bellamy and Nielsen, 1974; Douglas and Weetman, 1975; Sprent, 1976; Joel *et al.*, 1977). Assuming that such movement occurs, whether it occurs solely or predominantly at the GALT lymphoepithelium is speculative. Assuming that the frequency of radiolabeled lymphoid cells in lymphoepithelium as opposed to normal columnar epithelium is indicative of movement into the lumen (Joel *et al.*, 1972; Waksman, 1973), the lymphoepithelium seems to be a predominant site of migration into the lumen. The rabbit APP would appear to be an excellent model to investigate this phenomenon as it can be easily manipulated and there is suggestion of selective migration of lymphoid cells into its lumen (Jassinowski, 1925, quoted by Nieuwenhuis, 1971, p. 88). This important area of mucosal immunology is unexplored and the significance of cells in the lumen remains to be determined.

The dome, immediately below the lymphoepithelium (Fig. 2) contains large and medium-sized lymphocytes with some blast cells, but few small lymphocytes (Waksman *et al.*, 1973). The corona is a zone of predominantly small lymphocytes lying between the follicle and the dome. It may be analogous to the mantle zone of a typical germinal center. The follicle is surrounded by connective tissue and consists of a central, sparsely populated zone composed of small lymphocytes, some larger cells, but with few dividing cells. The peripheral zone of the follicle is densely populated with lymphocytes, blast cells and numerous macrophages. Macrophages are particularly abundant in the central region of the follicle and they contain numerous bacteria, presumably of lumenal origin, which they appear to degrade (Friedenstein and Goncharenko, 1965). It is interesting (see below) that despite numerous lymphocytes and macrophages, antibody forming cells are not normally found in the APP or other GALT (Hanaoka and Waksman, 1970; Bienenstock and Dolezel, 1971).

Waksman *et al.* (1973) have described a plane of cleavage in the rabbit APP which separates the dome and corona from the follicle and divides the TDA about equally. They have used this technique to characterize the various cell populations further (Waksman and Ozer, 1976).

Cytokinetic studies using *in vivo* injection of ^{3}H-thymidine have shown that the basolateral regions of this peripheral zone have a high DNA synthetic rate (Meuwissen *et al.*, 1969; Faulk *et al.*, 1971; Bienenstock *et al.*, 1973b). At 1 h following ^{3}H-thymidine injection, highly labeled cells were abundant in the basolateral regions of the follicles but some labeled cells were present in the dome, TDA and lymphoepithelium (Faulk *et al.*, 1971; Bienenstock *et al.*, 1973b). By 24 h, labeling in the peripheral zone of the follicle and in the dome and lymphoepithelium was more extensive; the TDA was largely unchanged from the 1 h labeling period. No significant differences were detected in the distribution of labeled cells in the APP, PP, or SR (Bienenstock *et al.*, 1973b). Following 1 h labeling *in vivo*, the percentage of cells labeled in a single cell suspension of PP was 10·4%, of the APP it was 24·1% and of the SR it was 16·7%, whereas in the spleen, only 3·3% of the cells were labeled (Faulk *et al.*, 1971). Meuwissen *et al.* (1969) found similar ranking, albeit lower percentages, PP 7%, APP 17%, SR 14%.

These cytokinetic studies clearly show that the peripheral areas of the GALT follicles are sites of rapid cell proliferation. Moreover, cell proliferation does occur in the dome and lymphoepithelium, although at a lower rate.

The TDA is composed largely of small lymphocytes and, perhaps of most significance, it is the only area of GALT which contains high endothelial venules (HEV) and large lymphatic sinuses (Waksman *et al.*, 1973). HEV are major sites of lymphocyte migration from blood into tissues (Anderson *et al.*, 1976; Stamper and Woodruff, 1976). Few studies have been published on lymphocyte traffic in rabbit GALT or other tissues, whereas studies in other species, particularly in the mouse, rat and sheep have been extensive (e.g. Griscelli *et al.*, 1969; Parrott and Ferguson, 1974; Guy-Grand *et al.*, 1974; McWilliams *et al.*, 1975, 1977; Rose *et al.*, 1976a, b; Hopkins and Hall, 1976; Scollay *et al.*, 1976; Cahill *et al.*, 1977; Hall *et al.*, 1977; McDermott and Bienenstock, 1979).

In the rabbit, Durkin *et al.* (1975) have studied the migratory patterns of *in vitro* ^{3}H-adenosine labeled bone marrow, APP, mesenteric lymph node (MLN) and popliteal lymph node cells at various times after transfer to recipients and Perey and Milne (1975) investigated the 24-h localization of thoracic duct lymph (TDL) cells labeled *in vitro* with either ^{3}H-uridine or ^{3}H-thymidine. These two groups showed that the GALT TDA are sites of thymus-dependent cell localization in the rabbit as in other species. Moreover, and as distinct from other species, labeled cells localized in the dome and corona of GALT, which were identified as areas of B cell influx (Durkin *et al.*, 1975; Perey and Milne, 1975). The significance of this unique B cell localization in rabbit GALT is unclear.

2. *Peyer's patches*

Rabbit PP (Fig. 1) are found on the anti-mesenteric border of the jejunum and ileum but not in the duodenum (Sackmann, 1977). They number from 2 to 10 (Cooper *et al.*, 1966b; Faulk *et al.*, 1971; Sackmann, 1977) and each is composed of about 40-50 lymphoid nodules. In other species the numbers of PP in the small intestine are variable, with 6-13 in the mouse (Sobhon, 1971; Abe and Ito, 1977), 18-26 in the rat (Hummel, 1935), and from a peak of over 400 in adolescent man to near 100 in the aged (Cornes, 1965). The characteristics of this involution require further study particularly with reference to thymic and bursal or bursal-equivalent involution. Hummel (1935) described two PP in the rat colon. PP-like lymphoid aggregates are present in birds as well as mammals (Janković and Mitrović, 1967; Perey, 1971; Bienenstock *et al.*, 1973a; Firth, 1977; Befus *et al.*, 1980).

The adult PP contains the same basic elements as the APP (Fig. 2), but the follicles are less elongated and the TDA is enlarged (Faulk *et al.*, 1971; Waksman *et al.*, 1973). In addition, villi separating the neighbouring domes are not mushroom-shaped, as in the APP, but appear as normal villi. Blasts and mitoses are rare in the dome and upper follicle, an observation which has lead to the interpretation that PP contain an enlarged corona of small lymphocytes.

3. *Sacculus rotundus*

The SR of the rabbit encircles the ileocaecal junction (Fig. 1) and appears to be absent in other mammals. In the bird, however, there is a lymphoid aggregate, at the base of each caecum, called the *tonsilla caecalis* (e.g. Hoshi and Mori, 1973), which may be analogous to the SR. As with the APP and PP, many lymphoid nodules are present in the SR. Structurally, the SR appears to be a mixture of the APP and PP as the TDA is intermediate in size between that of the APP and PP, and the villi of the SR are mushroom-shaped as in the APP. The follicles are elongated as in the APP but the corona of small lymphocytes is large as in the PP.

4. *Solitary lymphoid nodules*

SLN have received little attention until recently (Keren *et al.*, 1978) because, although they had been well recognized by anatomists (Dukes and Bussey, 1926; Bloom and Fawcett, 1968; Kealy, 1976; Cole, 1978), there was little interest in their function. They are distributed throughout the small and large intestine and range up to about 3 mm in diameter (Bloom and Fawcett, 1968). SLN in the small intestine possess a lymphoepithelium (Keren *et al.*, 1978) and this appears to be so for those in the large bowel also (Cole, 1978). The relationship between these SLN in the large bowel and the two PP in the large bowel of the rat (Hummel, 1935) is unclear. Detailed studies of the morphology and function of SLN remain to be conducted.

B. ONTOGENY

In the early 1960s, a considerable literature appeared on the prenatal development of the thymus and other lymphoid tissues which showed that the thymus was the first lymphoid organ to develop in all mammalian species studied (Archer *et al.*, 1964). However, the timing of lymphoid development in the spleen, gut and lymph nodes varied considerably among species. Moreover, the effects of neonatal thymectomy differed, being most severe in the mouse and hamster and less so in the rabbit. Given these species differences, and the suggestion that GALT represented a mammalian bursal-equivalent, the ontogeny of rabbit GALT was investigated by a variety of authors.

Whereas in man the lymphoid nature of the APP and PP is clearly evident by 20-24 weeks of gestation (Cornes, 1965; Jones *et al.*, 1972), the rabbit, with a gestation period of 31-32 days, does not develop lymphoid nodules in the gut until about the 4th day after birth (Archer *et al.*, 1964; Friedenstein and Goncharenko, 1965; Ackerman, 1966; Stramignoni and Mollo, 1968; Nieuwenhuis, 1971). However, recognizable dome structures are present from about day 26 of gestation and lymphocyte accumulations from day 29; much later than the appearance of lymphoid organization in the thymus (days 18-20), spleen, popliteal and MLN (days 26-28) (Ackerman, 1966). The epithelium of the newborn APP is capable of pinocytotic uptake characteristic of the adult lymphoepithelium and by day 6 post parturition is infiltrated with lymphocytes (Bockman and Cooper, 1973; Nieuwenhuis, 1971). PP are not easily recognizable at or before birth (Faulk *et al.*, 1971; Bienenstock *et al.*, 1973a) but appear by day 4 (Archer *et al.*, 1964). The development of the SR is less completely studied but is said to be delayed 1-2 days relative to the APP (Ackerman, 1966).

Barg and Draper (1975), using intrathymic inoculation with ^{3}H-thymidine, followed the accumulation of thymocytes in the GALT and other lymphoid tissues of the neonatal rabbit through to 90 days of age. There was a pronounced migration of T cells to the developing GALT, especially in the neonate, but this had disappeared by 30 days of age. The migration to the PP, SR and MLN was greater than to the APP, which corresponded with the relative sizes of the TDA of these tissues (Waksman *et al.*, 1973). This also correlated well with the results of Richter *et al.* (1970) and Abdou and Richter (1970) who showed that the SR and PP, but not the APP, reconstituted immune competence to lethally irradiated rabbits.

To investigate the role of the thymus in the postnatal development of the APP, and other lymphoid tissue, neonatal thymectomy (Tx), was performed (Archer *et al.*, 1964). Such extirpative surgery clearly depressed follicular development in the spleen and peripheral lymph nodes (PLN), but the APP appeared normal. That the ontogeny of the APP was unaffected by Tx was considered evidence that it was a bursal-equivalent. Moreover, neonatal thymectomy-appendectomy (TxAPPx) caused long-term lymphoid depletion and depressed antibody production, further supporting the hypothesis that the APP played a central lymphoid role (Archer *et al.*, 1964; section II,C,3a).

Despite these results, the ontogenetic studies cited above suggest that the rabbit GALT is in large part dependent upon antigen stimulation for its development and maintenance (Perey and Good, 1968; Perey, 1971; Blythman and Waksman, 1973). Studies on germ-free animals (Pollard and Sharon, 1970; Perey, 1971) support the role of antigenic stimulation in GALT development. Despite the suggestion that two types of GALT exist, one which is antigen-independent and the other which is antigen-dependent (Perey, 1971), we feel that there is little evidence to support this contention. It appears that antigen is unnecessary for the initiation of the GALT, but may be essential for its maturation.

C. PHYSIOLOGICAL CHARACTERISTICS

1. *Rabbit thymus lymphocyte antigen (RTLA) and surface immunoglobulin (sIg) on GALT cells*

a. *Thymic Markers (RTLA)*

To characterize cells of the GALT, single cell suspensions have been tested for surface RTLA (Fradelizi *et al.*, 1973) and for sIg (Jones and Cebra, 1974; Fujiwara *et al.*, 1974; Rudzik *et al.*, 1975a; Craig and Cebra, 1975). Table 1 summarizes results of studies on the proportion

TABLE 1
Percentage of RTLA-bearing cells in various tissues of 14-18 week old rabbits

Cell source	Reference	
	Fujiwara *et al.* (1974)[a]	Rudzik *et al.* (1975)[b]
Thymus	94·5	94·0
Spleen	37·8	19·7
Peripheral blood	40·1	43·9
Popliteal lymph node	57·0	—[c]
Bone marrow	15·5	—
APP	23·3	—
PP	—	16·6
TDL	—	72·4
BALT	—	18·4
Small intestinal lamina propria (LP)	—	11·1

[a] determined by surface immunofluorescence.
[b] determined by lymphocytotoxicity.
[c] — not determined.

of RTLA positive (+ve) cells in various tissues of 14-18 week old rabbits. As expected RTLA +ve cells are abundant in the thymus and TDL, but less so in other organs. In the APP and PP such cells represented 17-23% of the total, and although SR was not studied, it would presumably fit into this range. The number of +ve cells at other mucosal sites, namely BALT and lamina propria (LP) of the small intestine will be discussed later (section III, A and B).

Fujiwara *et al.* (1974) also studied the changes with age of RTLA +ve cells in various organs. Of the organs they studied, the popliteal lymph nodes and APP showed significant changes with age. In 1·4-week-old rabbits, the APP contained 62·4% +ve cells but by 6 weeks and 18 weeks this had dropped to 19·5% and 23·3% respectively and had risen to 46·9% by 140 weeks. Similar trends occurred in the lymph node with higher values in the young and old animals, in contrast with rabbits of intermediate age.

b. *Cell Markers (sIg)*

The proportions of cells with various heavy chain markers on their surfaces varied from organ to organ also, but a consistent finding was that in GALT and other mucosa-associated tissues (e.g. BALT, section III, B), the proportion of IgA-positive cells was greater than at other sites (Table 2; Jones and Cebra, 1974; Rudzik *et al.*, 1975a; Craig and Cebra, 1975). IgD and IgE have not been studied.

Calkins *et al.* (1975) have used class specific anti-immunoglobulin sera to stimulate DNA synthesis in B cells of various rabbit tissues, including the APP. Whereas, in the popliteal lymph node, IgM-, IgG- and IgA-bearing cells were demonstrated, in the spleen only IgM- and IgG-bearing cells were stimulated. In the APP, on the other hand, only cells bearing IgM and IgA receptors were demonstrated. Moreover, by separating the APP cells along the plane of cleavage (see above, Waksman *et al.*, 1973; Waksman and Ozer, 1976), dome and corona cells responded well to the anti-immunoglobulin stimuli, whereas TDA cells were unresponsive. Potential responsiveness in follicular cells could not be detected as spontaneous DNA synthetic rates were high. These results emphasize the association of IgA with mucosal surfaces. It was puzzling that IgA-bearing cells were not demonstrated in the spleen or IgG-bearing cells in GALT, as surface fluorescence studies (using intact antisera and not $F(ab)_2$ reagents) had shown that cells bearing these isotypes were present (Rudzik *et al.*, 1975a). This may simply reflect the different techniques used and the relative insensitivity of anti-immunoglobulin induced DNA synthesis. Alternatively, cytophilic immunoglobulins, as opposed to ones endogenously synthesized, may have led to significant overestimates of the proportion of Ig-bearing cells seen by immunofluorescence. Jones and Cebra (1974) and Craig and Cebra (1975) showed that following pronase digestion of sIg and after a period for recovery, the proportion

TABLE 2
Percentage of surface immunoglobulin sIg-bearing cells in various tissues of 14-18-week-old rabbits[a]

Cell source	Fujiwara *et al.* (1974)	Rudzik *et al.* (1974a)		
	Surface immunoglobulin			
	Ig	IgM	IgG	IgA
Thymus	5·0	—[b]	—	—
Spleen	47·4	9·8	4·7	3·0
Peripheral blood	42·4	—	—	—
Popliteal lymph Node	37·3	—	—	—
Bone marrow	37·2	—	—	—
APP	53·0	—	—	—
PP	—	32·0	16·8	29·9
TDL	—	10·8	61·0	10·8
BALT	—	16·8	7·5	17·2
Small intestinal lamina propria (LP)	—	6·2	3·2	7·3

[a] determined by immunofluorescence using intact (not $F(ab)_2$) antigen.
[b] — not determined.

of cells expressing sIg was considerably less than before digestion. It may be that only cells synthesizing and also expressing a particular class of Ig on their surface are responsive in anti-immunoglobulin induced DNA synthesis.

Fujiwara *et al.* (1974) studying sIg +ve cells, rather than individual classes of immunoglobulin, showed that unlike the significant alterations in RTLA +ve cell numbers with age, there was no significant alteration in sIg +ve cell numbers in the APP. There was, however, a trend of increasing numbers from birth to at least 18 weeks. What was particularly interesting was the proportion of cells which showed neither classical T cell nor B cell markers. This null population must be heterogeneous and important areas of mucosal immunology will be exposed as we unravel its secrets. The above results of studies on rabbit GALT are similar to results in other species (for recent reviews see Waksman and Ozer, 1976; Lamm, 1976).

2. *Mitogenesis of GALT cells*

Rabbit GALT and lymphocytes from other organs have been extensively investigated for their responsiveness to various mitogens (e.g. Singhal *et al.*, 1968; Blythman and Waksman, 1973; Ozer and Waksman, 1974; Jones *et al.*, 1974; Waksman and Ozer, 1976; Bona *et al.*, 1977; Scheffel *et al.*, 1977). In summary, there are cells in rabbit GALT responsive to the classical T cell mitogens, phytohemagglutinin (PHA) and concanavalin A (Con A). Techniques which enrich for the relatively radioresistant TDA by selectively depleting the follicular region, such as manual separation, sublethal irradiation or sterilization of the lumen, enhance the responses to these T cell mitogens.

Lipopolysaccharide (LPS), considered to be a B cell mitogen in some species, does not induce extensive proliferation of rabbit GALT, or in rat, guinea pig or human B cells, as assessed by ratios of cpm of stimulated to control cultures (Waksman and Ozer, 1976). However, as mentioned above, the spontaneous DNA synthetic rate is high in APP, particularly in the follicle and hence the minimal stimulation with LPS may not reflect the potential of the cells to respond. Extracts from *Nocardia* spp. are potent B cell mitogens in rabbits (Bona *et al.*, 1975; Bona *et al.*, 1977) although they apparently have not been used with rabbit GALT cells. Pokeweed mitogen (PWM) clearly induces B cell mitogenesis and Jones *et al.* (1974) have shown that rabbit PP cells are stimulated to synthesize IgM and IgA; IgM by a surface IgM +ve cell population and IgA by a surface IgM -ve population presumably surface IgA +ve.

Hence, GALT contains cells responsive to both T and B cell mitogens as well as functional accessory cells (macrophages) which have been shown to be necessary for mitogenesis in many systems (e.g. Folch *et al.*, 1973) at levels of about 5% of the total cells (Nelson and Leu, 1975).

3. *Immunocompetence of GALT cells*

a. *Extirpation studies*

The early suggestion (Archer *et al.*, 1963) that GALT represented the mammalian bursal-equivalent was based upon observations that the development of the APP was apparently thymus independent (section II, B) and that the APP was morphologically similar to the bursa. From this hypothesis grew an array of studies attempting to characterize GALT functions using all the tools available. By 1964 it was clear that neonatal TxAPPx as compared to Tx or appendectomy (APPx) alone depressed antibody production following immunization (Sutherland *et al.*, 1964). Furthermore, in the TxAPPx group, lymphoid development was most severely depressed and lymphopenia was marked. Kondo and Harris (1966) combined Tx, APPx or TxAPPx with 450 rad in 3-week-old rabbits and depressed antibody production. Using adult rabbits in which the entire macroscopic GALT was extirpated, viz. SR, APP and PP (SAPPx rabbits) followed by 650 rad, Cooper *et al.* (1966b) showed that antibody production was significantly depressed, whereas the expression of delayed hypersensitivity and graft rejection was unaffected. This was considered to be strong circumstantial evidence that GALT represented a bursal-equivalent. Neonatal (4-weeks-old) removal of the GALT without irradiation resulted in depressed levels of circulating immunoglobulins and a depressed ability to produce antibody, as well as lymphopenia (Cooper *et al.* 1968; Perey *et al.*, 1968a). Allograft rejection and delayed hypersensitivity responses were unaffected, although SAPPx operations led to the development of the autoimmune processes as expressed by Coombs positive red cells. Moreover, neonatal SAPPx rabbits were clearly at a survival disadvantage as nearly all died within 98 days, whereas survival of APPx of splenectomized (SPx) rabbits was little affected. The controls for these extensively surgically manipulated animals (Cooper *et al.*, 1968; Perey *et al.*, 1968a) included sham SAPPx with removal of non-lymphoid intestinal tissue combined with SPx. These were subject to criticism because less lymphoid tissue was removed than by SAPPx; hence in subsequent studies (below) to answer this criticism control groups were subjected to sham SAPPx, SPx, and mesenteric lymphadenectomy (MLNx: Perey *et al.*, 1968b; Perey *et al.*, 1970).

The logical extension of these experiments, which had progressed from neonatal APPx, Tx, or APPxTx, to SAPPx operations in young or adult rabbits with or without sublethal irradiation, was the use of lethal irradiation and non-lymphoid fetal liver cell reconstitution of young (4 weeks) SAPPx operated rabbits (Perey *et al.*, 1968b). When such animals were immunized the antibody response was abolished in 9/14 and severely depressed in the other five. If only the APP and not the entire GALT was removed, the antibody response was delayed but not depressed. If SAPPx was not followed by irradiation, antibody production occurred suggesting that by 4 weeks of age plasma cell precursors had been widely distributed in the body and could respond to antigenic stimuli. The authors concluded that the differentiation of the B cell line was under strong influence of the GALT.

This study was confirmed and extended (Perey *et al.*, 1970). Whereas SAPPx with lethal irradiation and fetal liver reconstitution abolished a primary antibody response, secondary antibody responses were unaffected and, in fact, the secondary response to sheep erythrocytes was potentiated by irradiation and even more so by SAPPx or Tx coupled with irradiation. SAPPx in the absence of irradiation led to significantly elevated levels of IgM following immunization. SAPPx plus irradiation led to abrupt declines in circulating IgM, IgG and IgA. IgG levels recovered rapidly and were significantly elevated for as long as studied (10 weeks post irradiation), whereas IgM levels remained depressed in SAPPx irradiated animals for long periods. Recovery of normal serum IgA levels following irradiation was not influenced by the presence or absence of SAPP, but in Tx, irradiated, reconstituted rabbits low levels of IgA were persistent.

In all of these studies on the effects of SAPPx and irradiation on antibody production, only parenteral immunization protocols were used. It would have been most interesting if oral immunization had been incorporated for comparison and if antibody in secretions had been assessed, in addition to serum antibody.

The long-term depression of IgM in SAPPx, irradiated, reconstituted rabbits, concurrent with the rapid recovery of IgA and IgG and the subsequent significant elevation in IgG levels is curious. The authors concluded that "a significant component of newly sythesized IgM continuously derives from primary immune responses which cannot redevelop in the animal lacking the GALT. On the other hand, memory responses and secondary responses from which a major portion of IgG derives are not influenced by GALT once the peripheral lymphoid tissue has been well established". The elevation of IgM in immunized SAPPx rabbits not irradiated was considered due to the stimulation of differentiated but unsensitized cells. This dramatic IgM elevation might have reflected abnormal regulatory mechanisms in the absence of GALT.

In addition to these observations of immunoglobulin levels and antibody production, Perey *et al.* (1970) demonstrated that in SAPPx, irradiated, reconstituted rabbits the thymus-independent regions of lymphoid tissue did not repopulate. Moreover, in Tx, irradiated, reconstituted rabbits the TDA did not repopulate. The authors considered that their observations were consistent with the hypothesis that "new cells of the lymphoid plasma cell line develop in the GALT of the rabbit". They were careful, however, to state that, although the rabbit GALT functions are at least in part similar to the avian bursa of Fabricius, one cannot necessarily extrapolate to all other mammals or vertebrates. The rabbit GALT may represent a concentration of B cell differentiation sites which are more widely dispersed in other mammals. However, this suggestion simply emphasizes the usefulness of the rabbit as a model to study GALT and its functions.

b. *Reconstitution*

The corollary of the SAPP extirpation experiments reviewed above was the use of the intact GALT (shielded) or GALT cells to reconstitute irradiated rabbits (e.g. Jacobson *et al.*, 1950; Süssdorf and Draper, 1956; Süssdorf, 1960; Abdou and Richter, 1970; Hanaoka *et al.*, 1970; Hanaoka and Waksman, 1970; Ozer and Waksman, 1970, 1972; Richter *et al.*, 1970; Craig and Cebra, 1971; Nieuwenhuis, 1971; Blythman and Waksman, 1973; Nieuwenhuis *et al.*, 1974; Nieuwenhuis and Keuning, 1974).

Early studies (Jacobson *et al.*, 1950; Süssdorf and Draper, 1956; Süssdorf, 1960) showed that APP shielding during sublethal irradiation preserved the animal's ability to make antibodies, whereas spleen shielding was less effective. Moreover, if the shielded APP was removed within 3 h of irradiation, the animal maintained the ability to produce antibodies. Subsequent studies showed that APP and bone marrow shielding of rabbits given 900 rad led to a predominantly IgM antibody response to intravenous alum-precipitated bovine gamma globulin (BGG), a response which was enhanced by antigen administration into the appendiceal artery or lumen (Hanaoka *et al.*, 1970). Using another design, namely bone marrow shielding and APP cell reconstitution of irradiated (900 rad) APPx rabbits, it was shown that the early response to antigen was dependent upon both bone marrow and APP cells (Ozer and Waksman, 1970). APP cells cooperate with thymocytes as well (Ozer and Waksman, 1972). IgG antibody formation, unlike IgM, was unaffected by irradiation to the APP but was inhibited by bone marrow irradiation (Hanaoka *et al.*, 1970). Deaggregated BGG produced little response in rabbits and in fact appeared to inhibit antibody production in a challenge with alum-precipitated BGG. In animals producing anti-BGG antibody, cells containing the antibody were found, not in the APP, but primarily in the MLN draining the APP, in other lymph nodes and in the spleen (Hanaoka and Waksman, 1970). Other studies using *in vivo* cell labeling with ^{3}H-thymidine have clearly shown that cells migrate from GALT to various peripheral lymphoid tissues of the rabbit (Jacobson *et al.*, 1950; Süssdorf, 1960; Linna *et al.*, 1969; Nieuwenhuis, 1971; Nieuwenhuis *et al.*, 1974).

Waksman's group (Hanaoka and Waksman, 1970) concluded that: (a) the APP may function as the principle source of IgM precursor cells, and (b) these cells may be primed to gastrointestinal antigens and seed peripheral lymphoid structures, or are non-specifically stimulated by bowel contents such as endotoxin and are prepared to participate in IgM responses to any antigen in peripheral tissues. If they are sensitized to gut antigens, then the APP would simply be a very active peripheral lymphoid tissue, but if some are unsensitized, yet ready to respond to antigen, the APP would have some central lymphoid function.

The SR and PP presumably fulfil a similar role to that of the APP, although certainly the former has been less extensively studied. The PP have been studied in species such as the rat and mouse and they can be functionally lumped with the rabbit APP. For example, Cooper and Turner (1969) showed that rat PP are sources of IgM-producing cells that can be subsequently detected in the spleen. Craig and Cebra (1971) showed that in an irradiated allogeneic recipient rabbit, PP donor cells, but not popliteal lymph node cells, differentiate into IgA-containing cells in the recipient spleen, and gut LP. Bienenstock and his co-workers have extended these studies to include the recipient lung LP and the MLN (Rudzik *et al.*, 1975b; Befus *et al.*, 1978). It is now widely quoted that the PP represent an enriched source of IgA precursor cells. What is less well appreciated is that a similar precursor is present in the APP (Craig and Cebra, 1975) BALT (Rudzik *et al.*, 1975b, see below) and intestinal LP (Befus *et al.*, 1978); the SR has not been investigated for IgA precursors.

Although it would appear that the various GALT components have similar functions, there is some evidence, apart from the relative size differences in the TDA, that the SR differs functionally from the APP. As rabbits develop natural hemagglutinins against sheep erythrocytes (SRBC) (e.g. Henry *et al.*, 1970; Perey *et al.*, 1970; Scheffel and Draper, 1976), Richter *et al.* (1970) and Abdou and Richter (1970) surveyed various tissues of normal rabbits for anti-SRBC plaque-forming cells (PFC). They found that whereas transfer of SR as well as bone marrow and MLN cells into irradiated allogeneic recipients induced PFC activity, the APP did not. Henry *et al.* (1970) and Scheffel and Draper (1976) showed, however, that the APP developed anti-SRBC PFC *in vitro*, but this was dependent upon the age of the animals (Scheffel and Draper, 1977), as rabbits younger than 6 weeks or older than 6 months did not develop such PFC. Whether these age differences reflected either the absence of PFC precursors in young and old animals or the presence of regulatory cells (Kamin *et al.*, 1974; see below) was not determined. Normal PP developed such PFC, albeit the background levels were much less than in the APP or SR (Henry *et al.*, 1970). Following immunization, the PFC response in the PP rose, but to a lesser extent than that in the spleen (Henry *et al.*, 1970; Henry and Kodlin, 1971). To confuse the issue Süssdorf (1974), in the absence of reference to the work of Henry *et al.*, (1970), was unable to elevate PFC in the rabbit APP following immunization by various routes, including direct inoculation into the appendiceal tissue.

It is difficult to compare these studies, one with PP and one with APP, satisfactorily, and until APP, PP and SR are studied concurrently confusion will remain. The age of the animals must be carefully considered also (Scheffel and Draper, 1977). Whatever the cause, it is clear that the APP, PP and SR differ functionally by at least one characteristic: namely, in their response to SRBC. Unfortunately, too few studies have been conducted which compare these various GALT components and we hope that this review will stimulate such comparisons.

c. *IgA precursors*

Perhaps the most widely quoted function of the PP, apart from antigen uptake by the specialized lymphoepithelium, is as an enriched source of IgA precursor cells. Craig and Cebra (1971) first showed that PP cells were capable of repopulating the spleen and bowel LP of an irradiated allogeneic rabbit with IgA-containing cells. This IgA precursor cell population is present not only in the PP but also in the APP (Craig and Cebra, 1975), BALT (Rudzik *et al.*, 1975b; section III, B) and intestinal LP (Befus *et al.*, 1978). These precursors repopulate not only the spleen and intestinal LP but also the lung LP and the MLN (Rudzik *et al.*, 1975b; Befus *et al.*, 1978). The IgA precursor was shown to be a cell-bearing sIgA (Jones *et al.*, 1974; Jones and Cebra, 1974) and no sIgM. Moreover, the ability of a particular lymphoid tissue to produce IgA repopulation correlated well with the frequency of sIgA cells (Jones and Cebra, 1974; Befus *et al.*, 1978). Such studies predict that the precursor is present in the TDL and other studies support this hypothesis (e.g. Guy-Grand *et al.*, 1974; Williams and Gowans, 1975; Pierce and Gowans, 1975). *In vitro* stimulation with PWM induces the IgA precursor to synthesize IgA (Jones *et al.*, 1974).

Although many people have used the term "immediate" to describe the IgA precursor (Lamm, 1976; Waksman and Ozer, 1976; Cebra *et al.*, 1977a; Befus *et al.*, 1978) this term has not received widespread usage. It is an important qualification, however, as IgA cells can differentiate from sIgA cells but also from a more distant precursor, namely the sIgM cell (Cooper *et al.*, 1972).

As it could be said that the allogeneic transfer system used to demonstrate the IgA precursor in the rabbit was unphysiological, and indeed Rudzik *et al.* (1975c) showed that IgA repopulation was greater in allogeneic as opposed to autologous recipients, Cebra and his co-workers conducted similar experiments in congenic mice. Using anti-allotype sera they clearly showed that IgA repopulation of intestinal LP occurred with PP cells of donor origin (Cebra *et al.*, 1977a; Cebra *et al.*, 1977b). In experiments using adoptive transfer of PP cells into sublethally irradiated (600 rad) syngeneic mice they have shown that antigen-reactive cells are present in the PP and will produce not only IgA antibody but also IgM, IgG_1 and IgG_2 (Cebra *et al.*, 1977a, b). The frequency of antigen reactive cells in the PP is similar to that in the spleen, but the PP cells have a much greater capacity to produce IgA (Cebra *et al.*, 1977a, b; Cebra *et al.*, 1977c) and specifically IgA reactive with antigens found on gut organisms (Gearhart and Cebra, 1978). It has been suggested that these IgA precursor cells are previously primed cells (Cebra *et al.*, 1977c; Befus *et al.*, 1978; Gearhart and Cebra, 1979) as they express their potential in allogeneic systems. Allogeneic effect factors are not effective in the induction of virgin cells but merely augment the proliferation of already sensitized cells (Feldman and Basten, 1972). The abundant supply of antigens in the gut would facilitate the sensitization of GALT cells.

To investigate *in vivo* the role of PP in intestinal immune responses, Robertson and Cebra (1976), Cebra *et al.* (1977a, c) and Keren *et al.* (1978) established isolated, ileal (Thiry-Vella) loops with or without PP. Following immunization, IgA antibody appeared in the loop washings. The levels of antibody were higher in immunized loops containing a PP than in loops without PP. The same was true of isolated loops not given antigen but in animals with loops which had been immunized. These results emphasize the role of the PP in immune responses of the gut. The role of the SLN in loops not containing an obvious PP remains to be determined (Keren *et al.*, 1978). "The observations are consistent with antigen-stimulated B cell division in the patch follicles followed by departure of these cells via the mesenteric lymph nodes, through the circulation and back to the lamina propria of all sections of the gut." (Cebra *et al.*, 1977a.)

Another method has been used recently to demonstrate IgA precursors in mouse lymphoid tissues, which substantiates the above migratory pathway of these cells. Using isotype specific immunofluorescence combined with autoradiography of ^{3}H-thymidine labeled cells (Guy-Grand *et al.*, 1974; McWilliams *et al.*, 1977; McDermott and Bienenstock, 1979) MLN blast and TDL blasts migrated to the LP of the bowel and synthesized IgA within 24 hours. Therefore, in various phases of differentiation, cells of the IgA lineage have been demonstrated in the PP, APP, BALT, LP, MLN and TDL. This close association of IgA cells with mucosal lymphoid tissues must not channel our concepts so far to the extreme that we neglect the existence, albeit of lesser magnitude, of IgA cells in various phases of differentiation in non-mucosal lymph nodes and the spleen (Nakamura *et al.*, 1973; McDermott and Bienenstock, 1979; see section IV).

d. *IgE responses*

The nature of the association of IgE-mediated responses with mucosal surfaces has received much attention (Waksman and Ozer, 1976). This association could reflect local IgE synthesis with accumulation of effector cells (mast cells and basophils) at mucosal sites as in some parasitic infections (Mayrhofer *et al.*, 1976). Amid much speculation and controversy some clarification has occurred since the review by Waksman and Ozer (1976).

The rabbit made an early contribution to this aspect of mucosal immunity when Stannegård and Yurchison (1969) showed that at least a portion of rabbits fed antigen developed serum reaginic antibodies. Subsequently, it has been shown that rats will also develop IgE antibodies when fed antigens (Jarrett *et al.*, 1976; Bazin and Platteau, 1976). Moreover, high levels of circulating IgE antibody are a hallmark of many parasitic infections, including those of the bowel such as the nematode, *Nippostrongylus brasiliensis* (Ogilvie, 1967; Ogilvie and Jones, 1969).

To determine the distribution of IgE-producing cells in various tissues, immunofluorescence studies have been performed. Tada and Ishizaka (1971) first demonstrated the abundance of putative IgE-forming plasma cells in the respiratory and gut mucosa and in their regional lymph nodes. Thereafter, numerous reports of IgE-containing cells at various mucosal sites appeared (e.g. Brown *et al.*, 1975; Lloyd *et al.*, 1975; Shiner *et al.*, 1975; Heatley *et al.*, 1975; Halliwell, 1975). Whereas many of these workers indicated that IgE-containing cells were abundant and above normal in number in the mucosa, particularly in inflammatory bowel conditions, others (Baklien and Brandtzaeg, 1975, 1976; Brandtzaeg and Baklien, 1976a, b) did not find large numbers of IgE-containing cells or any consistent increase in their number. Brandtzaeg and Baklien (1976c) discussed these differences and suggested that many reports of IgE immunofluorescence may be misleading as the quality of reagents used could be seriously questioned. Furthermore, Halliwell (1973, 1975) had shown IgE fluorescence in mast cells, and Mayrhofer *et al.* (1976) and Mayrhofer (1977) showed in *N. brasiliensis* infected rats that IgE-containing cells were abundant in the small bowel, but these were predominantly mast cells. Plasma cells producing IgE were found in the MLN and axilliary lymph node, the latter near the site of larval injection. Few, if any, IgE plasma cells were seen in the PP, intrapulmonary lymphoid tissue or spleen. Ishizaka *et al.* (1976) noted a similar abundance of IgE-forming cells in the MLN of infected rats.

The apparent concentration of IgE and not other immunoglobulins by mast cells at mucosal and other sites (Halliwell, 1973, 1975; Mayrhofer *et al.*, 1976; Mayrhofer, 1977) opened an area of immediate hypersensitivity which requires considerable exploration as, for example, Padawer (1974) speculated that IgE stored in mast cell granules could act as a sort of immunological memory. Initially, the existence of IgE in mast cells must be confirmed by others, as previous reports suggested that mast cells bind various immunoglobulins and fluoresceniated reagents, and not specifically IgE, by poorly understood non-specific mechanisms (Young and Cowan, 1965; Todorov *et al.*, 1968; Simson *et al.*, 1977). What proportion of the IgE-containing cells described in earlier immunofluorescence studies were IgE plasma cells, as opposed to IgE-containing mast cells or a result of contaminants in the reagents, must be evaluated before the relationship between IgE and mucosal sites can be clarified.

It is clear, however, that the MLN can synthesize IgE (Halliwell, 1975; Ishizaka, 1976; Ishizaka *et al.*, 1976; Mayrhofer *et al.*, 1976; Mayrhofer, 1977). Attempts to demonstrate IgE precursor cells in rat PP using an allogeneic irradiated recipient system similar to the IgA model (see above) were unsuccessful (Befus and Bienenstock, unpublished). However, this negative result probably reflected the resistance of IgE precursors to allogeneic stimuli (Katz *et al.*, 1974) rather than to an absence of IgE precursors, as cells capable of producing IgE have been uncovered in PP populations (Ngan and Kind, 1976; Gerbrandy and Bienenstock, 1976). Cells capable of regulating such responses also occur in PP (see below; Jarrett, 1977; Ngan and Kind, 1978). It is tempting to speculate that lung lymph nodes and lymphoid aggregates (BALT) influence IgE responses in ways similar to PP. Indeed, IgE responses have been stimulated by aerosol and intratracheal immunization (Van Hout and Johnson, 1972; Gerbrandy and Bienenstock,

1976) and a recent presentation documented suppression of such responses by nebulized antigen (Fox and Siraganian, 1981). An attractive direction of pursuit is the obvious similarity between IgA and IgE responses at mucosal sites. Undoubtedly, the sensitive technique of combining immunofluorescence and radiolabeling of cells (Guy-Grand *et al.*, 1974; McWilliams *et al.*, 1977; McDermott and Bienenstock, 1979) will extend our understanding of these similarities.

The rabbit has not been a major model in the above advances but skin-sensitizing IgE and IgGa in the rabbit have been characterized (Zvaifler and Becker, 1966; Stux and Ovary, 1976) and there is no reason why the relationship between IgE and mucosal lymphoid tissue cannot be pursued in the rabbit. The unique ability to produce high amounts, and almost exclusively IgE following neonatal sensitization in the rabbit (Pinckard *et al.*, 1972) as well as reports of fatal anaphylactic shock in infant rabbits (Coates and O'Donoghue, 1967) may provide interesting models. These reports have been followed by other studies showing an early postnatal ability to produce IgE antibodies, rather than antibodies of other classes (Imada *et al.*, 1977). In addition, the nature of the predominant effector cell of IgE responses in the rabbit, namely the basophil, rather than the mast cell as in rodents, makes the rabbit an appealing model for comparison with the human in whom circulating basophils are abundant.

e. *T cell functions*

T cell function of rabbit GALT cells has received little attention. Ozer and Waksman (1974), as noted above, demonstrated mitogenic responses by GALT cells to the T cell mitogens Con A and PHA. T cells functional in mixed lymphocyte cultures occur in the PP (Singal *et al.*, 1976) and APP TDA (Ozer and Waksman, 1974). Killer cell activity has also been shown (Behelak and Richter, 1974).

Studies have been much more extensive in other species, notably the mouse, rat and guinea pig. In these species responses to mitogens have been documented (e.g. Levin *et al.*, 1973; Nelson *et al.*, 1976; Doenhoff *et al.*, 1976). Controversy has surrounded the capacity of GALT cells to function in graft versus host (GVH) reactions, although it now seems that such reactivity exists if assayed appropriately (Perey and Gutmann, 1972; Heim *et al.*, 1972; Katz and Perey, 1973; Levin *et al.*, 1974; Eloy *et al.*, 1975; Vuitton *et al.*, 1977; MacDonald and Carter, 1978). GALT T cells can act as carrier-primed helper cells (Katz and Perey, 1973; Kagnoff, 1975) and as antigen-specific killer cells (Kagnoff and Campbell, 1974; Kagnoff, 1978) as well as mitogen-induced killer cells (Nelson *et al.*, 1976; Arnaud-Battandier *et al.*,

1978). On the other hand, effector cells for antibody-dependent cellular cytotoxicity (ADCC) reactions are absent from GALT (Nelson *et al.*, 1976; Kagnoff and Campbell, 1976; Arnaud-Battandier *et al.*, 1978).

PP lymphocytes respond to PPD (purified tuberculin protein) following oral immunization with BCG (Müller-Schoop and Good, 1975). More recently, macrophage migration inhibition factor (MIF) activity has been shown in cell suspensions of swine bowel LP following viral infection (Frederick and Bohl, 1976). The role of cell-mediated immunity in the maintenance of mucosal integrity is only beginning to be explored and the extent of its significance promises to be an exciting area (Ferguson and MacDonald, 1977).

One such area, which we have neglected to discuss to this point, is the immunoregulatory function of GALT cells. Needless to say, this area has received little attention until recently, but the literature is expanding rapidly. One of the earliest demonstrations of suppressor cells in GALT was that of Kamin *et al.* (1974). Normal rabbit APP cells suppressed the secondary *in vitro* response to a variety of antigens. Suppression was non-specific and affected IgG responses to a greater extent than IgM responses. Suppressor cells were associated with T cell fractions and were present in the PP and spleen as well as the APP. Behelak and Richter (1972) and Behelak *et al.* (1973) showed a similar suppression of *in vitro* antibody responses using rabbit GALT cells (APP, PP, SR) in allogeneic systems, but not with autologous cells as shown by Kamin *et al.* (1974). The age-related changes in spontaneous anti-SRBC PFC activity in the APP discussed before (Scheffel and Draper, 1977) may reflect alterations in suppressor activity. In this regard, it is interesting that Perey *et al.* (1970) showed very high anti-SRBC PFC activity in SAPPx, irradiated reconstituted rabbits—procedures which could very well have removed suppressor activity.

Recently, Asherson *et al.* (1977) showed that mice fed the contact-sensitized agents oxazolone or picryl chloride by stomach tube developed specific suppressor activity in PP and in MLN, and later in the PLN and spleen. The suppressor cells were characterized as including both putative B cells (formed rosettes with red cells coated with antibody and complement and resistant to anti-thy 1 and complement) as well as T cells. In rats, antigen-specific suppressor cells were first seen in the PP and MLN within 2 days of antigen feeding and thereafter appeared in the spleen and thymus (Mattingly and Waksman, 1978). Indeed, unresponsiveness to antigen challenge following earlier feeding is not uncommon and recently reports of inhibition of homocytotropic antibody responses have been published (e.g. David,

1977; Hanson *et al.*, 1977; Jarrett, 1977; Vaz *et al.*, 1977). This unresponsiveness most likely reflects the occurrence of antigen-specific suppressor cells for IgE and IgG in the PP following antigen feeding (Ngan and Kind, 1978). Clearly, immunoregulation (suppression) may be a key role of GALT, which is constantly flooded by large quantities of immunogenic materials and yet pathological responses are infrequent occurrences.

D. IS GALT A BURSAL EQUIVALENT?

We have previously stated that much of the interest in rabbit GALT was stimulated by the pursuit of a mammalian equivalent of the avian bursa of Fabricius with its apparently unique capacity as a site of early B cell differentiation. Strictly speaking, the bursa is a primary, or central, lymphoid organ (see Nossal and Ada, 1971) with the fundamental role of providing the microenvironment for the differentiation of pluripotent stem cells into immunocompetent B lymphocytes. The thymus provides a similar function for T cell differentiation. These central lymphoid organs exhibit intense lymphopoiesis which is largely antigen-independent and have an epithelial component. By contrast, peripheral lymphoid organs such as the spleen and lymph nodes show antigen-dependent proliferation and differentiation of cells previously processed by the central organs. In the search for the mammalian bursal-equivalent, an organ with morphological, antigenic and functional characteristics similar to the bursa was sought. These characteristics included:

1. Immigration of stem cells and their differentiation into B lymphocytes, ultimately capable of differentiation to plasma cells following migration to a peripheral site. Such an organ would be the first site of B cell differentiation during ontogeny.
2. Intense, early and largely antigen-independent, lymphopoiesis in follicular structures similar to the bursa.
3. Organogenesis independent of the thymus.
4. An epithelial cell component, i.e. lymphoepithelial organ derived from the embryonic gut.
5. The capability of repopulation of the B cell areas in irradiated animals.
6. The lack of ability to express any recognizable T cell functions such as GVH reactions.

Clearly, although all of these are characteristics of the bursa, the mammalian equivalent would not necessarily have to express all of them to fulfil the fundamental role of providing the appropriate microenvironment for B cell differentiation from pluripotent stem cells. This list of characteristics was extensively reviewed by Perey (1971) and Cooper and Lawton (1972). Perey (1971) concluded that GALT possessed bursa-like attributes but also immunocompetent T and B cells characteristic of peripheral lymphoid tissue. Cooper and Lawton (1972) stated that "a large body of circumstantial evidence decidedly favors the concept that lymphoid follicles of GALT are sites in which lymphoid differentiation is induced along plasma cell lines in mammals". There was insufficient evidence to state categorically whether B lymphocytes differentiate from stem cells in GALT.

However, it is now accepted that fetal liver, bone marrow and spleen, as well as adult bone marrow are sites of B cell differentiation (Nossal and Pike, 1973; Owen *et al.*, 1974; Owen *et al.*, 1975; Melchers *et al.*, 1975; Raff *et al.*, 1976; Owen *et al.*, 1977). In the current model being tested, a pluripotent stem cell, in for example the fetal liver, differentiates into a large, rapidly dividing cell which contains low levels of cytoplasmic IgM (cIgM + ve), but lacks surface IgM (sIgM-ve); this cell has been called a pre-B cell (Raff *et al.*, 1976). Such cells are present by day 12 of gestation in the mouse fetal liver, 4 to 5 days prior to the appearance of sIgM + ve, recognizable B cells (Owen, 1977). They appear in fetal liver of the rabbit by 23 days of gestation, well before the development of GALT (see section II, B) and in man by day 60 of a 280-day gestation period. The B cells are found also in fetal spleen and bone marrow and in adult bone marrow but not adult spleen or lymph nodes (Lawton *et al.*, 1977; Owen, 1977). We have been unable to find a statement of whether adult GALT contains pre-B cells and until this is clarified, whether adult GALT is a site of B lymphocyte differentiation from stem cells, as is bone marrow, remains an open question.

There remain, however, many similarities between the bursa and mammalian GALT such as extensive lymphopoiesis; an amplification function (Perey, 1971; Cooper and Lawton, 1972). Waksman and Ozer (1976) have attempted to explain these similarities on a functional basis by comparison with the studies of Toivanen and Toivanen (1973) and Toivanen *et al.* (1974) on bursal and post-bursal cells. In the chicken there are: (1) pluripotent stem cells of the yolk sac and fetal liver; (2) bursal cells capable of differentiation only in the presence of the bursa; (3) early post-bursal cells which can independently of the bursa, restore germinal centers in the spleen and antibody formation; and (4) late postbursal cells capable of antibody production but not of germinal center formation. In the mammal it is suggested that stem cells from fetal tissues or adult marrow differentiate into B cells *in situ*, move to GALT where they are capable of germinal center formation and can further differentiate through a switch mechanism (Cooper *et al.*, 1972) from IgM production to production of other immunoglobulins, predominantly IgA and perhaps IgE (sections II, C, 3 and D). Early post-bursal cells could be equated with unprimed B cells of GALT and late post-bursal cells with sensitized B cells leaving GALT. GALT and lymphoid aggregates of other mucosal sites are not totally unique in these processes as Nieuwenhuis and Keuning (1974) showed that spleen and lymph nodes perform a similar function as an antigen-dependent amplification system for B cells. One of the fundamental questions that remains is why GALT cells become largely IgA and perhaps IgE-producing cells, whereas the spleen and non-mucosal lymph nodes generate predominantly IgG-producing cells. This relative compartmentalization could reflect differential localization of immunoglobulin class precursors or different microenvironmental stimuli leading to specific antibody class expression.

Although it is well established that the chicken possesses Peyer's patches (section II, A,2) in addition to the bursa, the function of these patches is unknown. Bursectomy (Bx), but particularly BxTx at hatching, produces IgA deficiency in the chicken (Perey and Bienenstock, 1973) and major disorganization of the BALT while preserving the organization of the caecal tonsil (Bienenstock *et al.*, 1974). We have looked at Peyer's patches from birds rendered selectively IgA deficient by Dr R. M. Blaese (Blaese *et al.*, 1977), but have been unable to detect any morphological differences between PP from normal or IgA-deficient birds. We can only conclude that much work must be done in the chicken to establish the role of PP in an animal possessing a bursa (Befus *et al.*, 1980).

Thus, although GALT is not a bursal-equivalent in the strictest sense, the original hypothesis stimulated much investigation largely in the rabbit which improved our understanding of GALT and other lymphoid tissues. Therefore, in summary, GALT is a major B cell amplification site which provides largely IgM, IgA and perhaps IgE precursors to other predominantly mucosal sites. A selection of T cell functions including regulation and cytotoxicity are also expressed by GALT cells. The roles of GALT cells in the differentiation of the normal and lymphoepithelium is unexplored as the question of cell traffic into the lumen. GALT holds many secrets yet to be uncovered.

III. Lymphoid tissue at other mucosa-associated sites

A. CELLS OF THE INTESTINAL LAMINA PROPRIA (LP) AND EPITHELIUM

Despite the vast literature on the characteristics and functions of GALT, remarkably little has been published on the adjacent lymphoid cells in the intestinal LP. The LP undoubtedly contains cells of fundamental importance in mucosal immunity as evidenced by so many IgA-producing cells, and presumably cells of other types which originate in GALT or elsewhere. At least until recently, the paucity of information on LP cells could be attributed to the lack of appropriate techniques for isolating such cells free of mucus and other intestinal contaminants.

However, rabbit LP cells have now been isolated by a non-enzymatic mechanical procedure and many of their characteristics determined (Rudzik and Bienenstock, 1974; Rudzik *et al.*, 1975a; Singal *et al.*, 1976; Befus *et al.*, 1978). This technique yields a suspension of small, medium and large lymphocytes with few macrophages and few plasma cells (about 1%) containing IgA or other immunoglobulins, despite the apparently high proportion of IgA-producing plasma cells *in situ* in the LP (Rudzik and Bienenstock, 1974). About 1% of the cells incorporated ^{3}H-thymidine over 24 h of culture, although most utilized ^{3}H-uridine within 1 h. About 25% (16-43) of the lymphocytes contained metachromatic cytoplasmic granules (Rudzik and Bienenstock, 1974); *in situ* such granulated cells are seen largely within the epithelium and not in the LP itself (Collan, 1972). This implies that a large proportion of the isolated cells are from within the epithelium. The function of these granulated lymphocytes is undetermined but, histochemically and ultrastructurally, the granules resemble those found in mast cells and basophils. Whether they contain vasoactive amines and/or other chemical mediators and, moreover, what might stimulate them to release such mediators, remains a pivotal question in our quest for understanding of mucosal immune responses.

The cell suspensions contain 11% RTLA +ve cells (T cells) and 16% B cells as assessed by sIg (Tables 1 and 2; Rudzik *et al.*, 1975a). The cells can function both as stimulators and responders in MLC (Singal *et al.*, 1976). IgA precursors can be demonstrated in 6-day repopulation studies of irradiated allogeneic recipients. A large proportion of the cells (about 73%) do not carry T or B cell markers. Undoubtedly, this null population is heterogeneous and hides many important unknowns. At present, these suspensions of rabbit cells must include both intraepithelial (IE) as well as true LP cells. What proportion of the LP cells are of SLN origin has yet to be determined. Assuming that SLN cells are similar to PP cells, the observation that radiolabeled LP blast cells specifically localize back in the LP, whereas PP cells do not (Bienenstock *et al.*, 1978) suggests that few LP cells are of SLN origin.

Studies on LP cells in other species have been less extensive but are beginning to contribute to our knowledge of this important compartment of the mucosal lymphoid system. For example, PFC have been demonstrated in otherwise poorly characterized LP suspensions by Werner *et al.* (1971: host not stated but probably the mouse), Robertson and Cooper (1972: rat) and Olson and Waxler (1977: bovine). Macrophage inhibition factor (MIF) was produced by swine LP cells following oral (14/15 animals positive) but not subcutaneous (1/10 positive) immunization (Frederick and Bohl, 1976). Coccidia-infected LP cells have been isolated from chickens and some of their characteristics determined (Fernando and Pasternak, 1977).

Recent studies on the guinea pig are particularly interesting, especially from the standpoint of IE versus LP cells (Arnaud-Battandier *et al.*, 1978). Using the mechanical (rubbing) technique of Rudzik and Bienenstock (1974), albeit less vigorously, these authors isolated a population containing about 40% granulated lymphocytes which they called an IE population. The bowel remaining was then subjected to collagenase digestion as described by Bull and Bookman (1977) for human bowel (see below). This yielded a cell population (LP) with only 4% granulated lymphocytes, or minimal IE cell contamination. The IE and LP populations were then assayed for cytotoxic activity as were PP, MLN and spleen populations. The assays included spontaneous cell mediated cytotoxicity (SCMC), mitogen-induced cell cytotoxicity (MICC) and ADCC. The effector cells for SCMC and ADCC bear Fc receptors, whereas MICC is effected by polyclonally activated T cells. SCMC, MICC and ADCC were expressed by IE and spleen cells, whereas MLN, PP and LP cells expressed essentially only MICC and to a limited extent. Thus, although cytotoxic activity was present in all gastrointestinal cell populations, IE cells were most active and contained a diversity of effector cells. Other functions of IE cells remain to be elucidated (Ferguson, 1977). IE cells and LP cells must be characterized further, not only in the normal animal, but also in various disease states.

In this regard, recent studies using either mechanical or enzymatic techniques, have examined human LP cells in various diseases (Clancy, 1976; Bull and Bookman, 1977; Clancy and Pucci, 1878; Machado and Falchuk, 1978; Goodacre *et al.*, 1979). It is of interest that Bull and Bookman (1977), using a collagenase digestion, found few null cells in human colon, whereas Rudzik and Bienenstock (1974) found many in rabbit small intestine. Moreover, IgA positive cells were abundant in human LP cells (Bull and Bookman, 1977; Goodacre *et al.*, 1979) but scarce in rabbit suspensions (Rudzik and Bienenstock, 1974; Rudzik *et al.*, 1975a). Mitogenic responses occur to PHA and Con A (Bull and Bookman, 1977; Machado and Falchuk, 1978; Goodacre *et al.*, 1979), although these have been difficult to induce in rabbit or rat LP cells (unpublished, Befus, Bienenstock, Clancy and O'Neill). Bookman *et al.* (1977) and Clancy and Pucci (1978) could not detect effectors of ADCC responses in human LP cells. As pointed out by Arnaud-Battandier *et al.* (1978), this difference between the human and guinea pig could reflect species or tissue differences, but most likely reflects that in the human studies few IE cells are harvested relative to LP cells. Despite the increasing attention being paid to IE lymphocytes in human disease (Ferguson, 1977), it appears unclear whether or not granulated lymphocytes occur in any numbers in the human bowel epithelium. If it is true that they do not, then a convenient marker for distinguishing IE from LP cells is absent in man.

Given the obvious importance of the IE and LP cells in mucosal immune responses, it is unrealistic to speak of GALT independently of IE and LP. It is more rational to consider the gut-associated lymphoid system (Guy-Grand *et al.*, 1974) as a unit which includes not only the PP, SR, APP but also the draining nodes (MLN), the thoracic duct, circulation and the LP and IE cells (see below).

B. BRONCHUS-ASSOCIATED LYMPHOID TISSUE (BALT)

Careful examination with the unaided eye of longitudinally opened bronchi and larger bronchioles may reveal areas in the bronchial wall of greater density than the surrounding tissue. These mucosal patches can be more readily seen following fixation in 2% acetic acid (Fig. 3; e.g. Bienenstock *et al.*, 1973a; Rácz *et al.*, 1977). Upon microscopic study, these patches are seen to be well-organized aggregates of lymphoid tissue and have been called the bronchus-associated lymphoid tissue (BALT; Bienenstock *et al.*, 1973a). BALT has been seen in all species studied including rabbits, guinea pigs, chickens, rats, dogs, pigs, mice, monkeys and man (Brundelet, 1965; Bienenstock *et al.*, 1973a, b, 1974; Chamberlain *et al.*, 1973; Rácz *et al.*, 1977; Fournier *et al.*, 1977) but not as yet in the golden hamster (Bienenstock *et al.*, 1973a).

Microscopically BALT has remarkable similarity to GALT (Fig. 4; compare with Fig. 2). The epithelium over the BALT is a lymphoepithelium as that over GALT, with a heavy infiltrate of lymphocytes in an epithelium of nearer cuboidal rather than columnar type

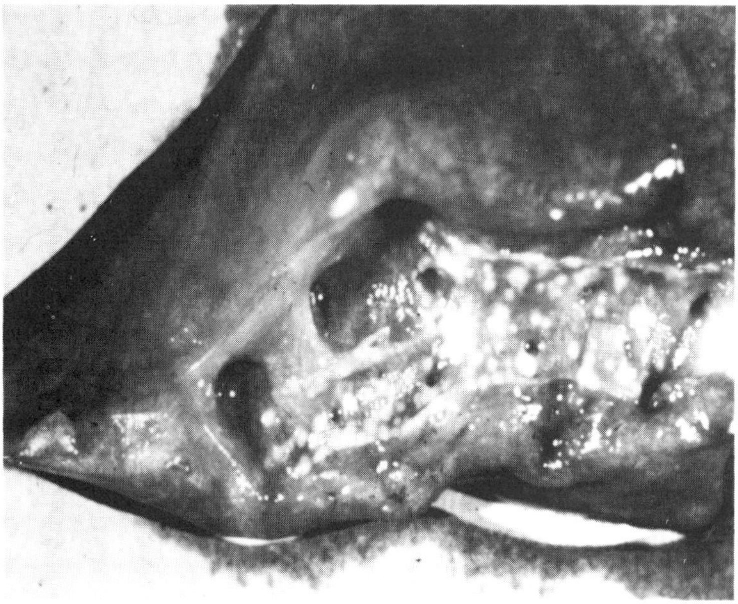

FIG. 3 Bronchus-associated lymphoid tissue (BALT) in the rabbit lung.

(Bienenstock *et al.*, 1973a; Fournier *et al.*, 1977). This lymphoepithelium lacks the goblet and ciliated cells of the surrounding epithelium but the flattened epithelial cells have microvilli reminiscent of M cells of the PP (Owen and Jones, 1974; Owen, 1977). Fournier *et al.* (1977) have shown that this respiratory lymphoepithelium is a major site of antigen transport as is the case in the GALT lymphoepithelium (Bockman and Cooper, 1973; Owen and Jones, 1974; Owen, 1977; Bockman and Stevens, 1977). Following intratracheal challenge of previously BCG sensitized animals, extensive hyperplasia of the BALT and lymphoepithelium occurred (Rácz *et al.*, 1977). This suggests that reactive changes occur in BALT and its lymphoepithelium. As discussed above with regard to GALT, understanding the mechanisms which induce such changes is crucial in our progress towards manipulation of mucosal immune mechanisms.

Underneath the lymphoepithelium (Fig. 4) there is a dome area (Bienenstock *et al.*, 1973a; Rácz *et al.*, 1977) composed largely of small lymphocytes. In cell-mediated immune reactions the dome may contain lymphoblasts and medium-sized lymphocytes as well as the occasional plasma cell. In the normal animal the follicle beneath the dome (Fig. 4) does not contain germinal centers (Bienenstock *et al.*, 1973a; Rácz *et al.*, 1977), but following stimulation by BCG, germinal centers with cap-like accumulations of lymphocytes and sparsely populated cores with more densely populated peripheral regions appear (Rácz *et al.*, 1977). The parafollicular area is composed of small lymphocytes but contains plasma cells also. HEV occur in this parafollicular region which appears to be the major reason that Rácz *et al.* (1977) considered this a thymus-dependent area comparable to the TDA in GALT. TDA of BALT, if one exists, remains to be clearly shown. Indeed, histological examination of BALT in neonatally Tx rats and chickens failed to show any significant differences between the Tx and sham operated animals (Bienenstock *et al.*, 1973b). It is interesting, but the significance is unclear, that adult Tx or Bx alone caused no changes in BALT, whereas combined TxBx led to dramatic depletion and disorganization of BALT, even though germinal centers in caecal tonsils remained prominent (Bienenstock *et al.*, 1974). It is tempting to speculate that this reflected the IgA deficiency in these surgically manipulated animals but no firm conclusions can be reached (see section II,D).

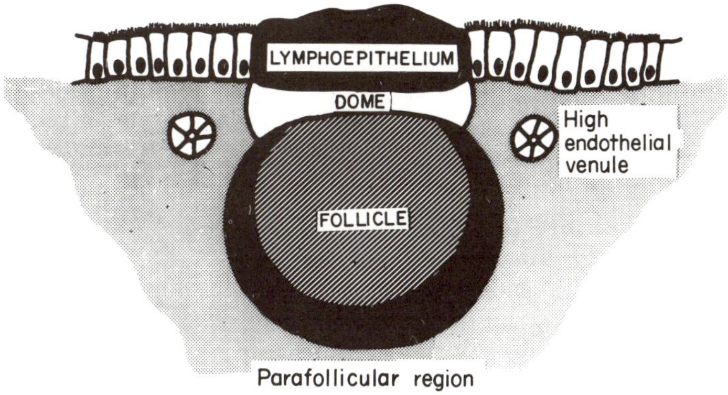

FIG. 4 Diagrammatic representation of BALT.

To return to the HEV, Rácz *et al.* (1977) showed that they "proliferate and are activated" during intense reactions to antigen challenge. As with the lymphoepithelium, perhaps HEV are under lymphocyte regulation and knowledge of the factors regulating the differentiation and activities of HEV is essential.

Cytokinetic studies utilizing *in vivo* injections of ^{3}H-thymidine (Bienenstock *et al.*, 1973b) showed that at 1 h, heavily labeled cells were scattered throughout the follicles and parafollicular regions. At 24 h, the pattern of labeling was similar, albeit caplike areas of labeled cells appeared in about half of the follicles, often at the lumenal edge. The lymphoepithelium contained few labeled cells. This distribution of labeled cells in BALT was not unlike that in GALT (see above, Meuwissen *et al.*, 1969; Faulk *et al.*, 1971; Bienenstock *et al.*, 1973b), although in GALT the basolateral aspects of the follicles contained more marked areas of DNA synthetic activity than seen in BALT.

Six prenatal rabbits removed from the uterus, 1 day preparturition, lacked BALT (Bienenstock *et al.*, 1973a) as well as GALT (see section II, B). However, germ-free adult rats possessed recognizable, albeit hypoplastic, BALT (Bienenstock *et al.*, 1973a), similar to the nature of GALT in adult germ-free animals (Pollard and Sharon, 1970). Moreover, just as GALT (Ferguson and Parrott, 1972; Milne *et al.*, 1975), BALT developed in fetal pulmonary tissue transplanted to ectopic sites in adult syngeneic mice (Bienenstock *et al.*, 1973b; Milne *et al.*, 1975).

As noted above, plasma cells were seen in small numbers in the lymphoepithelium, dome and parafollicular areas. Most of these cells contained IgG as shown by immunofluorescence (Bienenstock *et al.*, 1973a). Recent studies by Bienenstock *et al.* (1979) and McDermott and Bienenstock (1979) have shown that as with the small intestine, blast cells from the MLN, when compared with those of the PLN, will selectively lodge in the lung and often near BALT. Blasts from the mediastinal lymph nodes appear to be similar to those of the MLN. Moreover, about 60% of the MLN blasts which localize in the lung synthesize IgA and another 25% IgG. Of the fewer PLN blasts which localize in the lung, about equal proportions (30-35%) synthesize IgA or IgG. These results confirm that cells from one mucosal site, such as the MLN draining the bowel, can selectively lodge in another site such as the lung. IgA precursor cells represent a large proportion of those cells which exhibit this pattern. However, IgG cells in the lung can originate from both PLN and MLN sources.

Further characterization of BALT necessitated creation of single cell suspensions of this tissue. However, unlike GALT components such as PP, APP and SR which are largely and easily dissected relatively free of surrounding LP, the isolation of BALT aggregates is difficult. They are numerous, small, widely distributed and, in fresh material, contrast little with surrounding tissue. In fact, they could be equated with SLN of the bowel, although many BALT aggregates are larger than SLN. These difficulties must be taken into account in interpretation of this type of experiment. Notwithstanding this qualification, single cell suspensions of BALT were created by dissecting the bronchial mucosa free of the underlying lung parenchyma and dissociating it with homogenizers (Clancy and Bienenstock, 1974; Rudzik *et al.*, 1975b). This produced a suspension composed not only of cells of BALT but also cells of the adjacent bronchial LP. It must be recognized that in these suspensions the portions of BALT and bronchial LP cells is unknown.

Rudzik *et al.* (1975a) characterized these cells using RTLA antiserum and antisera to immunoglobulin heavy chain markers. In 14-18-week-old rabbits the proportion of RTLA +ve cells (18·4%) was similar to that of PP (16·6%) and intestinal LP (11·1%) (see Table 1). The BALT cell suspensions also contained a large proportion of sIgA +ve cells (17·2%), a value intermediate between that of PP (29·9%) and LP (7·3%) (see Table 2). This intermediate value is consistent with the hypothesis that the suspension was a mixture of BALT and bronchial LP cells, assuming that BALT and GALT, and lung and bowel LP are analogous. This assumption is not unjustified as in addition to the morphological and functional similarities listed above, the BALT cells repopulated allogeneic irradiated rabbits with IgA-containing cells as PP cells did (Rudzik *et al.*, 1975b). Indeed, as discussed above, Cebra and his co-workers have shown that the IgA precursor is a sIgA +ve cell (Jones *et al.*, 1974; Jones and Cebra, 1974). By reanalyzing the data of Rudzik *et al.* (1975b), we have shown that the ability of BALT cell suspensions to repopulate with IgA-containing cells is less than the ability to PP cells (Befus *et al.*, 1978), which further corresponds with the number of sIgA +ve cells in the two cell suspensions (Table 2). One of the most significant observations of Rudzik *et al.* (1975b) was that both BALT and PP cells repopulated the bronchial and intestinal LP as well as the spleen. This was the first direct demonstration that cells from one mucosal site could move to and perhaps differentiate at another mucosal site (see section IV).

Given the large number of RTLA and sIg +ve cells in BALT as in GALT, it was surprising that attempts to induce proliferation of BALT cells with mitogens such as PHA and PWM were unsuccessful

(Bienenstock *et al.*, 1974); a phenomenon reminiscent of the difficulty inducing mitogenesis with bowel LP cells (Befus, Bienenstock, Clancy, and O'Neill, unpublished; section III, A). This may reflect a dominant action by some suppressive factor associated with the mucosal site. Such phenomena are being investigated by many laboratories (see section II, C, 3, e). Despite the difficulty with non-specific mitogens, BALT cells and cells obtained by bronchial lavage were responsive to antigen following intratracheal but not foot pad immunization. The response was measured by ^{3}H-thymidine incorporation in the presence of antigen (Clancy and Bienenstock, 1974). A high spontaneous rate of incorporation characterized BALT and lavage cells in these intratracheal immunized animals. This corresponds with the hyperplasia of BALT in intratracheally immunized rabbits reported by Rácz *et al.* (1977).

There seems to be little doubt that BALT and GALT are analogous components of their respective environments. Their morphology, antigen sampling, cell kinetics, composition and function are almost indistinguishable. Future studies will clarify further the fundamental significance of these lymphoid aggregates in immunization of mucosal sites. It is the rabbit, with its extensive GALT, that has been the source of much of our knowledge of BALT. With this knowledge, it was concluded in 1973 that "this lymphoid tissue might be part of a more universal mucosal lymphoid system" (Bienenstock *et al.*, 1973a). Today we are experiencing a rapid increase of interest in this common mucosal immunological system (Parmely and Beer, 1977; Bienenstock *et al.*, 1978, 1979).

C. OTHER MUCOSA-ASSOCIATED LYMPHOID TISSUE (MALT)

Whether mucosa-associated lymphoid aggregates similar to GALT and BALT occur at other sites has not been adequately explored. One such aggregate, the tonsil, has received considerable attention and has been extensively reviewed recently (Waksman and Ozer, 1976). In brief, the tonsils appear to be similar to GALT and BALT in the association with the mucosal surface and with many of their other characteristics such as lymphopoiesis. They differ strikingly, however, in that unlike GALT and BALT, they have a large plasma cell component which appears to be generated locally and is predominantly IgG rather than IgA. For further details see Waksman and Ozer (1976).

Apart from the gut and respiratory tract, the mammary glands have received the most attention recently with regard to mucosal immunity.

Studies in rabbits (Montgomery *et al.*, 1974) demonstrated IgA antibodies to orally administered antigens in the milk and it was hypothesized that this was due to (a) antigen entering the circulation and inducing a response in the mammary glands; (b) IgA antibody produced in the gut being transferred into the milk; or (c) cells sensitized in the GALT or draining lymph nodes entering the circulation and seeding the mammary gland where they produce IgA antibody. Ahlstedt *et al.* (1975) and Goldblum *et al.* (1975) showed an abundance of IgA antibody-producing cells in human milk with specificity for intestinal antigens and argued in support of the migration of sensitized cells from gastrointestinal tract to the mammary gland. It has now been clearly shown that blast cells from the MLN can localize specificity in the mammary gland and produce IgA within 24 h (Roux *et al.*, 1977; Bienenstock *et al.*, 1978, 1979; McDermott and Bienenstock, 1979).

However, this demonstration of cell localization does not exclude possibility (b) above (Montgomery *et al.*, 1974) that IgA produced in the gut or elsewhere is specifically transported into secretions such as the milk as suggested by Bienenstock and Strauss (1970) for 11S IgA. Indeed, Montgomery *et al.*, (1977) have shown that oligomeric IgA is selectively transported into canine saliva. Furthermore, rat bile contains a large amount of secretory IgA and free secretory component (Lemaître-Coelho *et al.*, 1977) and obstruction of the bile duct induces dramatic elevation in serum levels of these molecules (Lemaître-Coelho *et al.*, 1978) suggesting that oligomeric serum IgA and free secretory component are normally transported into bile. Orlans *et al.* (1978) confirmed this suggestion by showing selective transport (as compared with IgG) of radiolabeled oligomeric IgA from serum to bile. Monomeric IgA was selectively transferred also, but to a lesser extent. The distribution and significance of this phenomenon at mucosal sites throughout the body remains to be determined.

To return to the mammary gland, it has been shown that colostrum and milk are rich sources of T cells (Diaz-Jouanen and Williams, 1974; Parmely *et al.,* 1976; Smith and Schultz, 1977; Parmely *et al.*, 1977). These T cells do not appear to be a random sample of peripheral T cells but are a selective sample of cells reactive to antigens encountered at mucosal sites such as the bowel and respiratory tract (see Parmely and Beer, 1977). This repertoire of antigen sensitivity along with the absence of any morphological evidence of mammary-associated lymphoid aggregates comparable to BALT and GALT led to the conclusion that "local humoral and cell-mediated immunity in the mammary gland depend upon inductive events at distant mucosal sites (Parmely and Beer, 1977) such as the bowel and respiratory tract.

What of other mucosal sites such as the salivary glands? Parmely and Beer (1977) suggested that the salivary glands are like the mammary glands and lack organized lymphoid aggregates. However, reports of intraparotid "lymph nodes" exist and Fichtelius (1969) referred to this lymphoid tissue as the "intraparotid lymphoepithelial micro-organ" which he grouped with PP. It is clear that these lymphoid aggregates must be investigated further to determine more precisely their nature. Salivary gland-associated lymphoid tissue, comparable to GALT and BALT, may exist. It may be that such aggregates develop *de novo* following long standing antigenic stimulation such as infection or neoplasia (Godwin, 1952; Bernier and Bhaskar, 1958), or it may be present at all times but most evident after infection which induces intense lymphopoiesis or lymphoid infiltration. With a view towards protecting various mucosal sites through immunization, it is of central importance to know if effector mechanisms can be generated locally by lymphopoiesis, for example, or whether effectors can be most efficiently generated elsewhere and induced to migrate to the desired site. This basic question must be answered not only for salivary glands but for many other mucosal sites such as the ear, eye, nose and urogenital tract. Meticulous studies must be conducted in search of lymphoepithelial aggregates in these sites in health and disease. There is indeed some evidence for aggregates in the urogenital tract (Marsh *et al.*, 1974) and controversy exists as to whether they are present in normal or only diseases states (see Kretschmer, 1952). Lymphoid aggregates have been described also in the paraocular and paranasal glands of chickens (Bang and Bang, 1968); whether they exist in mammals remains to be determined.

It is clear from the above that currently there is little understanding of the extent of MALT, apart from the BALT and GALT. It could be that MALT is widespread and represents antigen-dependent lymphopoietic sites where sensitized cells are generated and clones expanded. Alternatively, MALT may be restricted to BALT and GALT, and all other mucosal sites are seeded by cells sensitized and generated in lung and bowel. A third alternative intermediate between the above extremes would suggest that BALT and GALT are predominant components of MALT, largely through their chronic antigenic stimulation, but that mucosal aggregates could be generated elsewhere, especially following infection, and would serve as sites of generation and amplification of sensitized cells which could function locally or at distant mucosal sites. The differences between various

MALT would be quantitative, not qualitative, and would be dynamic, dependent upon recent antigenic challenge.

IV. The common mucosal immunologic system

We have described the contributions which studies on the rabbit have made to our current knowledge of the mucosal immune system. It is clear that this species has been of fundamental importance in our progress to date. At this point we do not wish to underrate its significance, but we feel that rather than reemphasize the rabbit as a model system, we would like to focus upon our current conceptual synthesis of existing information of the mucosal immune system. In brief, four areas will be discussed:

a. the nature of GALT;
b. that to consider GALT in isolation is conceptually restricting and we must consider the whole tissue distribution of the gut-associated immune system;
c. other mucosal lymphoid tissue, such as BALT, exists and the true extent of mucosa-associated lymphoid tissue (MALT) remains to be explored;
d. despite the evidence for a common mucosal immunologic system, it is evident that mucosal and systemic immune responses are not completely separable; they are integrated to an extent which is variable and knowledge of the factors controlling the extent of integration will be crucial as we attempt to manipulate immune responses.

GALT includes the APP, PP, SR and SLN, components which have morphologic and functional similarities. They contain a mixture of T and B cells and, although the T cell proportion is small and variable, the cells are functional in a variety of T cell assays. The occurrence of immunoregulatory cells, largely but not exclusively T cells, in GALT will receive much attention in the next few years. Such regulatory influences must be of crucial consequence in maintaining normal physiology amid constant antigen exposure.

Indeed, antigen uptake is a specialized function of GALT. These antigens prime B cells which in the follicle undergo intensive proliferation and differentiation. Despite the intense B cell proliferation in GALT, plasma cells are infrequently seen. IgA precursors are particularly prominent in this amplification site and IgM and IgG precursor cells are also present. Like IgA, precursors of IgE cells appear to be enriched in GALT, but the evidence is inconclusive. B cells from GALT must migrate to other sites before they are induced to complete their differentiation to antibody-producing plasma cells. This has been most clearly shown for IgA precursors which a number of days after transfer, are detected in the gut and respiratory lamina propria, MLN and spleen, where they appear to have differentiated into IgA-containing cells. Therefore, although GALT does not appear to perform the primary bursal function of inducing the differentiation of B lymphocytes from pluripotent stem cells, it does perform other important functions characteristic of the avian bursa such as vigorous B cell proliferation and seeding to distant lymphoid tissues. The exact nature of the relationship between GALT and IgA precursors and their seeding to mucosal sites remains one of the prime challenges to be unraveled by students of mucosal immunity.

From this summary it is clear that in considering intestinal immunity, one must survey tissues other than GALT, since although it may be a site of antigen uptake and initial B cell proliferation and differentiation, it is not the site where plasma cells differentiate or whether other effector cells are abundant. It is widely held that IgA precursors sensitized in the PP migrate to the MLN where they undergo further maturation. A large proportion then move through the TDL to the circulation and selectively localize in mucosal LP where they mature into IgA-producing plasma cells. B lymphoblasts from the MLN have a tendency to return to the GALT (viewed as the whole intestinal lymphoid system). Such cells also seed other mucosal sites and make predominantly IgA but the largest number selectively lodge in the GALT. Similarly, B blasts from the mediastinal lymph nodes draining the lungs tend to return to the lungs where they make mostly IgA (Bienenstock *et al.*, 1979; McDermott and Bienenstock, 1979). Antigen does not appear to be the prime attractant for such localization since fetal lungs, transplanted subcutaneously into syngeneic hosts, are populated by IgA-containing cells (Milne *et al.*, 1975). Moreover, Pierce and Gowans (1975) have shown in elegant studies that antigen is not necessary for localization of IgA cells in the intestine, although it appears to amplify this localization.

Despite the localization of both mesenteric and mediastinal B blasts in mucosal tissues other than that which they drain (common mucosal immunologic system: Bienenstock, 1974), the factors causing cell proliferation at these sites are not known. Candidates for this proliferation drive in mucosal tissues must include:

a. antigen;
b. sex hormones in their target tissues such as the breast (Weisz-Carrington *et al.*, 1978) and female reproductive tract (Bienenstock *et al.*, 1979; McDermott and Bienenstock, 1979); and
c. substances such as secretory component (Strober *et al.*, 1976).

The LP is the site where non-lymphoid cells, also thought to be direct or indirect effectors or mucosal immunity, exist. These include mast cells and eosinophils which are found in such elevated numbers in parasitic infections (see Befus and Podesta, 1976; Wakelin, 1978). Modified mast cells (globule leucocytes) and various cells mediating cytotoxicity are found in the epithelium, although they are virtually absent in GALT. Whether such effector cells found in LP and IE sites originate from precursors in GALT is unexplored, but *a priori* there is no reason to assume that GALT generates only precursors of antibody-forming cells. Certainly, we have previously described the presence in rabbit bronchial epithelium of basophil-like cells (Bienenstock and Johnston, 1976) similar to the basophiloid cells found in washings of the bronchial tract by Patterson and colleagues (Patterson *et al.*, 1974; Ts'ao *et al.*, 1977). Further, we described the presence of similar cells in the BALT and have speculated on their significance (Bienenstock *et al.*, 1976). Hence, in mucosal immunity one must view not only the GALT and BALT but also the draining lymph nodes, thoracic duct, circulation, LP and mucosal epithelia as an integrated mucosa-associated lymphoid system (Fig. 5). It is logical to assume that a variety of factors in each site could influence the ultimate expression of mucosal immune responses.

Although GALT and BALT have been emphasized throughout this article, other MALT have been described. The extent and nature of MALT is unclear but as outlined above (section III, C) three possibilities should be considered:

a. MALT is ubiquitously distributed at mucosal sites but has not been adequately investigated in sites other than the bowel and bronchus.
b. MALT is represented by only GALT and BALT and all other mucosal sites are seeded by cells sensitized and generated in the bowel and lung; or
c. although GALT and BALT are the predominant components of MALT, largely through their chronic antigenic stimulation, mucosal aggregates can be generated elsewhere, especially following infection, and would serve as sites of generation and amplification of sensitized cells which could function locally or at distant mucosal sites.

As complete maturation of GALT and BALT are unmistakably antigen-dependent, other MALT must be so also and at mucosal sites where antigenic stimulation is small, relative to the lung or bowel, local MALT could be small and easily overlooked. Given intense antigenic stimulation such as during acute infection, local MALT might become hyperplastic and easily recognizable (e.g. Godwin, 1952; Bernier and Bhaskar, 1958; Kretschmer, 1952; Marsh *et al.*, 1974).

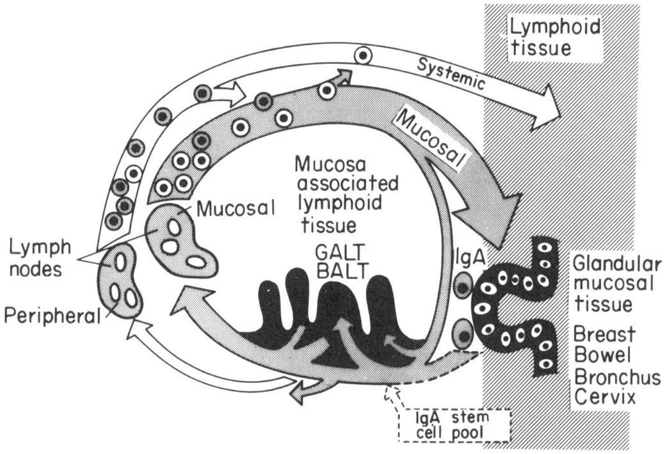

FIG. 5 The common mucosal immunologic system and its integration with systemic immune responses.

Hence, we conclude that MALT, as exemplified by GALT and BALT, would be an antigen-dependent site of predominantly, but not exclusively, IgA B cell differentiation and proliferation (Fig. 6). The degree of structural organization of MALT might depend upon the extent of antigen exposure, so that sites such as GALT would have highly organized B cell generation components with recognizable T cell areas. At the other extreme there might be isolated follicles and lymphoepithelial aggregates without recognizable T cell compartments. It seems likely that, given elevated antigenic stimulation, isolated follicles and lymphoepithelial aggregates might differentiate towards more organized MALT with specialized lymphoepithelium, generalized hyperplasia and perhaps even HEV. This differentiation might depend upon the existence of, for example, lymphocyte-derived factors which would influence the differentiation of epithelial cells and vascular endothelial cells. The observations of Rácz *et al.* (1977) on BALT lymphoepithelial hyperplasia and "activated" HEV in the rabbit suggests that such factors exist. The selective advantage of

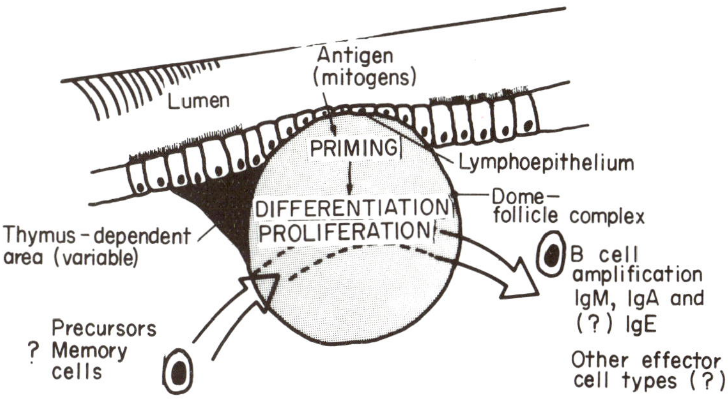

FIG. 6 Diagrammatic representation of mucosa-associated lymphoid tissue (MALT).

control over the differentiation of MALT would be that sites such as salivary glands, lacrimal glands, or the urinary bladder, which do not normally receive the same degree of antigenic stimulation as the GALT or BALT, could generate a response adequate to resist local mucosal infection. Enhanced IgA production from local precursors, not due simply to the emigration of IgA precursors from GALT or BALT, would distinguish local MALT from a localized inflammatory response characterized by IgG antibody.

In considering mucosal immunity we cannot be conceptually restricted to the local MALT but must also take into account the draining lymph nodes, lymphatics, circulation and local LP. Whether IgA precursors from all MALT go through an extensive migration before they localize in mucosal tissues, as documented for precursors from GALT, is unknown. From the teleologic standpoint of economy of energy, it seems reasonable that in salivary glands, for example, local IgA precursors (assuming that they exist) would move directly into local LP. Indeed, some IgA precursors from PP may migrate directly into local intestinal LP, as suggested by Crabbé *et al.* (1970)

and Parrott and Ferguson (1974). The reason that so many IgA precursors from PP follow the more indirect pathway through the MLN, TDL and circulation may be that this provides a more efficient dispersal of cells to all mucosal tissue LP, particularly that distant from any GALT.

So far this discussion has neglected the migration of cells from sites like GALT, MLN or BALT to lymph nodes or LP at other mucosal sites. For example, it is well documented (see sections III, B and C) that IgA precursors from BALT suspensions will repopulate gut LP and those from the MLN localize in the mammary glands, lungs, cervix and vagina. This extensive network of mucosal migrations occurs with T cells as well, as evidenced by T cells sensitive to bowel or lung antigens appearing in colostrum and milk (Parmely and Beer, 1977). Moreover, Cahill *et al.* (1977) suggested that there are T cell populations which selectively lodge in mucosal and others in non-mucosal sites, as documented for B cell homing patterns (e.g. Guy-Grand *et al.*, 1974; McWilliams *et al.*, 1975; McDermott and Bienenstock, 1979), although this has been recently questioned (Freitas *et al.*, 1977). Such interactions between various mucosal sites suggested that a cooperative mucosal immune system exists (Bienenstock *et al.*, 1973a; Bienenstock, 1974; Montgomery *et al.*, 1974; Lamm, 1976; Bienenstock *et al.*, 1978, 1979; Parmely and Beer, 1977).

The extent to which cells at one mucosal site are locally generated or have emigrated from distant sites might be variable. To be specific, bowel and lung might contain a large proportion of cells generated in GALT and BALT respectively, whereas sites such as the salivary glands might proportionately contain a mixed population from various mucosal sites, perhaps in ratios which would reflect the extent of cell proliferation throughout the entire mucosal system in the recent past.

In summary, GALT and BALT, due to their constant antigenic stimulation, are functionally dominant components of MALT. They serve as sites where priming occurs leading to differentiation and proliferation. Their products become effectors at various mucosal sites but also act in surveillance throughout the entire mucosal system. Some priming occurs at other MALT and contributes to the system, but quantitatively this is probably only a portion of the GALT and BALT contributions. The system is dynamic however, and given infections or other stimuli the relative contributions from various MALT might shift.

This model of the mucosal system lacks one critical component. If one accepts as a generalization that IgA responses are normally mucosal-associated and IgG responses are non-mucosal, then it is clear that a degree of integration of the two occurs normally, as evidenced by IgG precursors found in PP (e.g. Cebra *et al.*, 1977a, b) and IgA precursors in systemic sites such as the spleen (Nakamura *et al.*, 1974) and PLN (McDermott and Bienenstock, 1979). The mixing of IgA and IgG precursors and their differential migratory properties to various mucosal and non-mucosal sites has been extensively documented (McDermott and Bienenstock, 1979). What is missing from the model is that the mucosal immunologic system is not exclusive of what are generally considered to be systemic immune responses, but that integration of mucosal system and systemic responses occurs (Fig. 5). In the extreme, such as chronic inflammatory responses at mucosal sites (e.g. inflammatory bowel disease), tremendous infiltration of IgG-producing cells can occur (Brandtzaeg and Baklien, 1976a, b). Presumably, IgA production can be enhanced in non-mucosal lymph nodes or the spleen under appropriate conditions. The observation of Pierce and Gowans (1975) in rats and Pierce *et al.* (1977) in dogs, that parenteral priming with antigen followed by oral boosting induces the best mucosal response suggests that IgA precursors in peripheral tissues can be sensitized and migrate to local mucosal sites where they might function.

Normally, these mucosal and systemic systems maintain their separate identities, at least quantitatively, through differential migratory properties of their respective cell types. The reasons for their abnormal integration, particularly in pathological states, are unclear but probably reflect an inability of the normal state to cope with a particular challenge. Understanding the mechanisms of this integration would be significant in attempts to modulate immunopathologic processes.

In conclusion, with the rabbit as a principle contributor, our concepts of mucosal immunity have evolved through GALT, BALT and MALT to a common mucosal immunologic system which interacts with systemic responses. This evolution has unveiled as yet unexplored approaches to protection against infectious diseases.

Abbreviations

ADCC	antibody-dependent cell cytotoxicity
APP	appendix
APPx	appendectomy
BALT	bronchus-associated lymphoid tissue

BGG	bovine gamma globulin
Bx	bursectomized
BxTx	bursectomized-thymectomized
cIgM	cytoplasmic IgM
Con A	concanavalin A
GALT	gut-associated lymphoid tissue
GVH	graft versus host
HEV	high endothelial venules
IE	intraepithelial
LP	lamina propria
LPS	lipopolysaccharide
MALT	mucosa-associated lymphoid tissue
M cell	microfold cell
MICC	mitogen-induced cell cytotoxicity
MIF	macrophage inhibition factor
MLN	mesenteric lymph node
MLNx	mesenteric lymph nodectomy
-ve	negative
PFC	plaque-forming cell
PHA	phytohemagglutinin
PLN	peripheral lymph nodes
+ ve	positive
PP	Peyer's patches
PPD	purified tuberculin protein
PWM	pokeweed mitogen
RTLA	rabbit thymus lymphocyte antigen
SAPPx	combined surgical extirpation of sacculus rotundus, appendix and Peyer's patches
SCMC	spontaneous cell-mediated cytotoxicity
sIg	surface immunoglobulin
sIgM	surface IgM
SLN	solitary lymphoid nodule
SPx	splenectomy
SR	sacculus rotundus
SRBC	sheep red blood cells
TDA	thymus-dependent area
TDL	thoracic duct lymph
Tx	thymectomized

References

ABDOU, N. I. and RICHTER, M. (1970). *J. Immun.* **104**, 1087-1093.

ABE, K. and ITO, T. (1977). *Archs Histol. Jap.* **40**, 407-420.

ACKERMAN, G. A. (1966). *Anat. Rec.* **154**, 21-40.

AHLSTEDT, S., CARLSSON, B., HANSON, A. and GOLDBLUM, R. M. (1975). *Scand. J. Immun.* **4**, 535-539.

AMBRUS, C. M. and AMBRUS, J. L. (1959). *Ann. N.Y. Acad. Sci.* **77**, 445-486.

ANDERSON, N. D., ANDERSON, A. O. and WYLLIE, R. G. (1976). *Immunology,* **31**, 455-473.

ARCHER, O. K., SUTHERLAND, D. E. R. and GOOD, R. A. (1963). *Nature,* **200**, 337-339.

ARCHER, O. K., SUTHERLAND, D. E. R. and GOOD, R. A. (1964). *Lab. Invest.* **13**, 259-271.

ARNAUD-BATTANDIER, F., BUNDY, B. M., O'NEILL, M., BIENENSTOCK, J. and NELSON, D. L. (1978). *J. Immun.* **121**, 1059-1065.

ASHERSON, G. L., ZEMBALA, M., PERERA, M. A. C. C., MAYHEW, B. and THOMAS, W. R. (1977). *Cell. Immun.* **33**, 145-155.

BAKLIEN, K. and BRANDTZAEG, P. (1975). *Clin. exp. Immun.* **22**, 197-209.

BAKLIEN, K. and BRANDTZAEG, P. (1976). *Scand. J. Gastroent.* **11**, 447-457.

BANG, B. G. and BANG, F. B. (1968). *Am. J. Path.* **53**, 735-751.

BARG, M. and DRAPER, L. R. (1975). *Cell. Immun.* **20**, 177-186.

BAZIN, H. and PLATTEAU, B. (1976). *Immunology,* **30**, 679-683.

BEFUS, A. D., JOHNSTON, N., LESLIE, G. A. and BIENENSTOCK, J. (1980). *J. Immun.* **125**, 2626-2632.

BEFUS, A. D., O'NEILL, M. and BIENENSTOCK, J. (1978). *Immunology,* **35**, 901-906.

BEFUS, A. D. and PODESTA, R. B. (1976). *In* "Ecological Aspects of Parasitology" (Ed. C. R. Kennedy), pp. 303-325, North-Holland Publishing Company, Amsterdam.

BEHELAK, Y. and RICHTER, M. (1972). *Cell. Immun.* **3**, 542-558.

BEHELAK, Y. and RICHTER, M. (1974). *Transplantation,* **18**, 229-238.

BEHELAK, Y., SHIBATA, H. and RICHTER, M. (1973). *Cell. Immun.* **7**, 108-117.

BELLAMY, J. E. C. and NIELSEN, N. O. (1974). *Infect. Immun.* **9**, 615-619.

BERNIER, J. L. and BHASKAR, S. N. (1958). *Cancer,* **11**, 1156-1179.

BIENENSTOCK, J. (1974). *In* "Progress in Immunology II" (Eds L. Brent and J. Holborow), vol. 4, pp. 197-207. North-Holland Publishing Company, Amsterdam.

BIENENSTOCK, J. and DOLEZEL, J. (1971). *J. Immun.* **106**, 938-945.

BIENENSTOCK, J. and JOHNSTON, N. (1976). *Lab. Invest.* **35**, 343-348.

BIENENSTOCK, J. and STRAUSS, H. (1970). *J. Immun.* **105**, 274-277.

BIENENSTOCK, J., JOHNSTON, N. and PEREY, D. Y. E. (1973a). *Lab. Invest.* **28**, 686-692.

BIENENSTOCK, J., JOHNSTON, N. and PEREY, D. Y. E. (1973b). *Lab. Invest.* **28**, 693-698.

BIENENSTOCK, J., RUDZIK, O., CLANCY, R. L. and PEREY, D. Y. E. (1974). *In* "The Immunoglobulin A System" (Eds J. Mestecky and A. R. Lawton), pp. 47-56. Plenum Publishing Corporation, New York.

BIENENSTOCK, J., CLANCY, R. L. and PEREY, D. Y. E. (1976). *In* "Immunologic and Infectious Reactions in the Lung" (Eds C. H. Kirkpatrick and H. Y. Reynolds), vol. 1, pp. 29-58. Marcel-Dekker, New York and Basel.

BIENENSTOCK, J., MCDERMOTT, M., BEFUS, D. and O'NEILL, M. (1978). *In* "Secretory Immunity and Infection" (Eds J. R. McGhee, J. Mestecky and J. L. Babb), pp. 53-59. Plenum Publishing Corporation, New York.

BIENENSTOCK, J., MCDERMOTT, M. and BEFUS, D. (1979). *In* "The Immunology of Breast Milk" (Eds P. L. Ogra and D. Dayton), pp. 91-104. Raven Press, New York.

BLAESE, R. M., MUCHMORE, A. V., KOSKI, I. and DOOLEY, N. J. (1977). *In* "Avian Immunology" (Ed. A. A. Benedict), pp. 155-159. Plenum Publishing Corporation, New York.

BLOOM, W. and FAWCETT, D. W. (1968). "A Textbook of Histology". W. B. Saunders, Philadelphia, London, Toronto.

BLYTHMAN, H. E. and WAKSMAN, B. H. (1973). *J. Immun.* **111**, 171-182.

BOCKMAN, D. E. and COOPER, M. D. (1973). *Am. J. Anat.* **136**, 455-478.

BOCKMAN, D. E. and STEVENS, W. (1977). *J. Reticuloendothel. Soc.* **21**, 245-254.

BONA, C., CHEDID, L., DAMAIS, C., CIORBARU, R., SHEK, P. N., DUBISKI, S. and CINADER, B. (1975). *J. Immun.* **114**, 348-353.

BONA, C., CINADER, B. and DUBISKI, S. (1977). *Ann. Immun.* **128**, 572-598.

BOOKMAN, M. A., HELMS, R. A. and BULL, D. M. (1977). *Gastroenterology,* **72**, 1155.

BRANDTZAEG, P. and BAKLIEN, K. (1976a). *Clinic Gastroent.* **5**, 251-269.

BRANDTZAEG, P. and BAKLIEN, K. (1976b). *Scand. J. Gastroent.* **36**, 5-45.

BRANDTZAEG, P. and BAKLIEN, K. (1976c). *Lancet,* **2**, 1297-1298.

BROWN, W. R., BORTHISTLE, B. K. and CHEN, S.-T. (1975). *Clin. exp. Immun.* **20**, 227-237.

BRUNDELET, P. N. (1965). *Acta. path. microbiol. scand.* **175**, 31-45.

BULL, D. M. and BOOKMAN, M. A. (1977). *J. clin. Invest.* **59**, 966-974.

CAHILL, R. N. P., POSKITT, D. C., FROST, H. and TRNKA, Z. (1977). *J. exp. Med.* **145**, 420-428.

CALKINS, C. E., OZER, H. and WAKSMAN, B. H. (1975). *Cell. Immun.* **18**, 187-198.

CEBRA, J. J., KAMAT, R., GEARHART, P., ROBERTSON, S. M. and TSENG, J. (1977a). *In* "Immunology of the Gut" (Eds R. Porter and J. Knight), pp. 5-28. Ciba Foundation Symposium 46 (new series). Elsevier Excerpta Medica, North-Holland, Amsterdam, Oxford, New York.

CEBRA, J. J., GEARHART, P. J., KAMAT, R., ROBERTSON, S. M. and TSENG, J. (1977b). *Cold Spring Harb. Symp. quant. Biol.* **41**, 201-215.

CEBRA, J. J., GEARHART, P. J., KAMAT, R., ROBERTSON, S. M. and TSENG, J. (1977c). *Biochem. Soc. Trans.* **5**, 1565-1569.

CHAMBERLAIN, D. W., NOPAJAROONSRI, C. and SIMON, G. T. (1973). *Am. Rev. respir. Dis.* **108**, 621-631.

CLANCY, R. (1976). *Gastroenterology,* **70**, 177-180.

CLANCY, R. and BIENENSTOCK, J. (1974). *J. Immun.* **112**, 1997-2001.

CLANCY, R. and PUCCI, A. (1978). *Gut,* **19**, 273-276.

Coates, M. E. and O'Donoghue, P. N. (1967). *Nature,* **213**, 307-308.
Cole, F. M. (1978). *Radiology,* **128**, 41-43.
Collan, Y. (1972). *Scand. J. Gastroent.* **7**, Suppl. 18.
Cooper, M. D. and Lawton, A. R. (1972). *Contemp. Top. Immunobiol.* **1**, 49-68.
Cooper, M. D., Peterson, R. D. A., South, M. A. and Good, R. A. (1966a). *J. exp. Med.* **123**, 75-102.
Cooper, M. D., Perey, D. Y., McKneally, M. F., Gabrielsen, A. E., Sutherland, D. E. R. and Good, R. A. (1966b). *Lancet,* **1**, 1388-1391.
Cooper, M. D., Perey, D. Y., Gabrielsen, A. E., Sutherland, D. E. R.. McKneally, M. F. and Good, R. A. (1968). *Int. Archs Allergy appl. Immun.* **33**, 65-68.
Cooper, M. D., Lawton, A. R. and Kincade, P. W. (1972). *Clin. exp. Immun.* **11**, 143-149.
Cooper, G. N. and Turner, K. (1969). *J. Reticuloendothel. Soc.* **6**, 419-434.
Cornes, J. S. (1965). *Gut,* **6**, 225-233.
Crabbé, P. A., Nash, D. R., Bazin, H., Eyssen, H. and Heremans, J. F. (1970). *Lab. Invest.* **22**, 448-457.
Craig, S. W. and Cebra, J. J. (1971). *J. exp. Med.* **134**, 188-200.
Craig, S. W. and Cebra, J. J. (1975). *J. Immun.* **114**, 492-502.
David, M. F. (1977). *J. Allergy,* **60**, 180-187.
Diaz-Jouanen, E. and Williams, R. C. (1974). *Clin. Immun. Immunopath.* **3**, 248-255.
Doenhoff, M. J., Janossy, G. and Kerbel, R. S. (1976). *Immunology,* **30**, 367-378.
Douglas, A. P. and Weetman, A. P. (1975). *Digestion,* **13**, 344-371.
Dukes, C. and Bussey, H. J. R. (1926). *J. Path. Bact.* **29**, 111-116.
Durkin, H. G., Caporale, L. and Thorbecke, G. J. (1974). *Cell. Immun.* **16**, 285-300.
Eloy, R., Vuitton, D., Vaultier, J.-P. and Grenier, J. F. (1975). *Eur. J. Immun.* **5**, 502-504.
Faulk, W. P., McCormick, J. N., Goodman, J. R., Yoffey, J. M. and Fudenberg, H. H. (1971). *Cell. Immun.* **1**, 500-520.
Feldmann, M. and Basten, A. (1972). *J. exp. Med.* **136**, 722-736.
Ferguson, A. (1977). *Gut,* **18**, 921-937.
Ferguson, A. and Parrott, D. M. V. (1972). *J. Path.* **106**, 95-101.
Ferguson, A. and MacDonald, T. T. (1977). *In* "Immunology of the Gut" (Eds R. Porter and J. Knight), pp. 305-327. Ciba Foundation Symposium 46 (new series). Elsevier Excerpta Medica, North-Holland, Amsterdam, Oxford, New York.
Fernando, M. A. and Pasternak, J. (1977). *Parasitology,* **74**, 19-26.
Fichtelius, K. E. (1969). *In* "Lymphatic Tissue and Germinal Centers in Immune Response" (Eds L. Fiore-Donati and M. G. Hanna), pp. 9-20. Plenum Press, New York.
Fichtelius, K. E., Finstad, J. and Good, R. A. (1968). *Lab. Invest.* **19**, 339-351.

FIRTH, G. A. (1977). *Vet. Bull.* **47**, 167-179.

FOLCH, H., YOSHINAGA, M. and WAKSMAN, B. H. (1973). *J. Immun.* **110**, 835-839.

FOURNIER, M., VAI, F., DERENNE, J. P. H. and PARIENTE, R. (1977). *Am. Rev. respir. Dis.* **116**, 685-694.

FOX, P. C. and SIRAGANIAN, R. (1981). *Immunology,* **43**, 227-234.

FRADELIZI, D. P., CHOU, C.-T., CINADER, B. and DUBISKI, S. (1973). *Cell. Immun.* **7**, 484-501.

FREDERICK, G. T. and BOHL, E. H. (1976). *J. Immun.* **116**, 1000-1004.

FREITAS, A. A., ROSE, M. L. and PARROTT, D. M. V. (1977). *Nature,* **270**, 731-733.

FREIDENSTEIN, A. and GONCHARENKO, I. (1965). *Nature,* **206**, 1113-1115.

FUJIWARA, S., ARMSTRONG, R. M. and CINADER, B. (1974). *Immun. Commun.* **3**, 275-284.

GEARHART, P. J. and CEBRA, J. J. (1979). *J. exp. Med.* **149**, 216-227.

GLICK, B., CHANG, T. S. and JAAP, R. G. (1956). *Poultry Sci.* **35**, 224-225.

GODWIN, J. T. (1952). *Cancer,* **5**, 1089-1103.

GOLDBLUM, R. M., AHLSTEDT, S., CARLSSON, B., HANSON, A., LIDIN-JANSON, G. and SOHL-ÅKERLUND, A. (1975). *Nature,* **107**, 797-799.

GOOD, R. A. and FINSTAD, J. (1967). *In* "Germinal Centers in Immune Responses" (Eds H. Cottier, N. Odartchenko, R. Schindler and C. C. Congdon), pp. 4-27. Springer-Verlag, New York.

GOOD, R. A., DALMASSO, A. P., MARTINEZ, C., ARCHER, O. K., PIERCE, J. C. and PAPERMASTER, B. W. (1962). *J. exp. Med.* **116**, 773-796.

GOODACRE, R., DAVIDSON, R., SINGHAL, D. and BIENENSTOCK, J. (1979). *Gastroenterology,* **76**, 300-308.

GRISCELLI, C., VASSALLI, P. and MCCLUSKEY, R. T. (1969). *J. exp. Med.* **130**, 1427-1451.

GUY-GRAND, D., GRISCELLI, C. and VASSALLI, P. (1974). *Eur. J. Immun.* **4**, 435-443.

HALL, J. G., HOPKINS, J. and ORLANS, E. (1977). *Eur. J. Immun.* **7**, 30-37.

HALLIWELL, R. E. W. (1973). *J. Immun.* **110**, 422-430.

HALLIWELL, R. E. W. (1975). *Ann. N.Y. Acad. Sci.* **254**, 476-488.

HANAOKA, M. and WAKSMAN, B. H. (1970). *Cell. Immun.* **1**, 316-332.

HANAOKA, M., NOMOTO, K. and WAKSMAN, B. H. (1970). *J. Immun.* **104**, 616-625.

HANSON, D. G., VAZ, N. M., MAIA, L. C. S., HORNBROOK, M. M., LYNCH, J. M. and ROY, C. A. (1977). *Int. Archs Allergy appl. Immun.* **55**, 526-532.

HEATLEY, R. V., RHODES, J., CALCRAFT, B. J., WHITEHEAD, R. H., FIFIELD, R. and NEWCOMBE, R. G. (1975). *Lancet,* **2**, 1010-1012.

HEIM, L. R., MCGARRY, M. P., MONTGOMERY, J. R., TRENTIN, J. J. and SOUTH, M. A. (1972). *Transplantation,* **14**, 418-423.

HENRY, C. and KODLIN, D. (1971). *Cell. Immun.* **2**, 521-540.

HENRY, C., FAULK, W. P., KUHN, L., YOFFEY, J. M. and FUDENBERG, H. H. (1970). *J. exp. Med.* **131**, 1200-1210.

HEREMANS, J. F. (1974). *In* "The Antigens" (Ed. M. Sela), vol. 2, pp. 365-522. Academic Press, New York and London.
HEREMANS, J. F., HEREMANS, M. T. and SCHULTZE, H. E. (1959). *Clin chim. Acta,* **4**, 96-102.
HOPKINS, J. and HALL, J. G. (1976). *Nature,* **259**, 308-309.
HOSHI, H. and MORI, T. (1973). *Tohoku J. exp. Med.* **111**, 309-322.
HUMMEL, K. P. (1935). *Am. J. Anat.* **57**, 351-383.
IMADA, Y., NOMOTO, K., YAMADA, H. and TAKEYA, K. (1977). *Int. Archs Allergy appl. Immun.* **53**, 50-55.
ISKIZAKA, K. (1976). *in* "The Role of Immunological Factors in Infectious, Allergic, and Autoimmune Processes" (Eds R. F. Beers Jr. and E. G. Bassett), pp. 199-221. Raven Press, New York.
ISHIZAKA, T., URBAN, J. F. and ISHIKZAKA, K. (1976). *Cell. Immun.* **22**, 248-261.
JACOBSON, L. O., ROBSON, M. J. and MARKS, E. K. (1950). *Proc. Soc. exp. Biol. Med.* **75**, 145-152.
JACOBSON, L. O., MARKS, E. K., SIMMONS, E. L. and GASTON, E. O. (1961). *Proc. Soc. exp. Biol. Med.* **108**, 487-492.
JANKOVIĆ, B. D. and MITROVIĆ, K. (1966). *In* "Germinal Centers in Immune Responses" (Eds H. Cottier, N. Odartchenko, R. Schindler and C. C. Congdon), pp. 34-37. Springer-Verlag, New York.
JARRETT, E. E. E. (1977). *Lancet,* **2**, 223-225.
JARRETT, E. E. E., HAIG, D. M., MCDOUGALL, W. and MCNULTY, E. (1976). *Immunology,* **30**, 671-677.
JOEL, D. D., HESS, M. W. and COTTIER, H. (1972). *J. exp. Med.* **135**, 907-923.
JOEL, D. D., CHANANA, A. D., COTTIER, H., CRONKITE, E. P. and LAISSUE, J. A. (1977). *Cell Tissue Kinet.* **10**, 57-69.
JONES, P. P. and CEBRA, J. J. (1974). *J. exp. Med.* **140**, 966-976.
JONES, P. P., CRAIG, S. W., CEBRA, J. J. and HERZENBERG, L. A. (1974). *J. exp. Med.* **140**, 452-469.
JONES, W. R., KAYE, M. D. and ING, R. M. Y. (1972). *Biol. Neonate,* **20**, 334-345.
KAGNOFF, M. F. (1975). *J. exp. Med.* **142**, 1425-1435.
KAGNOFF, M. F. (1978). *J. Immun.* **120**, 395-399.
KAGNOFF, M. F. and CAMPBELL, S. (1976). *Gastroenterology,* **70**, 341-346.
KAMIN, R. M., HENRY, C. and FUDENBERG, H. H. (1974). *J. Immun.* **113**, 1151-1161.
KATZ, D. H. and PEREY, D. Y. E. (1973). *J. Immun.* **111**, 1507-1513.
KATZ, D. H., HAMAOKA, T., NEWBURGER, P. E. and BENACERRAF, B. (1974). *J. Immun.* **113**, 974-983.
KEALY, W. F. (1976). *J. clin. Pathol.* **29**, 241-244.
KEREN, D. F., HOLT, P. S., COLLINS, H. H., GEMSKI, P. and FORMAL, S. B. (1978). *J. Immun.* **120**, 1892-1896.
KONDA, S. and HARRIS, T. N. (1966). *J. Immun.* **97**, 805-814.
KOTANI, M., YAMASHITA, A., RAI, F., SEIKI, K. and HORII, I. (1967). *Blood,* **29**, 616-627.

KRETSCHMER, H. L. (1952). *J. Urol.* **68**, 252-260.

LAMM, M. E. (1976). *In* "Advances in Immunology" (Eds F. J. Dixon and H. G. Kunkel), vol. 22, pp. 223-290. Academic Press, New York, San Francisco and London.

LAWTON, A. R., KEARNEY, J. F. and COOPER, M. D. (1977). *In* "Progress in Immunology III" (Eds T. E. Mandel, C. Cheers, C. S. Hosking, I. F. C. McKenzie and G. J. V. Nossal), pp. 171-182. Australian Academy of Science, Canberra City.

LEMAÎTRE-COELHO, I., JACKSON, G. D. F. and VAERMAN, J.-P. (1977). *Eur. J. Immun.* **8**, 588-590.

LEMAÎTRE-COELHO, I., JACKSON, G. D. F. and VAERMAN, J.-P. (1978). *J. exp. Med.* **147**, 934-939.

LEVIN, D. M., ROSENSTREICH, D. L. and REYNOLDS, H. Y. (1973). *J. Immun.* **111**, 980-983.

LEVIN, D. M., ROSENSTREICH, D. L., WAHL, S. M. and REYNOLDS, H. Y. (1974). *J. Immun.* **113**, 1935-1941.

LINNA, T. J., BRENNING, T. and HEMMINGSSON, E. (1969). *In* "Lymphatic Tissue and Germinal Centres in Immune Response" (Eds L. Fiore-Donati and M. G. Hanna), pp. 133-142. Plenum Press, New York.

LLOYD, G., GREEN, F. H. Y., FOX, H., MANI, V. and TURNBERG, L. A. (1975). *Gut,* **16**, 861-866.

MACDONALD, T. T. and CARTER, P. B. (1978). *Transplantation,* **26**, 162-165.

MACHADO, I. and FALCHUK, Z. M. (1978). *Gastroenterology,* **74**, 1059.

MARSH, F. P., BANERJEE, R. and PANCHAMIA, P. (1974). *J. clin. Path.* **27**, 297-307.

MATTINGLEY, J. A. and WAKSMAN, B. H. (1978). *J. Immun.* **121**, 1878-1883.

MAYRHOFER, G. (1977). *In* "Immunology of the Gut" (Eds R. Porter and J. Knight), pp. 155-182. Ciba Foundation Symposium 46 (new series) Elsevier Excerpta Medica, North-Holland, Amsterdam, Oxford, New York.

MAYRHOFER, G., BAZIN, H. and GOWANS, J. L. (1976). *Eur. J. Immun.* **6**, 537-545.

MCDERMOTT, M. and BIENENSTOCK, J. (1979). *J. Immun.* **122**, 1892-1898.

MCKNEALLY, M. F., SUTHERLAND, D. E. R. and GOOD, R. A. (1971). *Surgery,* **69**, 345-353.

MCWILLIAMS, M., PHILLIPS-QUAGLIATA, J. M. and LAMM, M. E. (1975). *J. Immun.* **115**, 54-58.

MCWILLIAMS, M., PHILLIPS-QUAGLIATA, J. M. and LAMM, M. E. (1977). *J. exp. Med.* **145**, 866-875.

MELCHERS, F., VON BOEHMER, H. and PHILLIPS, R. A. (1975). *Transplant. Rev.* **25**, 27-58.

MEUWISSEN, H. J., KAPLAN, G. T., PEREY, D. Y. and GOOD, R. A. (1969). *Proc. Soc. exp. Biol. Med.* **130**, 300-304.

MILLER, J. F. A. P. (1961). *Lancet,* **2**, 748-749.

MILNE, R. W., BIENENSTOCK, J. and PEREY, D. Y. E. (1975). *J. Reticuloendothel. Soc.* **17**, 361-369.

MITCHISON, N. A. (1953). *Quart. J. exp. Physiol.* **38**, 139-150.
MONTGOMERY, P. C., ROSNER, B. R. and COHN, J. (1974). *Immun. Commun.* **3**, 143-156.
MONTGOMERY, P. C., KHALEEL, S. A., GOUDSWAARD, J. and VIRELL, G. (1977). *Immun. Commun.* **6**, 633-642.
MÜLLER-SCHOOP, J. W. and GOOD, R. A. (1975). *J. Immun.* **114**, 1757-1760.
NAKAMURA, I., RAY, A. and MÄKELÄ, O. (1973). *J. exp. Med.* **138**, 973-988.
NELSON, D. L., BUNDY, B. M., BLAESE, R. M. and STROBER, W. (1976). *Cell. Immun.* **22**, 165-175.
NELSON, R. D. and LEU, R. W. (1975). *J. Immun.* **114**, 606-609.
NGAN, J. and KIND, L. S. (1976). *Int. Archs Allergy appl. Immun.* **51**, 311-319.
NGAN, J. and KIND, L. S. (1978). *J. Immun.* **120**, 861-865.
NIEUWENHUIS, P. (1971). "On the Origin and Fate of Immunologically Competent Cells". Wolters-Noordhoff, Groningen.
NIEUWENHUIS, P. and KEUNING, F. J. (1974). *Immunology,* **26**, 509-519.
NIEUWENHUIS, P., VAN NOUHUIJS, C. E., EGGENS, J. H. and KEUNING, F. J. (1974). *Immunology,* **26**, 497-507.
NOSSAL, G. J. V. and ADA, G. L. (1971). "Antigens, Lymphoid Cells, and the Immune Response". Academic Press, New York and London.
NOSSAL, G. J. V. and PIKE, B. L. (1973). *Immunology,* **25**, 33-45.
OGILVIE, B. M. (1967). *Immunology,* **12**, 113-131.
OGILVIE, B. M. and JONES, V. E. (1969). *In* "Cellular and Humoral Mechanisms in Anaphylaxis and Allergy" (Ed. H. Z. Movat, ed), pp. 13-22. Karger, Basel.
OLSON, D. P. and WAXLER, G. L. (1977). *Am. J. vet. Res.* **38**, 1177-1181.
ORLANS, E., PEPPARD, J., REYNOLDS, J. and HALL, J. (1978). *J. exp. Med.* **147**, 588-592.
OWEN, J. J. T. (1977). *in* "Progress in Immunology III" (Eds T. E. Mandel, C. Cheers, C. S. Hosking, I. F. C. McKenzie and G. J. V. Nossal), pp. 153-154. Australian Academy of Science, Canberra City.
OWEN, J. J. T., COOPER, M. D. and RAFF, M. C. (1974). *Nature,* **249**, 361-363.
OWEN, J. J. T., RAFF, M. C. and COOPER, M. D. (1975). *Eur. J. Immun.* **5**, 468-473.
OWEN, J. J. T., WRIGHT, D. E., HABU, S., RAFF, M. C. and COOPER, M. D. (1977). *J. Immun.* **118**, 2067-2072.
OWEN, R. L. (1977). *Gastroenterology,* **72**, 440-451.
OWEN, R. L. and JONES, A. L. (1974). *Gastroenterology,* **66**, 189-203.
OZER, H. and WAKSMAN, B. H. (1970). *J. Immun.* **105**, 791-792.
OZER, H. and WAKSMAN, B. H. (1972). *J. Immun.* **109**, 410-421.
OZER, H. and WAKSMAN, B. H. (1974). *J. Immun.* **113**, 1780-1792.
PADAWER, J. (1974). *Am. J. Anat.* **141**, 299-302.
PARMELY, M. J. and BEER, A. E. (1977). *J. dairy Sci.* **60**, 655-665.

PARMELY, M. J., BEER, A. E. and BILLINGHAM, R. E. (1976). *J. exp. Med.* **144**, 358-370.

PARMELY, M. J., REATH, D. B., BEER, A. E. and BILLINGHAM, R. E. (1977). *Transplant. Proc.* **9**, 1477-1483.

PARROTT, D. M. V. (1976). *Clins. Gastroent.* **5**, 211-228.

PARROTT, D. M. V. and FERGUSON, A. (1974). *Immunology,* **26**, 571-588.

PATTERSON, R., TOMITA, Y., OH, S. H., SUSKO, I. M. and PRUZANSKY, J. J. (1974). *Clin. exp. Immun.* **16**, 223-234.

PEREY, D. Y. E. (1971). *In* "Cellular Interactions in the Immune Response" (Eds S. Cohen, G. Cudkowicz and R. T. McCluskey), pp. 13-24. Karger, Basel.

PEREY, D. Y. E. and BIENENSTOCK, J. (1973). *J. Immun.* **111**, 633-637.

PEREY, D. Y. E. and GOOD, R. A. (1968). *Lab. Invest.* **18**, 15-26.

PEREY, D. Y. E. and GUTTMANN, R. D. (1972). *Lab. Invest.* **27**, 427-433.

PEREY, D. Y. E. and MILNE, R. W. (1975). *Lab. Invest.* **33**, 678-686.

PEREY, D. Y. E., COOPER, M. D. and GOOD, R. A. (1968a). *Surgery,* **64**, 614-621.

PEREY, D. Y. E., COOPER, M. D. and GOOD, R. A. (1968b). *Science,* **161**, 265-266.

PEREY, D. Y. E., FROMMEL, D., HONG, R. and GOOD, R. A. (1970). *Lab. Invest.* **22**, 212-227.

PIERCE, N. F. and GOWANS, J. L. (1975). *J. exp. Med.* **142**, 1550-1563.

PIERCE, N. F., SACK, R. B. and SIRCAR, B. K. (1977). *J. infect. Dis.* **135**, 888-896.

PINCKARD, R. N., HALONEN, M. and MENG, A. L. (1972). *J. Allergy,* **49**, 301-310.

POLLARD, M. and SHARON, N. (1970). *Infect. Immun.* **2**, 96-100.

PORTER, R. and KNIGHT, J. (1977). "Immunology of the Gut". Ciba Foundation Symposium 46 (new series). Elsevier Excerpta Medica, North-Holland, Amsterdam, Oxford, New York.

RÁCZ, P., TENNER-RÁCZ, K., MYRVIK, Q. N. and FAINTER, L. K. (1977). *J. Reticuloendothel. Soc.* **22**, 59-83.

RAFF, M. C., MEGSON, M., OWEN, J. J. T. and COOPER, M. D. (1976). *Nature,* **259**, 224-225.

RICHTER, M., ROSE, B. and ABDOU, N. I. (1970). *Int. Archs Allergy appl. Immun.* **38**, 269-281.

ROBERTSON, P. W. and COOPER, G. N. (1972). *Aust. J. exp. Biol. med. Sci.* **50**, 703-714.

ROBERTSON, S. M. and CEBRA, J. J. (1976). *La Ricerca in Clinica e in Laboratorio,* **6**, Suppl. 3, 105-119.

ROSE, M. L., PARROTT, D. M. V. and BRUCE, R. G. (1976a). *Immunology,* **31**, 723-730.

ROSE, M. L., PARROTT, D. M. V. and BRUCE, R. G. (1976b). *Cell. Immun.* **27**, 36-46.

ROUX, M. E., MCWILLIAMS, M., PHILLIPS-QUAGLIATA, J. M., WEISZ-CARRINGTON, P. and LAMM, M. E. (1977). *J. exp. Med.* **146**, 1311-1322.

RUDZIK, O. and BIENENSTOCK, J. (1974). *Lab. Invest.* **30**, 260-266.

RUDZIK, O., CLANCY, R. L., PEREY, D. Y. E., BIENENSTOCK, J. and SINGAL, D. P. (1975a). *J. Immun.* **114**, 1-4.

RUDZIK, O., CLANCY, R. L., PEREY, D. Y. E., DAY, R. P. and BIENENSTOCK, J. (1975b). *J. Immun.* **114**, 1599-1604.

RUDZIK, O., PEREY, D. Y. E. and BIENENSTOCK, J. (1975c). *J. Immun.* **114**, 40-44.

SACKMAN, W. (1977). *Acta. anat.* **97**, 109-113.

SCHEFFEL, J. W. and DRAPER, L. R. (1976). *Cell. Immun.* **26**, 54-67.

SCHEFFEL, J. W. and DRAPER, L. R. (1977). *Cell. Immun.* **30**, 183-187.

SCHEFFEL, J. W., KREUTZER, D. L., ROBERTSON, D. C. and DRAPER, L. R. (1977). *Infect. Immun.* **16**, 493-499.

SCOLLAY, R., HOPKINS, J. and HALL, J. (1976). *Nature,* **260**, 528-529.

SHINER, M., BALLARO, J. and SMITH, M. E. (1975). *Lancet,* **1**, 136-140.

SIMSON, J. A. V., HINTZ, D. S., MUNSTER, A. M. and SPICER, S. S. (1977). *Expl. mol. Path.* **26**, 85-91.

SINGAL, D. P., O'NEILL, M., CLANCY, R. and BIENENSTOCK, J. (1976). *Gut,* **17**, 325-327.

SINGHAL, S. K., DAGUILLARD, F. and RICHTER, M. (1968). *Int. Archs Allergy appl. Immun.* **34**, 119-127.

SMITH, J. W. and SCHULTZ, R. D. (1977). *Cell. Immun.* **29**, 165-173.

SOBHON, P. (1971). *J. Morph.* **135**, 457-482.

SPRENT, J. (1976). *Cell. Immun.* **21**, 278-302.

STAMPER, H. B. and WOODRUFF, J. J. (1976). *J. exp. Med.* **144**, 828-833.

STANNEGARD, Ö., and YURCHISON, A. (1969). *Int. Archs Allergy appl. Immun.* **35**, 579-590.

STRAMIGNONI, A. and MOLLO, F. (1968). *Acta. anat.* **70**, 202-218.

STROBER, W., KRAKAUER, R., KLAEVEMAN, H. L., REYNOLDS, H. Y. and NELSON, D. L. (1976). *New Engl. J. Med.* **294**, 351-356.

STUX, S. V. and OVARY, Z. (1976). *Int. Archs Allergy appl. Immun.* **51**, 338-358.

SÜSSDORF, D. H. (1960). *J. infect. Dis.* **107**, 108-114.

SÜSSDORF, D. H. (1974). *Immunology,* **27**, 305-310.

SÜSSDORF, D. H. and DRAPER, L. R. (1956). *J. infect. Dis.* **99**, 129-142.

SUTHERLAND, D. E. R., ARCHER, O. K. and GOOD, R. A. (1964). *Proc. Soc. exp. Biol. Med.* **115**, 673-676.

TADA, T. and ISHIZAKA, K. (1970). *J. Immun.* **104**, 377-387.

TEIR, H., RYTÖMAA, T., CEDERBERG, A. and KIVINIEMI, K., (1963). *Acta. path. microbiol. scand.* **59**, 311-324.

TODOROV, D. M., WILKINSON, P. C. and WHITE, R. G. (1968). *Immunology,* **15**, 51-64.

TOIVANEN, P. and TOIVANEN, A. (1973). *Eur. J. Immun.* **3**, 585-595.

TOIVANEN, P., TOIVANEN, A. and TAMMINEN, P. (1972). *Eur. J. Immun.* **4**, 405-410.

TOMASI, T. B. (1976). "The Immune System of Secretions". Prentice-Hall, New Jersey.

Tomasi, T. B. and Zigelbaum. (1963). *J. clin. Invest.* **42**, 1552-1560.
Ts'ao, C., Patterson, R., McKenna, J. M. and Susko, I. M. (1977). *J. Allergy,* **59**, 320-326.
Van Hout, C. A. and Johnson, H. G. (1972). *J. Immun.* **108**, 834-836.
Vaz, N. M., Maia, L. C. S., Hanson, D. G. and Lynch, J. M. (1977). *J. Allergy,* **60**, 110-115.
Vuitton, D., Eloy, R., Gosse, F., Pousse, A. and Grenier, J. F. (1977). *Experientia,* **33**, 526-528.
Wakelin, D. (1978). *Nature,* **273**, 617-620.
Waksman, B. H. (1973). *J. Immun.* **111**, 878-884.
Waksman, B. H. and Ozer, H. (1976). *Prog. Allergy,* **21**, 1-113.
Waksman, B. H., Ozer, H. and Blythman, H. E. (1973). *Lab. Invest.* **28**, 614-626.
Weisz-Carrington, P., Roux, M. E., McWilliams, M., Phillips-Quagliata, J. M. and Lamm, M. E. (1978). *Proc. Natn. Acad. Sci. U.S.A.* **75**, 2928-2932.
Werner, H. J., Lefevre, H. and Raettig, H. (1971). *Nature,* **232**, 119-120.
Williams, A. F. and Gowans, J. L. (1975). *J. exp. Med.* **141**, 335-345.
Young, S. and Cowan, D. M. (1965). *Br. J. exp. Path.* **46**, 649-656.
Zvaifler, N. J. and Becker, E. L. (1966). *J. exp. Med.* **123**, 935-951.

6 *Comparative Aspects of Conglutinin and Immunoconglutinins*

D. G. INGRAM*

I. Introduction

Bovine serum contains a protein which will strongly aggregate immune complexes having complement bound to them. This serum protein was named conglutinin by Bordet and Streng (1909) and the aggregation reaction was called conglutinin. The first accurate description of this reaction was by Bordet and Gay (1906) who observed that guinea pig red blood cells were strongly clumped in the presence of fresh horse serum and heated bovine serum. They suggested that a heat stable component of bovine serum was responsible for the aggregation. Bordet and Streng (1909) concluded that three substances were necessary for the red blood cells to be conglutinated: (1) antibody to sensitize the cells, (2) complement of such a nature that its adsorption did not result in immediate lysis of the cells, and (3) conglutinin, a heat stable substance present in normal bovine serum. They showed that conglutinin was a discrete component of bovine serum since it could be adsorped from the serum by antigen-antibody-complement complexes.

Streng (1909) showed that bacteria, as well as red blood cells, could be conglutinated and that this reaction was identical to that with red blood cells in that it was dependent on the presence of specific antibody, complement and conglutinin. Using bacterial cells in the reaction, the complements from the guinea pig, rabbit, horse or man could be used since lysis of the bacteria did not occur. Streng (1909)

*This contribution is published posthumously and is dedicated to the memory of the author. [Editor] suggested that the reaction could be used for the detection of antibody. In developing this idea, Streng (1910) showed that it was possible to perform a conglutinating complement absorption test analogous to the hemolytic complement fixation test. He demonstrated that in the conglutinating complement absorption test horse, cat or pig complement could be used. The indicator system of sheep red blood cells and heat-inactivated bovine serum would aggregate or conglutinate to detect the presence of conglutinating complement if the complement had not been destroyed by previous exposure to a complement-fixing antigen-antibody reaction.

At about the same time, several reports (Moreschi, 1911; Perussia, 1911) showed that "anticomplement" was produced following the injection of complement-treated cells. These early researchers did not differentiate between the action of this "anticomplement" and antibodies to other serum proteins which also were present in antisera produced by this method. Streng (1930) inoculated rabbits with red blood cells or bacteria which had been treated with complement and produced a substance which reacted with complement in an analogous manner to the conglutinin in bovine serum. He named this substance immunoconglutinin (IK) and demonstrated that it reacted with cells treated with complements derived from a variety of animal species. Streng was the first to recognize that fixed or adsorbed complement had a common specificity regardless of the species of origin of the serum utilized as a complement source. He showed that the immunoconglutinin could be used in a conglutinating complement adsorption test and was not neutralized by serum containing complement which had not been activated.

Wartiovaara (1932) reported that intravenous inoculation of rabbits with untreated bacteria or a variety of other antigens resulted in the production of immunoconglutinin. It remained for Coombs (1947) to provide a possible explanation of the immunoconglutinin produced in response to the injection of antigens not treated with complement. He suggested that when complement was adsorbed onto an antigen-antibody complex the surface configuration of the complement proteins were altered to expose new antigenic determinants which were masked while the complement proteins remained in solution and it was these newly exposed determinants which react with conglutinin and immunoconglutinin. This was the first formulation of the concept "hidden determinants" and the validity of this concept now has been widely confirmed.

Following Wartiovaara's report, interest in the conglutinin reaction lagged until Hole and Coombs (1947a,b,c) reawakened interest in the reaction as a serological diagnostic test. They reported on the development of the conglutinating complement absorption test for the diagnosis of glanders infection. This investigation was continued using serum from various animal species as a source of complement for the detection of complement-fixing or complement-absorbing antibodies. The most useful serum for complement in several antigen–antibody systems was shown to be horse serum and the most sensitive test for the detection of antibodies was usually the conglutinating complement absorption test (Coombs and Hole, 1948; Blomfield *et al.*, 1949, 1950).

An excellent review of the literature on conglutinin and immunocon glutinins covering the first half of the twentieth century was published by Hole and Coombs (1947a). Coombs and his collaborators reinvestigated the reactions of conglutinin and immunoconglutinins and the results obtained, with a review of other relevant research, were published in a monograph by Coombs *et al.* (1961). Subsequent reviews on this subject have been presented by Lachmann and Coombs (1965), Lachmann (1967) Lachmann *et al.* (1972) and Ingram (1972).

II. Conglutinin

A. MOLECULAR CHARACTERISTICS

Bovine conglutinin is a non-immunoglobulin serum protein, a euglobulin which is precipitated by 33% saturated ammonium sulfate (Lachmann and Coombs, 1965). The amino acid composition of conglutinin has been determined (Lachmann and Coombs, 1965) and a feature of the protein is the relatively high content of glycine (18·4%) and proline (10·7%). These proportions are rather typical of fibrous proteins and may reflect the molecular asymmetry. The carbohydrate content of conglutinin was estimated to be less than one per cent.

Conglutinin has been purified and has been shown to be a highly asymmetrical molecule with a molecular weight of 750 000 (Lachmann, 1967). It is sedimented on a sucrose density gradient in the 7S region and is excluded from Sephadex G200. The molecule has been visualized under the electron microscope as a particle 450 Å by 30 to 60 Å. Purified conglutinin is antigenic in rabbits and on immunoelectrophoresis migrates in the IgM area. Sage *et al.* (1963) reported that optical rotary dispersion data showed that conglutinin had a very low γ-helix content.

The stability of bovine conglutinin is shown in Table 1. Chymotrypsin causes inefficient and incomplete breakdown of conglutinin. Treatment of conglutinin with sodium dodecyl sulfate and mercaptoethanol indicated that it is composed of eight polypeptide chains held together by a combination of disulfide and weak intermolecular bonds (Lachmann, 1967). The reaction of conglutinin with fixed complement is calcium dependent. Conglutinin will react with zymosan and requires calcium for this reaction although no complement is needed. Absorption studies and mixed agglutination have shown that the site of reaction on fixed complement is the same as the site of reaction on zymosan. Both these reactions are inhibited by *N*-acetyl-D-glucoasmine. Conglutinin also reacts with agar although the agar must be molten to show the reaction clearly.

TABLE 1
The stability of conglutinin

Treatment	Stability
Heating (56°C for 30 minutes)	stable
0·1 M ammonia	stable
Reduction with 0·1 M mercaptoethanol followed by alkylation or reoxidation	stable
Reduction and alkylation followed by 1 M acetic acid	stable
Na dodecyl sulfate	stable
Pepsin at pH 3	stable
Neuraminidase	stable
Cellulase	stable
Na dodecyl sulfate and mercaptoethanol	unstable
Trypsin (0·5%, 37°C for 15 minutes)	unstable
Papain	unstable

B. REACTION OF CONGLUTININ WITH ADSORBED COMPLEMENT

Of the nine recognized components of the complement system, six have been separated from bovine serum: C1, C5, C6, C7, C8 and C9 (Barta *et al.*, 1976). Bovine complement is not markedly hemolytic when titrated in the usual system of sheep red blood cells sensitized with rabbit or horse antibody although it is a good conglutinating complement in this system. However, bovine complement is highly hemolytic for guinea pig erythrocytes sensitized with bovine antibody (Barta and Barta, 1972).

Activation and adsorption of the early acting components of complement, C1, C4, C2 and C3, are required for the reaction of immune complexes with conglutinin. The complement components C5 to C9 do not participate in the conglutination reaction although the presence of these components does not appear to interfere with the conglutination reaction.

The activation, fixation and subsequent fate of C3 are complex and involve a sequence of reactions. C3 in serum is activated by the complex C142 which forms as a result of antigen-antibody interaction. This complex splits the C3 molecule to form a small fragment, C3a, which is released into the surrounding fluid and a large fragment C3b which becomes attached to the cell membrane or antigen-antibody complex. The adsorbed C3b, in turn, is acted upon by the conglutinogen-activating factor (KAF or C3 inactivator) and is broken down into C3c and C3d which are no longer active in hemolysis or immune adherence. These C3 fragments form the substrate for the reaction with conglutinin (Lachmann and Muller-Eberhard, 1968). KAF is an enzyme acting on C3b to produce a configurational change which results in the bound C3 fragment acquiring the ability to react with conglutinin.

The conglutination reaction is usually demonstrated by aggregation of red blood cells which have been treated with (a) non-agglutinating, or subagglutinating amounts of antibody and (b) non-hemolytic, or sublytic amounts of complement. Conglutinin detects an alteration on the cell membrane brought about by the physical attachment of complement components — specifically the attachment of a fragment of C3.

C. PURIFICATION OF CONGLUTININ

1. *Zymosan method*

Conglutinin is relatively easy to purify from bovine serum by taking advantage of its reactivity with zymosan as was first demonstrated by Fesce (1961). In this procedure, normal bovine serum is first heated at 56°C for 30 minutes to destroy complement activity since, if this is not done, complement components also react with zymosan. The heat-inactivated normal bovine serum is mixed with zymosan and incubated for 30 to 60 minutes. The treated zymosan then is well washed to remove other serum proteins and the conglutinin is eluted from the washing zymosan by centrifugation from the conglutinin which is released into solution. The conglutinin may then be separated from other contaminating proteins by precipitation as a euglobulin by dialysis against phosphate buffer pH 5·4, ionic strength 0·02. To remove lipid contaminants the precipitate can be centrifuged at 20 000 g for one hour. A second cycle of adsorption and elution from zymosan results in further purification. The conglutinin prepared by this method gives a single line on immunoelectrophoresis against anti-bovine serum.

2. *Chromatographic method*

A second precedure for the purification of conglutinin has been described by Lachmann (1967). This method involves the treatment of normal bovine serum with 0·1 M mercaptoethanol and fractionation on Sephadex G200 equilibrated with a buffer containing 0·01 and 0·025 M mercaptoethanol. Conglutinin is present in the elution peak whereas all immunoglobulins are eluted later in the fractionation. The exclusive peak is precipitated as a euglobulin, washed and redissolved at physiological pH and ionic strength. This procedure removes most of the contaminating lipid. The conglutinin preparation is reoxidized by dialysis against saline through which air is bubbled.

Conglutinin may also be purified by a combination of these

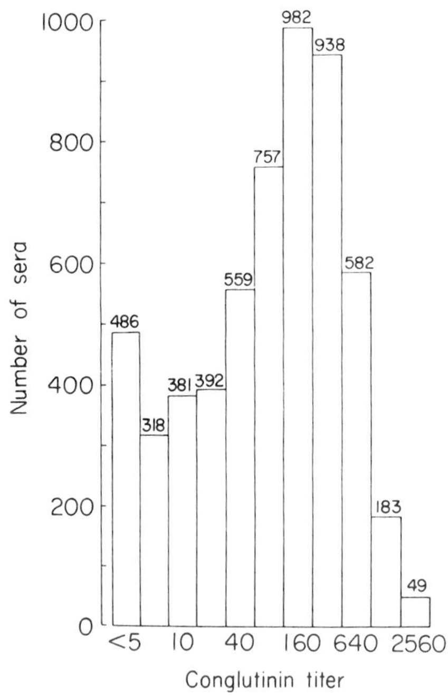

FIG. 1 Distribution of titers of conglutinin in sera from normal cattle.

A few cows calved without showing any marked changes in the serum level of conglutinating activity. Cows which had no significant change in serum conglutinin levels at one calving, did show the characteristic drop in levels at another calving time.

Serum titers of conglutinating activity in cows of different ages were very similar in mid to late gestation. However, the characteristic low levels of serum conglutinating activity at calving was lower in older cows and these older cows also required a longer period than younger cows to return to the levels of conglutinin which characterized the period of mid to late gestation (Ingram and Mitchell, 1970).

4. *Fetal and calf serum*

Detectable levels of conglutinin have been observed in sera obtained from some bovine fetuses as early as 80 to 90 days of gestation although the majority of fetuses of this age had no conglutinating activity in their serum. The average titer increases steadily during the second and third trimester of pregnancy and conglutinin was detected in sera from all fetuses over 160 days of age. At birth the average titer of conglutinin in the serum of calves was 5 (Barta, 1969; Ingram, 1972; Barta and Barta, 1973a). There was no correlation between the titer of conglutinating activity in a fetus and the titer in the dam.

After birth, calves had a decrease in the serum conglutinin titer with the lowest levels at about 5 to 10 days of age (Barta and Barta, 1973a). From this time the conglutinin titers rose slowly and reached a mean titer of 5 at about two months of age. This pattern of change in conglutinin levels in young calves is not affected by the feeding of colostrum. Although conglutinin can be demonstrated in some colostrum and milk (Ingram and Mitchell, 1970), it is apparent that the conglutinin is not absorbed through the calf intestine in an active form as occurs with immunoglobulins. The conglutinin titer in calf serum gradually rises with increasing age and titers typical of adult cattle are attained at about 6 to 12 months of age (Barta and Barta, 1973a; Kakoma and Kinyanjui, 1974).

III. Immunoconglutinins

A. MOLECULAR CHARACTERISTICS

Immunoconglutinins are antibodies which react with antigenic determinants exposed when complement components are fixed on an antigen-antibody complex but which do not react with non-activated complement components free in solution. The predominant immunoconglutinins which are demonstrated by the usual technique of immunoconglutinin titration (Coombs *et al.*, 1961) are of the IgM class. These immunoconglutinins sediment in the 19S region in zone centrifugation, are excluded from Sephadex G200, are mercaptoethanol sensitive and have IgM antigenicity. Immunoconglutinins do not require calcium ions for reaction with fixed complement components and are not inhibited by *N*-acetyl-D-glucosamine (Lachmann and Coombs, 1965; Bienenstock and Block, 1966).

However, not all immunoconglutinins are of the IgM class. Henson (1968) used non-agglutinating anti Forssman antibodies to fix complement and developed an anti-globulin test for the detection of immunoconglutinins of various Ig classes. All human and rabbit sera tested by this method had IgG immunoconglutinins with titers comparable to those of the IgM immunoconglutinins. Immunoconglutinins of the IgA class were also detected in three human sera.

B. REACTION OF IMMUNOCONGLUTININS WITH ADSORBED COMPLEMENT

In the classical complement activation process, C4 and C3 become firmly attached to erythrocyte membranes at or near the site of the antigen-antibody interaction. Quantitatively the C3 fragments form the largest number of bound components and the great majority of immunoconglutinins react with this bound C3.

The formation and decay of the bound complement complexes with which conglutinin and immunoconglutinin react were investigated by Ingram (1962h). He showed that there was a direct relationship between the amount of complement used to prepare the cells for conglutination and the sensitivity of the cells to conglutinin or immunoconglutinins. Maximum sensitivity was detected by allowing the horse complement to react with the antigen-antibody complex at 35°C for 5 to 10 minutes. At 5°C it required 180 minutes to attain maximum sensitivity. At 0°C horse complement showed only a slight reaction at 24 hours whereas guinea pig complement showed no reaction. The rate of decay of the complement complex with which conglutinin and immunoconglutinins react is also temperature dependent with a half life of about 60 minutes at 35°C and about 160 minutes at 25°C. The decay rate for the bound complement complex is different from those of the recognized complement intermediates of the hemolytic system.

Ingram (1962h) also studied the formation and decay of the conglutinated complex, i.e. the interaction of the bound complement complex with conglutinin or immunoconglutinins. The rate of the conglutination reaction was also temperature dependent and maximum reactions occurred at 35°C in 30 minutes. At 0°C reactions were observed at 30 minutes and maximum reaction was at 210 to 240 minutes. The optimum temperature for reaction with conglutinin was 25°C whereas optimum temperature for immunoconglutinins was 35°C. The rate of decay of the conglutinated complex was similar to the rate of decay of the complement complex with which conglutinin and immunoconglutinins react. It appears that reaction with conglutinin or immunoconglutinins does not protect the complement complex from decay. Lachmann and Liske (1966) confirmed that the stability of the complement complex, C1423, was much greater for conglutination than for hemolysis.

Lachmann (1966), using the sedimentation technique for the detection of immunoconglutinins, found that immunoconglutinins with a specificity for bound C4 were common in human serum. However, most immunoconglutinins were shown to react with bound C3 components. Henson (1968) using the antiglobulin technique confirmed that immunoconglutinins in rabbit and human serum have a specificity for either bound C4 or bound C3 and can be either IgM or IgG class. Bound C3 must be acted upon by KAF before it can react with conglutinin but KAF is not required for bound C3 to react with immunoconglutinins (Lachmann and Muller-Eberhard, 1968). Some immunoconglutinins react more strongly with bound C3 which has not been acted on by KAF whereas others react more strongly with bound C3 which has been acted on by KAF. Therefore, the specificities of conglutinin and immunoconglutinins for C3, while similar, are not identical.

Immunoconglutinins differ from conglutinin in that they do not react with zymosan, are not inhibited by *N*-acetyl-D-glucosamine or antrypolol and do not require calcium ions for activity. Some immunoconglutinins react with bound C4 but this reaction is relatively weak, possibly because of the low numbers of C4 molecules bound on antigen-antibody-complement complexes.

C. EXPERIMENTAL PRODUCTION OF IMMUNOCONGLUTININS

1. *Heterostimulation*

The production of immunoconglutinins in rabbits following the injection of sensitized bacteria which had adsorbed complement, then were washed free of unbound serum components was demonstrated by

Streng (1930). He suggested that complement was the specific stimulus for immunoconglutinin production and demonstrated that immunoconglutinins produced in this manner reacted with bound complement from several species of animals. He concluded that all complements tested had a common antigenic factor. Because of the similarity of the reaction to that of bovine conglutinin, he named this substance "immunokonglutinin".

Heterostimulation (Coombs and Coombs, 1953) refers to the technique of producing immunoconglutinins by the injection of complement from a heterologous species of animal adsorbed either on an antigen-antibody complex or on the surface of an active particle such as kaolin. Immunoconglutinins (heterostimulation) are readily produced in high titers by the injection of a suspension of sensitized bacteria or of kaolin which has been exposed to complement (Ingram 1962a). However, if the serum used as a source of complement has been heat-inactivated, 56°C for 45 minutes, no immunoconglutinins are produced.

Antisera produced by the injection of sensitized bacteria coated with complement may contain (1) immunoconglutinins, antibodies against bound complement components, (2) antibacterial antibodies, (3) antibodies against the proteins of the serum used for sensitization and (4) antibodies against the proteins of the serum used as a source of complement. Each of these antibody specifications are distinct and each can be specifically removed from the serum without affecting the other antibodies (Ingram, 1962a). Similarly antisera produced by the injection of activated kaolin treated with fresh serum and then washed will contain (1) immunoconglutinins and (2) antibodies against proteins of the serum used as a source of complement.

The route of inoculation has a pronounced effect on the production of immunoconglutinins by heterostimulation. In increasing order of efficacy for immunoconglutinin production the routes of inoculation are subcutaneous, intraperitoneal, intramuscular and intravenous (Ingram, 1962b). The intravenous route of inoculation is much more effective than other routes.

By combining the kaolin-complement complex with Freund's complete adjuvant, an increased and prolonged response occurs. In this instance, the intramuscular route of inoculation gives the highest and most persistent titers of immunoconglutinin although the attainment of peak titers is delayed as compared to intravenous inoculation (Ingram, 1962f).

The heterostimulation technique with bacteria provides a very high titer of immunoconglutinins but the serum also contains antibodies of other specificity which may be undesirable. By utilizing kaolin in this procedure some of these undesirable antibodies are avoided. Cortisone treatment during the series of inoculations does not suppress production of immunoconglutinins by heterostimulation (Ingram, 1962g). Immunoconglutinin serum produced by heterostimulation usually contains both IgM and IgG immunoconglutinins.

2. *Autostimulation*

Immunoconglutinins appear in the serum following most strong antigenic challenges. Wartiovaara (1932) found that inoculation of many antigens which had not been treated with complement stimulated the production of immunoconglutinins to a moderate degree. Coombs and Coombs (1953) suggested that in this instance it is the animal's own complement which is adsorbed *in vivo* to display the changed surface pattern and the production of immunoconglutinins is stimulated by the animal's own altered serum proteins. They proposed that the production of immunoconglutinins in response to antigenic challenges which do not involve injection of heterologous complement be referred to as autostimulation.

A number of bacteria, proteins, carbohydrates and other substances with biophysically active surfaces stimulate the production of immunoconglutinins by autostimulation. (Ingram, 1962c). Fesce *et al.* (1962) showed that rabbits injected with BCG produced high titers of immunoconglutinins. In general, particulate antigens were more effective than soluble antigens and enhanced immunoconglutinin responses followed a second course of injections. Multiple inoculations and the presence of complement-fixing antibodies in the animal at the time of inoculation resulted in greater immunoconglutinin responses and the intravenous route of inoculation was the most efficacious (Ingram, 1962d).

With the autostimulation technique, the incorporation of Freund's complete adjuvant results in reduced immunoconglutinin responses regardless of route of inoculation. Cortisone treatment during the period of inoculations markedly suppresses the production of immunoconglutinins by autostimulation (Ingram, 1962f,g).

The autostimulation technique can provide moderate to high titers of immunoconglutinins and the serum normally does not contain undesirable antibodies against heterologous serum proteins.

3. *Persistence of serum immunoconglutinins*

In experimental stimulation of the production of immunoconglutinins, the immunoconglutinin titers reach a peak a few days after the last inoculation then usually decreased quite rapidly and returned to the normal low levels within four weeks (Ingram, 1962b,d). This occurred in both autostimulation and heterostimulation. However, rabbits inoculated with the kaolin-complement complex in adjuvant maintained high titers of immunoconglutinins for 4 to 5 months and rabbits inoculated intramuscularly with this material reached peak titers of immunoconglutinins at 8 weeks and had very high titers for over 6 months.

D. PURIFICATION OF IMMUNOCONGLUTININS

Some degree of purification of immunoconglutinins by dissociation of IgM antibodies at low pH was described by Lachmann (1967). With this technique, an antigen-antibody precipitate is prepared at optimal proportions and is exposed to complement then mixed with serum containing immunoconglutinins. The conglutinated complex is washed, then eluted at pH 4·5 to dissociate the bulk of the immunoconglutinins without dissolving the precipitate. This procedure can achieve a 50- 100-fold purification.

A similar technique for the purification of immunoconglutinins was developed by Quinn (1970) and this procedure is illustrated schematically in Fig. 4. *Salmonella typhimurium* was used as antigen and an antiserum prepared in rabbits was used to sensitize the bacteria. The sensitized bacteria were washed, then exposed to a serum containing complement for 30 minutes at 37°C. The bacteria were washed three times and resuspended in saline. A 2 ml volume of these complement-coated bacteria was treated with 0·2 ml of 2% gluteraldehyde and washed again. This complex was exposed to the serum containing immunoconglutinins at room temperature for 1 to 2 hours, then washed. The immunoconglutinins were eluted by exposure to glycine HCl buffer pH 2·1 and were separated by centrifugation.

A variation of this procedure utilizing column chromatography was also developed (Quinn, 1970) with bovine serum albumen as antigen instead of bacteria. The soluble antigen-antibody complex was prepared at optimal proportions and resuspended in veronal buffer to give 4 mg of precipitate per ml. The antigen-antibody complex was exposed to serum containing complement for 30 minutes at 37°C then washed three times and resuspended to approximately 4 mg ml^{-1}.

The antigen-antibody-complement complex was treated with 0·2 ml of 2% gluteraldehyde per ml of suspension. The complexes were washed again, then mixed with an equal amount of Sephadex G25

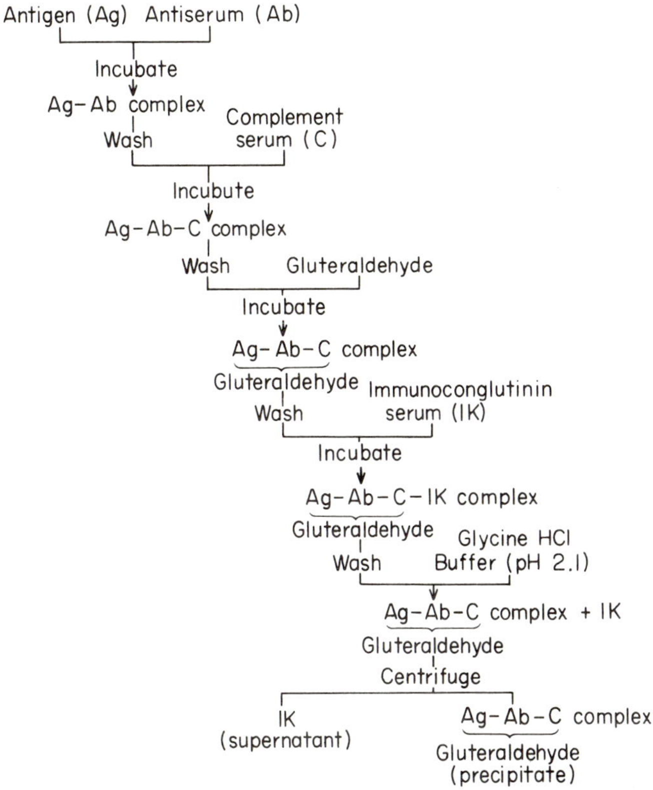

FIG. 4 Schematic procedure for purification of immunoconglutinins.

(up to 200 ml of each). In preparing the chromatography tube, Sephadex G50 was added to a vertically mounted tube as a slurry and allowed to settle to form a layer a few centimetres deep. The mixture of the immune complex and Sephadex G25 was poured into the column and allowed to settle. The immunoconglutinin serum (10 ml) was applied to the column and allowed to enter the gel. The outlet was closed and the serum held in contact with the gel-immune complex mixture for up to 75 minutes. The serum was washed through the column with veronal buffer and the optical density of the eluate was recorded at 280 μ. When all unbound protein had been washed from the gel, 0·2 M glycine HCl buffer pH 2·1 was added and fractions were collected. Two peaks of activity were found in the eluate. The collected fractions were pooled and concentrated by dialysis against Ficoll. Immunodiffusion and immunoelectrophoresis showed that the eluates were gammaglobulins and with heterostimulated immunoconglutinins were primarily IgG.

The column was washed with veronal buffer and could be re-used repeatedly over several days. It seems that in this procedure the bound complement was not denatured by gluteraldehyde treatment of the antigen-antibody-complement complex but the bound complement configuration with which immunoconglutinins react was preserved.

The latter procedure can be utilized to purify bovine conglutinin by using either the glycine HCl buffer or Na_2EDTA for elution. However, for the purification of bovine conglutinin it is preferable to use an antigen other than bovine serum albumen since the antibody may react with components in the bovine serum.

IV. Biological significance of conglutinin and immunoconglutinins

A. CONGLUTININ AND IMMUNOCONGLUTININS IN VARIOUS ANIMAL SPECIAL AND BODY FLUIDS

1. *Conglutinin*

Conglutinating activity has been observed in the serum of most animal species (Coombs *et al.*, 1961) but the differentiation between conglutinin and immunoconglutinin was based largely on whether it was in normal or immune serum. Lachmann (1962) clearly differentiated the two proteins and the usual screening method now employed is based on the requirement of conglutinin for calcium. The easiest method for distinguishing these two proteins is to mix the conglutinated complex with EDTA — only conglutination due to immunoconglutinins remains aggregated.

Conglutinin has been reported in cattle and a number of African ruminants including the African buffalo, water buck, Uganda kob, Kenya kob, dik-dik, topi and Jackson's hartebeest (Lachmann, 1967). Mittal and Jaiswal (1973) recorded conglutinin in India buffalo and Zebu cattle and Bhatnagar (1976) confirmed the presence of conglutinin in the India buffalo. Kakoma and Kinyanjui (1974) reported that higher and more consistent titers of conglutinin were present in Zebu cattle than in Hereford cattle.

A conglutinin has been reported to be present in newborn swine but not in adult swine (Tlaskalova and Barta, 1968; Barta *et al.*, 1970). This swine conglutinin is unusual in that it has a molecular weight similar to IgM but is not sensitive to 2-mercaptoethanol. It requires calcium ions for its activity but does not react with zymosan nor is it inhibited by *N*-acetyl-D-glucosamine.

Conglutinating activity in milk was detected irregularly by Ingram and Mitchell (1970) but it was not determined whether this was conglutinin or immunoconglutinins. Cerny *et al.* (1970) reported that in cattle the conglutinin titer in lymph from the efferent vessels of the supra-mammary lymph node was one half to one quarter the titer in blood.

2. *Immunoconglutinins*

Immunoconglutinins, as well as conglutinin, have been demonstrated in the serum of European and Canadian cattle (Barta and Barta, 1973b) and in Zebu cattle (Mittal and Jaiswal, 1973; Kakoma and Kinyanjui, 1974) as well as in buffalo (Mittal and Jaiswal, 1973).

Only immunoconglutinins have been found in the serum of mice, rabbits, guinea pigs, dog, sheep, goat, camel, adult swine, chickens and man (Bienenstock and Bloch, 1966; Lachmann, 1967; Mittal and Jaiswal, 1973; Mittal and Ingram, 1974). No conglutinating activity has been demonstrated in the serum of horses, donkeys nor mules.

An unusual immunoconglutinin which occurs in human saliva has been described by Lachmann *et al.* (1972). They were of the IgA class and were found in all human saliva examined. The salivary immunoconglutinins require calcium for their activity but they do not react with zymosan and are not inhibited by *N*-acetyl-D-glucosamine. These immunoconglutinins were not destroyed by 2-mercaptoethanol and they had the distinctive characteristic of being inhibited by fresh normal serum. Williams *et al.* (1975) reported that high titers of salivary immuno-conglutinins occur in parotid, sublingual and submaxillary saliva of most human subjects but that lower titers are present in mixed saliva, probably due to neutralization by C3 arising from crevicular fluid.

B. EFFECTS OF INFECTION ON SERUM TITERS OF CONGLUTININ AND IMMUNOCONGLUTININS

1. *Conglutinin*

The level of conglutinating activity in the serum of healthy and sick cattle was studied by von Jettmar (1923). He found that the conglutinating activity of bovine serum decreased during infections with *Mycobacterium tuberculosis* and that it returned to normal levels when the cattle recovered.

During the study of two herds of dairy cows to find the fluctuations of serum conglutinin levels (Ingram and Barnum, 1965; Ingram and Mitchell, 1971b) an accurate record of occurrence of disease was maintained. Minor or local infections, such as mild forms of mastitis or foot rot, did not have a significant effect on the level of serum conglutinating activity. Routine tuberculin tests also did not cause any change in conglutinin in the serum. On the other hand, acute systemic infections, such as metritis and pneumonia, caused marked decrease in titers of conglutinin: the mean titers dropped from about 80 to less than 5. By approximately four weeks after infection the titers had returned to normal levels. In cows which aborted, the pattern of conglutinin levels in the serum was similar to that occurring during and after normal calving.

In adult cows, the titers of conglutinating activity in the serum was not altered by mild or localized infections but abortion and acute systemic infections caused significant decreases in the level of serum conglutinin. This decrease was not due to the formation of inhibitory substances in the serum (Ingram and Mitchell, 1971b).

The passive transfer of conglutinin to the serum of mice was reported by Ingram (1959a) and the conglutinating activity of the recipient was detectable for 10 to 12 days. However, if the mice with passively transferred conglutinin were challenged with *Salm. typhimurium*, the conglutinating activity in their serum dropped to undetectable levels within 4 to 8 hours indicating that the conglutinin was involved in the reaction to the bacteria in infected mice.

2. *Immunoconglutinins*

The passive transfer of rabbit immunoconglutinins to the serum of mice was also demonstrated by Ingram (1959a). These mice also showed a rapid drop in serum conglutinating activity following challenge with *Salm. typhimurium*. Similarly, Ingram *et al.* (1959) reported that rabbits which had immunoconglutinins in the serum showed a drop in the serum level of conglutinating activity within a few hours after experimental infection with *Salm. typhimurium* or *Listeria monocytogenes*. Similar responses in rabbits injected intravenously with killed bacteria were observed by Ingram (1962e).

Marks and Coombs (1957) reported that the level of immunoconglutinins was raised in infectious diseases of man and in other disease where an antigen-antibody interaction was incriminated in the etiology. In extending this observation to experimental infections of laboratory animals Ingram *et al.* (1959) and Ingram (1965a,b) showed that immunoconglutinins were produced in experimental animals following challenge with a number of bacterial, viral or trypanosomal microorganisms. In experimental infections the highest titers of immunoconglutinin were produced in response to Trypanosome infections. The infections and diseases which have been reported to stimulate immunoconglutinin production in animals are listed in Table 2 and the list for man is shown in Table 3. These data indicate that a broad range of antigenic challenges can stimulate production of immunoconglutinins. The low level of immunoconglutinins present in the serum of some of the animals (Ingram *et al.*, 1959) and in the serum of man (Marks and Coombs, 1957; Jasser and Bragiel, 1962; Ingram, 1974) appear to be a response to continuous natural exposure to low levels of antigenic stimulation.

C. ANTIMICROBIAL ACTIVITIES OF CONGLUTININ AND IMMUNOCONGLUTININS

An antibacterial effect of conglutinin was first demonstrated by Ingram (1959b) when he showed that mice injected with conglutinin preparations had higher survival rates following subsequent challenge with *Salm. typhimurium*. Using conglutinin purified by the zymosan method, Fesce and De Zulian (1961) showed similarly higher survival rate in mice challenged with *Salm. cholerasuis* and *Escherichia coli.* Ingram (1959a) reported that the rate of clearance of *Salm. typhimurium* from the blood circulation was markedly enhanced in mice which had been injected one day previously with conglutinin.

Subcutaneous inoculation of mice with rabbit immunoconglutinins followed by intraperitoneal challenge one day later resulted in enhanced rate of survival following infection with a number of Gram-positive and Gram-negative bacteria (Ingram, 1959b). The rate of survival and the rate of blood clearance of bacteria were both higher with immunoconglutinins than with conglutinin-treated mice. Ingram (1959a) also showed that in immunoconglutinin-treated mice there was enhanced killing of bacteria in the liver and spleen.

The effect of immunoconglutinins on bactericidal activity of serum was investigated by Mittal and Ingram (1969) who showed that immunoconglutinin rabbit serum had a higher titer of bactericidal activity than normal rabbit serum (Table 4). Utilizing a different technique they also showed a marked decrease in the number of sur-

TABLE 2
Diseases of animals characterized by production of immunoconglutinins

Disease or infection	Species	Reference
Salmonella typhimurium	rabbit, mouse	Ingram *et al.* (1959); Ingram (1965b)
Salmonella paratyphi	rabbit	Fesce *et al.* (1962)
Salmonella enteriditis	mouse	Ingram (1965a)
Pasteurella septica	rabbit, mouse	Ingram *et al.* (1959)
Pasteurella multocida	mouse	Ingram (1965a)
Pasteurella pseudotuberculosis	mouse	Ingram (1965a)
Klebsiella pneumoniae	mouse	Ingram *et al.* (1959); Ingram (1965a)
Escheria coli	mouse	Ingram *et al.* (1959)
Bordetella bronchiseptica	dog	Ingram (1963, 1965a)
Brucella abortus S19	mouse	Ingram (1965b)
Staphylococcus aureus	mouse	Ingram *et al.* (1959); Ingram (1965a)
Streptococcus pneumoniae	mouse	Ingram *et al.* (1959); Ingram (1965a)
Streptococcus pyogenes	mouse	Ingram (1965a)
Streptococcus agalactiae	mouse	Ingram (1965a)
Listeria monocytogenes	rabbit, mouse	Ingram *et al.* (1959)
Erysipelothrix rhusiopathiae	mouse	Ingram (1965a)
Mycobacterium tuberculosis	rabbit	Ingram *et al.* (1959)
Mycobacterium tuberculosis (human)	rabbit	Ingram (1965b)
Mycobacterium tuberculosis (avian)	rabbit	Ingram (1965b)
BCG	rabbit	Fesce *et al.* (1962)
Rickettsia burneti	guinea pig	Ingram *et al.* (1959)
Rickettsia phagocytophia	calf	Lachmann and Coombs (1965)
Contagious Bovine Pleuropneumoniae	cow	Kakoma and Masiga (1973)
Western Equine Encephalomyelitis virus	rabbit	Ingram *et al.* (1959)
Hammon Reeves virus	rabbit	Ingram *et al.* (1959)
Murray Valley Encephalitis virus	rabbit	Ingram *et al.* (1959)
Aedes trivittatus virus	rabbit	Ingram *et al.* (1959)
Infectious canine hepatitis virus	dog	Ingram (1963)
Canine distemper virus	dog	Ingram (1963)
Trypanosoma brucei	rabbit	Ingram *et al.* (1959)
Trypanosoma brucei	rabbit, cat, mouse	Ingram and Soltys (1960)
Dictycaulus filaria	lamb	Tewari *et al.* (1972)
Silicosis	rat	Jones and Heppelston (1961)

TABLE 3
Diseases of man characterized by production of immunoconglutinins

Diseases of infection	References
Acute bacterial infections	Marks and Coombs (1957)
Lobar pneumonia	Marks and Coombs (1957)
Bronchopneumonia	Marks and Coombs (1957)
Acute Streptococcal tonsilitis	Marks and Coombs (1957)
Acute appendicitis	Marks and Coombs (1957)
Streptococcal septicemia	Marks and Coombs (1957)
Acute meningitis	Marks and Coombs (1957)
Acute viral respiratory disease	Rytel and Lytle (1973)
Chronic bacterial infections	Marks and Coombs (1957)
Tuberculosis	Marks and Coombs (1957)
Bronchiectasis	Marks and Coombs (1957)
Chronic visceral abscess	Marks and Coombs (1957)
Subacute bacterial endocarditis	Marks and Coombs (1957); Williams and Kunkel (1962)
Acute viral infections	Marks and Coombs (1957)
Poliomyelitis	Marks and Coombs (1957)
Rheumatic disorders	Marks and Coombs (1957)
Acute active rheumatoid arthritis	Marks and Coombs (1957)
"Burnt-out" rheumatism	Marks and Coombs (1957)
Acute rheumatic fever	Marks and Coombs (1957)
Mitral stenosis	Marks and Coombs (1957)
Ankylosing spondylitis	Marks and Coombs (1957); Bienenstock and Block (1967)
Rheumatoid arthritis	Caspari and Ball (1962); Bienenstock and Block (1967)
Systemic lupus erytematosus	Marks and Coombs (1957); Bienenstock and Block (1967); Lachmann (1967)
Hodgkin's disease	Merucci *et al.* (1975)
Hashimoto's thyroiditis	Caspary and Ball (1962); Bienenstock and Block (1967)
Sjogren syndrome	Bienenstock and Block (1967)
Myasthesia gravis	Bienenstock and Block (1967)
Acute nephritis	Marks and Coombs (1957); Williams and Kunkel (1962)
Nephrotic syndrome	Ngu and Blackett (1970)
Renal transplant rejection	Ngu *et al.* (1971)
Kala-azar	Woodruff *et al.* (1972)
Malaria	Topley *et al.* (1973)
African trypanosomiasis	Lachmann (1967)
Anaphylactoid purpura	Marks and Coombs (1957)
Primary gout	Bienenstock and Block (1967)
Silicosis	Pernis *et al.* (1959)
Amyloidosis	Muckle (1968)
Myelomatosis	Muckle (1968)

TABLE 4
Comparative bactericidal activity of rabbit serum containing immunoconglutinins

Microorganism	Bactericidal titer of serum: Normal	Immunoconglutinin
Esch. coli	0	16
Salm. typhimurium	2	16
Salm. cholerasuis	2	32
Bacillus sp.	8	32
List. monocytogenes	4	32
Candida albicans	0	4

Normal serum: conglutinating titer 0.
Immunoconglutinin serum: conglutinating titer 640 (produced by heterostimulation with kaolin coated with horse complement).

TABLE 5
Bactericidal activity of normal and immunoconglutinin rabbit serum

Microorganism	Serum	Number of tests	Mean percentage surviving bacteria: 3 hours	6 hours
Salm. typhimurium	NS	3	48	94
	IKS	3	7	9
List. monocytogenes	NS	6	>100	>100
	IKS	6	10	70

NS, normal serum: conglutinating titer 0.
IKS, immunoconglutinin serum: conglutinating titer 640 (produced by heterostimulation with kaolin coated with horse complement).

TABLE 6
Enhancement of phagocytosis in the mouse peritoneal cavity by immunoconglutinins

Minutes after challenge	*Esch. coli* strain 078:K80		3662	
	NS[a]	IKS	NS	IKS
30	14[b]	85	27	88
60	31	85	61	100
120	29	77	29	23

[a] Injected subcutaneously 24 hours before intraperitoneal challenge.
[b] Percentage of peritoneal macrophages with ingested bacteria — mean of 3 tests.
NS, normal rabbit serum: conglutinating titer 0.
IKS, immunoconglutinin rabbit serum: conglutinating titer 640 (produced by heterostimulation with kaolin coated with horse complement).

surviving bacteria exposed to immunoconglutinins as opposed to normal rabbit serum (Table 5). Appropriate absorptions of these sera showed that natural antibodies probably had a role in this bactericidal activity and that complement was essential for the demonstration of any bactericidal activity.

D. ENHANCEMENT OF PHAGOCYTOSIS BY IMMUNOCONGLUTININS

The *in vivo* enhancement of phagocytosis by immunoconglutinins was investigated by Mittal (1970) utilizing the technique of Medearis and Kenny (1968). In this procedure the effect of injection of normal serum or immunoconglutinin serum on phagocytosis by macrophages in the peritoneal cavity of the mouse is measured. Table 6 shows that in normal mice previously injected with immunoconglutinins there was a significant increase in the number of peritoneal macrophages which were active in phagocytosis of two virulent strains of *Esch. coli*. By two hours after challenge with strain 3662, very few bacteria remained in the peritoneal cavity of immunoconglutinin-treated mice, whereas considerable numbers of strain 078:K80 were still present after two hours.

To determine whether natural antibodies in the normal or immunoconglutinin rabbit serum were important in this phagocytic activity, both sera were absorbed with *Esch. coli* 078:K80 and these absorbed sera were then utilized in a series of phagocytosis experiments. Table 7 illustrates that absorption of the normal rabbit serum reduced the phagocytosis, while removal of antibacterial antibodies from the

TABLE 7
Effect of absorption of serum on phagocytosis promoting activity in the mouse peritoneal cavity

Minutes after challenge	Rabbit serum[a]			
	NS	IKS	Abs NS	Abs IKS
30	22[b]	76	5	82
60	46	80	7	62
120	56	82	63	100

[a] Injected subcutaneously 24 hours before intraperitoneal challenge.
[b] Percentage of peritoneal macrophages with ingested bacteria — mean of 6 tests.
NS, normal rabbit serum: conglutinating titer 0.
IKS, immunoconglutinin rabbit serum: conglutinating titer 640 (produced by heterostimulation with kaolin coated with horse complement).
Challenge was *Esch. coli* strain 078:K80.

immunoconglutinin serum did not significantly alter its effect on phagocytosis in the mouse peritoneal cavity.

The *in vitro* phagocytosis-enhancing effect of immunoconglutinins was reported by Parappally and Ingram (1973). They found that phagocytosis of Gram-negative bacteria in coverslip cultures of peritoneal macrophages was increased by serum containing immunoconglutinins (Table 8). The enhanced phagocytosis was an effect of an increase in the opsonic index. These data indicate that immunoconglutinins potentiate the opsonic activity of serum.

TABLE 8
Enhancement of *in vitro* phagocytosis by immunoconglutinins

Bacteria	Serum	Phagocytic index	Opsonic index	P	Percentage phagocytosis	P
Esch. coli	3662 NS	1·66 ± 0·30	2·88	0·001	40·55 ± 4·01	0·001
	IKS	4·78 ± 0·85			67·33 ± 4·02	
Salm. typhimurium	NS	1·76 ± 0·27	2·61	0·02	36·28 ± 1·90	0·005
	IKS	4·59 ± 0·90			60·26 ± 3·22	
Esch. coli	S16 NS	1·57 ± 0·29	2·27	0·001	39·58 ± 4·23	0·02
		3·56 ± 0·25			59·59 ± 5·59	

NS, normal rabbit serum: conglutinating titer 0.
IKS, immunoconglutinin rabbit serum: conglutinin titer 1024 (produced by heterostimulation with kaolin coated with horse complement).

The results of the research on resistance enhancement by immunoconglutinins and on bactericidal and phagocytic activity indicate that immunoconglutinins play a significant role in enhancing resistance of the animal host against a broad variety of bacteria.

E. IMMUNOCONGLUTININS IN VIRAL INFECTIONS

Although immunoconglutinins are produced during a number of viral infections, very little research has been carried out on the influence of immunoconglutinins in viral diseases. Joshi *et al.* (1965) reported that immunoconglutinins protect tissue cultures against the cytopathic effect of a number of viruses; infectious bovine rhinotracheitis, equine herpes virus type 1 and swine enteroviruses. In these experiments, tissue cultures were grown into even sheets of cells adherent to the glass surface, then the culture medium was replaced by a mixture of culture medium and rabbit serum: either normal serum or immunoconglutinin serum. After a period, this mixture was replaced with normal nutrient medium and the culture was infected. The treatment of the cell cultures with immunoconglutinins delayed and/or reduced the development of cytopathic effects of the virus. These results were interpreted as a protective effect of immunoconglutinins against virus infections.

V. Conglutination as a serological tool

A. DIRECT CONGLUTINATION

Direct conglutination is the reaction in which an antigen is aggregated by the action of antibody, complement and conglutinin to bring about a visible clumping of the immune complex. This technique has been utilized primarily to aggregate particulate antigens although the reaction can be used to increase flocculation in immune precipitating systems (Coombs *et al.*, 1961).

Direct conglutination has been used in a number of blood group studies. Braend (1959) compared the direct conglutination reaction with the hemolytic test usually used to detect red blood cell antigens in cattle and found good agreement between the two methods. Sellei (1975) reported that with cattle red cells the degree of conglutinability was influenced by the particular blood group antigen-antibody combination. Franks (1959) employed the direct conglutination reaction in blood group studies in the horse. He found the reaction to be more sensitive than the hemolytic test but the red cells from some horses failed to conglutinate or to hemolyse although the presence of antigens could be demonstrated by an antiglobulin test. These differences in reaction were apparently a quantitative effect of antigen expression.

The detection of human blood group antibodies by direct conglutination, using either conglutinin or immunoconglutinins, was investigated by Mollison and Polley (1960). They reported that, provided a suitable complement was used, positive conglutination was obtained with all human sera which had been shown by other methods to contain complement-binding antibodies. When human complement was used, good reactions were obtained with rabbit immunoconglutinins but no reaction was obtained with conglutinin nor human immunoconglutinins.

The direct conglutination reaction utilizing sheep red blood cells and horse complement was used by Soulsby (1958) to measure the rise in heterophile antibodies in swine following infection with *Ascaria lumbricoides*. Barber (1955) used direct conglutination to detect antibodies to *Rick. burneti* and found that, with some human sera, the reaction was more sensitive than the hemolytic complement fixation test.

Bacterial antigens can also be conglutinated by the direct conglutination reaction (Coombs *et al.*, 1961). With the variety of techniques now available for the demonstration of antigens and antibodies the application of the direct conglutination test is not common.

In a study of the supplementing factor, Rose *et al.* (1974) showed that the modified card agglutination test for the detection of bovine anaplasmosis is a direct conglutinin reaction which is dependent on the presence of complement and conglutinin. The supplementing factor in the normal bovine serum is absorbed by zymosan, inactivated by Na_2EDTA and inhibited by *N*-acetyl-D-glucosamine and it was concluded that this factor is conglutinin.

B. THE CONGLUTINATING COMPLEMENT ABSORPTION TEST

Streng (1910) initially developed the conglutinating complement absorption test as an alternative to the hemolytic complement fixation test. Hole and Coombs (1947a,b,c) revived interest in the test and demonstrated that with many antigens, it is a sensitive and reliable technique. Coombs *et al.* (1961) reviewed the advantages and applications of the test and showed that it was the test-of-choice for a number of antigen-antibody systems. With this technique, serum from a variety of animal species can be used as a source of complement but horse complement is usually the most efficacious.

Stoker and Marion (1950) showed that the conglutinating complement absorption test was a sensitive technique for the diagnosis of influenza infection in man and Stoker *et al.* (1950) applied the test to the detection of antibodies against a number of viruses. Pautrizel *et al.* (1964) investigated the test for the diagnosis of schistosomiasis. They found that the test demonstrated anti-schistosome antibodies in the sera of all patients but interpretation was sometimes difficult because of a zone phenomenon.

In animal disease, Rice *et al.* (1952) recommended that the conglutinating complement absorption test be used as a supplementary test for the detection of antibodies in early *Bruc. abortus* infections since it was more sensitive than the routine testing procedures. Engelhard and Millian (1964) devised a modification of the conglutinating complement absorption test for the detection of antibodies to the hog cholera virus in pigs. Using this technique, antibody production was detected in vaccinated swine and in swine in contact with pigs which had been vaccinated with a live virus vaccine as well as in swine vaccinated with a bovine virus diarrhea vaccine. In these tests the prozone phenomenon was negligible. Norcross and Poppensiek (1961) adapted the conglutinating complement absorption test to the detection of antibodies to foot-and-mouth disease virus. The test was especially valuable for swine sera since it avoided a problem of procomplementary activity and with bovine serum it was more sensitive than the hemolytic complement fixation test. Singh (1972) showed that buffalo bulls vaccinated with rinderpest vaccine developed serum antibodies demonstrable by the conglutinating complement absorption test and the presence of these antibodies was associated with resistance to challenge infection with rinderpest.

The conglutinating complement absorption test is a versatile technique for the detection of antibodies to a great variety of infectious agents. In many antigen–antibody systems it is more sensitive than the hemolytic complement fixation test and it has the advantage that complements from a variety of species of animals are effective in the test thus adding to its flexibility.

C. OTHER REACTIONS OF CONGLUTININ AND IMMUNOCONGLUTININS

The mixed conglutination reaction utilizing purified conglutinin or bovine serum was developed and described by Lachmann *et al.* (1965). This is a mixed aggregation reaction of a cell or other structure reacting with an indicator particle to allow the recognition of antigens on various members of a mixed population. The technique may allow demonstration of a particular reactive area on a cell. The reaction detects complement fixing antibodies to antigens on cell surfaces and has been utilized to detect H-2 antibodies in the mouse, organ-specific isoantibodies in the mouse, Forssman antigen on tissue culture cells and auto-antibodylike factor in normal guinea pigs which reacts with their own testicular tissue.

Tomopoulos (1970) found that conglutinin protected sheep red blood cells from lysis by streptolysin 0 and suggested that the protection of red blood cells from lysis may be a natural function of conglutinin.

Conglutinin has been utilized to develop a solid phase radioimmune assay for complement-fixing immune complexes in human serum (Eisenberg and Theofilopoulous, 1976). Conglutinin bound to CNBr-activated agarose has been shown to specifically retain appreciable quantities of complement-fixing immune complexes from sera and permits their quantitative elution under relatively mild conditions with 0·01 M EDTA or 0·01 M *N*-acetyl-D-glucosamine. This technique may provide a powerful tool for investigation of immune complex diseases.

The serological activities of immunoconglutinins were reported by Ingram (1969). As with many other antibodies, immunoconglutinins, reacting with their specific antigen of bound complement components, can bring about agglutination or precipitation, complement fixation and hemolysis, enhanced bactericidal and phagocytic activities. Immunoconglutinins can be specifically absorbed from serum. The reaction of immunoconglutinins with autologous or isologous complement has been demonstrated repeatedly (Ingram, 1959a, 1962e, 1969; Lachmann and Coombs, 1965; Henson, 1968). It would appear that immunoconglutinins are antibodies which enhance a number of *in vivo* and *in vitro* reactions and increase the resistance of the host to a wide variety of infectious agents.

The role of immunoconglutinins in the *in vivo* and *in vitro* destruction of red blood cells was investigated by Tedesco and Corrocher (1972). They showed that in immunoconglutinin-producing rabbits which were complement-depleted, injection of red blood cells with fixed C43 resulted in minor sequestration of the cells and their return to the circulation in 20 to 30 minutes, whereas in the normal controls such cells returned to the circulation over a period of 3 to 4 hours. In the complement-depleted animals red blood cells with fixed C43 formed rosettes around Kupffer cells whereas cells with fixed C43 IK did not. This suggested that in this situation immunoconglutinins interferred with the interaction between C3 and C3-receptors on Kupffer cells. Injections of red cells with fixed C43 and with C43 IK into rabbits producing immunoconglutinins and with an active complement system resulted in marked lysis and erythrophagocytosis. Both *in vivo* and *in vitro* results indicated that bound immunoconglutinins caused the fixation of more C4 and C3 if these components were available. It was concluded that immunoconglutinins normally have an amplifying effect on complement fixation *in vivo* and potentiate the ability of complement to bring about red blood cell destruction.

In an investigation into the role of complement in the induction of immunological responses, Pepys (1976) found that the form of C3 which is recognized by lymphocyte complement receptors resembles the form of C3 with which immunoconglutinins react. In mice actively producing immunoconglutinins there was a significant suppression of the T-dependent, but not the T-independent, antibody responses. Pepys suggested that immunoconglutinins may have a regulatory role in a cooperative antibody formation.

VI. Summary

Conglutinin is a protein normally present in bovine serum which has a large molecular weight but is not an immunoglobulin although it can react specifically with bound C3 which has been acted upon by KAF. Conglutinin has antibody-like activities in that it can cause clumping of antigens which have reacted with complement and it is capable of activating complement fixation under appropriate conditions.

Conglutinin is produced during fetal life of the calf and most adult cattle have a titer of between 40 to 640. The serum level of conglutinin shows a seasonal variation and there is usually a marked decrease in the level of conglutinin at about the time of calving. Severe infections also cause a drop in the serum titer of conglutinin. Conglutinin appears to play a part in resistance of the animal against infectious diseases.

Immunoconglutinins are antibodies which may be induced by, and react with, autologous bound complement components. They are chiefly directed against C3 but some may be directed against other fixed complement components, especially C4. Immunoconglutinins have been demonstrated in the IgM, IgG and IgA classes of immunoglobulins and react with autologous, isologous or heterologous complements. The antigenic specificities with which immunoconglutinins react are shared by the complement systems of man and many species of animals.

Immunoconglutinins are produced in many animal species in response to infection or any strong and repeated antigenic stimulations. Production of immunoconglutinins has been demonstrated in man in many pathological conditions which are associated with antigen-antibody interactions. Immunoconglutinins enhance complement fixation and bactericidal activity of serum and increase phagocytosis of foreign antigenic particles. Immunoconglutinins increase resistance to infectious diseases and may aid the body in elimination of foreign particles and materials.

Conglutination is a useful serological tool for the detection and identification of a variety of antigens and antibodies. It has proved valuable as a sensitive and specific test for the diagnosis of numerous infectious diseases and newer techniques are showing its potential for the investigation of diseases such as those caused, or complicated, by immune complex formation.

References

BARBER, H. (1955). *J. Hyg., Camb.* **53**, 63-75.
BARTA, O. (1969). Ph.D. Thesis, University of Guelph, Guelph, Canada.
BARTA, O. and BARTA, V. (1972). *J. Immun. Meth.* **1**, 363-374.
BARTA, O. and BARTA, V. (1973a). *Zentbl. vet med. B,* **20**, 57-70.
BARTA, O. and BARTA, V. (1973b). *Zentbl. vet Med. B,* **20**, 71-82.
BARTA, O., BARTA, V., MINIATS, O. P. and INGRAM, D. G. (1970). *J. Immun.* **105**, 350-354.
BARTA, O., NELSON, R. A. and KUO, C. Y. (1976). *Immun. Commun.* **5**, 75-86.
BHATNAGAR, R. N. (1976). Ph.D. Thesis, Agra University, Agra, India.
BIENENSTOCK, J. and BLOCH, K. J. (1966). *J. Immun.* **96**, 637-645.
BIENENSTOCK, J. and BLOCH, K. H. (1967). *Arth. Rheumat.* **10**, 187-198.
BLOMFIELD, A. M., COOMBS, R. R. A. and HOLE, N. H. (1949). *J. Hyg., Camb.* **47**, 132-141.
BLOMFIELD, A. M., COOMBS, R. R. A. and HOLE, N. H. (1950). *J. Hyg., Camb.* **48**, 77-95.
BORDET, J. and GAY, F. P. (1906). *Annls Inst. Pasteur,* **20**, 467-498.
BORDET, J. and STRENG, O. (1909). *Zentbl. Bact. Parasitkde Abt. I Orig.* **49**, 260-276.
BRAEND, M. (1959). "Blood Groups of Cattle in Norway: Serological and Genetical Studies". Skandinavisk Bladforlag.
CASPARY, E. A. and BALL, E. J. (1962). *Br. Med. J.* **2**, 1514-1515.
CERNY, L., CELER, V. and JELINKOVA, E. (1970). *Zentbl. vet Med. B,* **17**, 977-981.
COOMBS, A. M. and COOMBS, R. R. A. (1953). *J. Hyg., Camb.* **51**, 509-531.
COOMBS, R. R. A. (1947). Ph.D. Thesis, University of Cambridge, Cambridge, England.
COOMBS, R. R. A. and HOLE, N. H. (1948). *J. Hyg., Camb.* **46**, 296-310.
COOMBS, R. R. A., COOMBS, A. M. and INGRAM, D. G. (1961). "The Serology of Conglutination and Its Relation to Disease". Blackwell, Oxford.
EISENBERG, R. and THEOFILOPOULOS, A. N. (1976). *Fedn Proc. Fedn Am. Socs exp. Biol.* **35**, 670.
ENGELHARD, W. E. and MILLIAN, S. J. (1964). *Am. J. vet. Res.* **25**, 1371-1375.
FESCE, A. (1961). *Boll. 1st Sieroter. Milanese,* **40**, 137-140.
FESCE, A. and DE ZULIAN, V. (1961). *Atti Soc. ital. Sci. vet.* **15**, 802-808.
FESCE, A. and PELIZZATTI, P., CECCARELLI, A., DE ZULIAN, V. and MARENZI, C. (1962). *Atti Soc. ital. Sci. vet.* **16**, 598-601.
FRANKS, D. (1959). *J. comp. Path.* **69**, 353-366.
HENSON, P. M. (1968). Immunology, **14**, 697-705.
HOLE, N. H. and COOMBS, R. R. A. (1947a). *J. Hyg., Camb.* **45**, 480-489.
HOLE, N. H. and COOMBS, R. R. A. (1947b). *J. Hyg., Camb.* **45**, 490-496.
HOLE, N. H. and COOMBS, R. R. A. (1947c). *J. Hyg., Camb.* **45**, 497-503.
INGRAM, D. G. (1959a). *Immunology,* **2**, 322-333.
INGRAM, D. G. (1959b). *Immunology,* **2**, 334-345.

Ingram, D. G. (1962a). *Can. J. Microbiol.* **8**, 297-306.
Ingram, D. G. (1962b). *Can. J. Microbiol.* **8**, 307-313.
Ingram, D. G. (1962c). *Can. J. Microbiol.* **8**, 335-344.
Ingram, D. G. (1962d). *Can. J. Microbiol.* **8**, 345-360.
Ingram, D. G. (1962e). *Can. J. Microbiol.* **8**, 461-471.
Ingram, D. G. (1962f). *Can. J. Microbiol.* **8**, 535-543.
Ingram, D. G. (1962g). *Can. J. Microbiol.* **8**, 703-708.
Ingram, D. G. (1962h). *Immunology,* **5**, 511-521.
Ingram, D. G. (1963). *Cornell Vet.* **53**, 167-180.
Ingram, D. G. (1965a). *Can. J. Microbiol.* **11**, 151-159.
Ingram, D. G. (1965b). *Can. J. Microbiol.* **11**, 161-165.
Ingram, D. G. (1969). *Can. J. Microbiol.* **15**, 981-987.
Ingram, D. G. (1972). *In* "Biological Activities of Complement" (Ed. D. G. Ingram), pp. 215-228. S. Karger, Basel.
Ingram, D. G. (1974). *In* "Microbiology of Easter Island" (Ed. G. L. Nogrady), pp. 121-125. G. L. Nogrady, Montreal.
Ingram, D. G., Barber, H., McLean, D. M., Soltys, M. A. and Coombs, R. R. A. (1959). *Immunology,* **2**, 268-282.
Ingram, D. G. and Barnum, D. A. (1965). *Can. vet. J.* **6**, 162-169.
Ingram, D. G. and Mitchell, W. R. (1970). *Am. J. vet. Res.* **31**, 487-492.
Ingram, D. G. and Mitchell, W. R. (1971a). *Am. J. vet. Res.* **32**, 23-28.
Ingram, D. G. and Mitchell, W. R. (1971b). *Am. J. vet. Res.* **32**, 875-878.
Ingram, D. G. and Soltys, M. A. (1960). *Parasitology,* **50**, 231-239.
Jasser, S. and Bragiel, I. (1962). *Arch. Immun. Ther. Exp.* **10**, 103-108.
von Jettmar, H. M. (1923). *Z. ImmunForsch. exp. ther.* **36**, 148-201.
Jones, J. H. and Heppleston, A. G. (1961). *Nature,* **191**, 1212-1213.
Joshi, N. N., Savan, M. and Ingram, D. G. (1965). *Can. J. Microbiol.* **11**, 1023-1025.
Kakoma, I. and Kinyanjui, M. (1974). *Res. vet. Sci.* **17**, 122-124.
Kakoma, I and Masiga, W. N. (1973). *Res. vet. Sci.* **15**. 101-105.
Lachmann, P. J. (1962). *Immunology,* **5**, 687-705.
Lachmann, P. J. (1966). *Immunology,* **11**, 263-271.
Lachmann, P. J. (1967). *In* "Advances in Immunology" (Eds F. J. Dixon and J. H. Humphrey), vol. 6, pp. 479-527. Academic Press, New York and London.
Lachmann, P. J. and Coombs, R. R. A. (1965). *In* "Complement" (Eds G. E. W. Wolstenholme and J. Knight), Ciba Foundation Symposium, pp. 242-273. Churchill, London.
Lachmann, P. J., Elias, D. E. and Moffett, A. (1972). *In* "Biological Activities of Complement" (Ed. D. G. Ingram), pp. 202-214. S. Karger, Basel.
Lachmann, P. J. and Liske, R. (1966). *Immunology,* **11**, 255-262.
Lachmann, P. J. and Muller-Eberhard, H. J. (1968). *J. Immun.* **100**, 691-698.
Lachmann, P. J., Sell, K. W. and Spooner, R. L. (1965). *Immunology,* **8**, 345-353.
Leon, M. A. (1957). *Proc. Soc. exp. Biol. Med.* **96**, 202-204.

Marks, J. and Coombs, R. R. A. (1957). *J. Hyg., Camb.* **55**, 81-90.
Medearis, D. N. and Kenny, J. F. (1968). *J. Immun.* **101**, 534-540.
Merucci, P., Abbolito, M. R. and Barduagni, A. (1975). Biomed. *int.* **23**, 52-54.
Mittal, K. R. (1970). Ph.D. Thesis, University of Guelph, Guelph, Canada.
Mittal, K. R. and Ingram, D. G. (1969). *Immunology,* **17**, 677-684.
Mittal, K. R. and Ingram, D. G. (1974). *Can. J. comp. Med.* **38**, 292-297.
Mittal, K. R. and Jaiswal, T. N. (1973). *Immunology,* **25**, 237-240.
Mollison, P. L. and Polley, M. J. (1960). *Immunology,* **3**, 11-18.
Moreschi, C. (1911). *Z. ImmunForsch. exp. Ther.* **11**, 275-287.
Muckle, T. J. (1968). *Ann. rheum. Dis.* **27**, 531-536.
Ngu, J. L. and Blackett, K. (1970). *J. trop. Med. Hyg.* **73**, 250-254.
Ngu, J. L., Barratt, T. M. and Hulme, B. (1971). *Clin. exp. Immun.* **9**, 477-482.
Norcross, N. L. and Poppensiek, G. C. (1961). *J. Bact.* **81**, 478-481.
Parappally, N. P. and Ingram, D. G. (1973). *Immunology,* **25**, 523-530.
Pautrizel, R., Tribouley, J., Szerznovicz, F. and Duret, J. (1964). *Annls Inst. Pasteur,* **107**, 863-872.
Pepys, M. B. (1976). *Transplantn Rev.* **32**, 93-120.
Pernis, B., Gambini, G. and Finalli, M. (1959). *Med. Lavoro,* **50**, 250-256.
Perussia, F. (1911). *Z. Immun Forsch. exp. Ther.* **11**, 287-294.
Quinn, P. J. (1970). Ph.D. Thesis, University of Guelph, Guelph, Canada.
Rose, J. E., Amerault, T. E. and Roby, T. O. (1974). *Am. J. vet. Res.* **35**, 1147-1151.
Rice, C. E., Boulanger, P., Mackie, C. and Moore, T. (1952). *Can. J. comp. Med.* **16**, 348-356.
Rytel, M. W. and Lytle, R. I. (1973). *Clin. expl. Immun.* **14**, 227-235.
Sage, H. J., Ransby, A. and Lion, M. A. (1963). *J. Immun.* **90**, 347-357.
Sellei, J. (1975). *Anim. Blood Gps. biochem. Genetics,* **6**, 31-40.
Singh, G. (1972). *Indian J. anim. Hlth.* **11**, 157-162.
Soulsby, E. J. L. (1958). *J. comp. Path.* **68**, 345-351.
Stoker, M. G. P. and Marion, B. P. (1950). *Br. J. Exp. Path.* **31**, 332-337.
Stoker, M. G. P., Coombs, R. R. A. and Bedson, S. P. (1950). *Br. J. exp. Path.* **31**, 217-232.
Streng, O. (1909). *Zentbl. Bakt. Parasitkde. Abt. I Orig.* **52**, 523-531.
Streng, O. (1910). *Finska LakSallsk. Handl.* **52**, 95-106.
Streng, O. (1930). *Acta. path. microbiol. scand. Suppl.* 3, **20**, 411-429.
Tedesco, F. and Corrocher, R. (1972). *Clin. exp. Immun.* **10**, 685-696.
Tewari, H. C., Mittal, K. R. and Gangadhara Rao, Y. V. B. (1972). *Indian vet. J.* **49**, 246-249.
Talskalova, H. and Barta, O. (1968). *Folia microbiol., Praha,* **13**, 450-458.
Tomopoulos, D. S. (1970). *Res. vet. Sci.* **11**, 596-597.
Topley, E., Knight, R. and Woodruff, A. W. (1973). Trans. R. *Soc. trop. Med. Hyg.* **67**, 51-54.
Wartiovaara, T. W. (1932). *Acta Soc. Med.* A 14, No. 15. 1-143.

WILLIAMS, B. D., CHALLACOMBE, S. J., SLANEY, J. M., LACHMANN, P. J. and LEHNER, T. (1975). *Clin. exp. Immun.* **19**, 423-433.
WILLIAMS, R. C. and KUNKEL, H. G. (1962). *J. clin. Invest.* **41**, 666-675.
WOODRUFF, A. W., TOPLEY, E., KNIGHT, R. and DOWNIE, C. G. B. (1972). *Br. J. Haemat.* **22**, 319-329.

7 *Aspects of Amphibian Immunity*

B. F. EDWARDS and L. N. RUBEN

I. Introduction

Studies of immunity in lower (poikilotherm) vertebrates have been justified on several grounds. The rationale generally offered is that an understanding of relatively "simple" systems should aid in unraveling the more "complex" mechanisms of mammalian immunity. A related arguement is that a comparative phylogenetic approach should distinguish those features of immunity that are basic to all species from those that have evolved uniquely in the adaptations of particular species. However, the most compelling reason for not restricting research to higher vertebrates is that in many instances an organism from a lower phylogenetic level may provide the best possible system for investigating an aspect of immunity that is of universal interest and applicability.

As a group, Class Amphibia is the most extensively studied of the poikilotherms and there now exists a wealth of knowledge on the anatomy and physiology of immunity in a number of representative species. Current interest in amphibian immunity is not due merely to it popularity as a laboratory animal system, but rather because the amphibia represent a key transitional step in vertebrate evolution — the emergence from a totally aquatic environment. The transition from aquatic to terrestrial environments is accompanied by dramatic advances in both the organization and functional sophistication of the amphibian immune system. The extent of these modifications and advances is emphasized when one compares the immune system of a primitive aquatic urodele (*e.g.* Axolotl) with that of a phylogenetically more advanced anuran (*e.g.* Ranid frogs).

The immune system of most urodeles can be characterized as follows:

1. Thymus glands lack clear demarcation into cortical and medullary regions.
2. The spleen is not organized into red pulp and white pulp areas.
3. They lack lymphopoietic bone marrow, gut-associated lymphoid tissue (GALT), and lymph nodes.
4. They synthesize and secrete only a single class of serum immunoglobulin (IgM).
5. Allograft responses are chronic and mixed lymphocyte reactions (MLR) stimulation indices are relatively low.

In contrast, advanced representatives of the Order Anura display the following:

1. The structural organization of the thymus and spleen is more like that of the mammal.
2. Adults possess lymphopoietic bone marrow, definite accumulations of GALT, and lymph-node like bodies in the throat region.
3. They synthesize at least two antigenetically distinct classes of immunoglobulins.
4. Allograft responses are acute.

It should not be inferred from these comparisons that urodeles are immunologically deficient. They synthesize specific antibodies against a large number of antigens, show immunologic memory to at least some antigens, and react specifically against allogeneic cells and tissue grafts. Furthermore, they display the equivalent of some mammalian B cell and T cell functions such as carrier-specific "helper" activity, characteristic of cell cooperation in anti-hapten responses of mammals, and differential blastogenic responses to T cell and B cell mitogens.

It is clear that the more advanced anura possess an immune system similar in its basic features to that of mammals. What makes the amphibia of particular interest is that it is within this class that we see the initial expression of key immunologic advances: multiple classes of immunoglobulin; lymph-node like structures; acute allograft responses; and therefore a major histocompatibility complex.

The many practical and theoretial advantages offered by amphibia as a laboratory tool have been well documented and need only brief review here. Large numbers of siblings can be obtained and easily raised at any time of the year. Syngeneic animals are now available through both inbreeding and nuclear transplantation. Larvae develop free from maternal influence and their environment (water temperature, population density) can be manipulated to control developmental rate. The immune system begins to function very early (the thymus is immunocompetent 6-7 days post-fertilization and the spleen 12-14 days in *Xenopus laevis*) and is susceptible to a variety of surgical manipulations. Both natural (nucleolar mutants) and laboratory induced (polyploidy) cell markers are available. Cultures of cell suspensions and intact tissues thrive for long periods of time with minimal maintenance and primary immune responses can be generated *in vitro* from fragments of lymphoid tissue. Amphibians respond to a variety of soluble and particulate antigens as evidenced by the production of antigen-specific binding cells (ABC), secretory antibody-producing cells (APC), and both lytic and agglutinating serum antibodies. Finally, it should be noted that anuran metamorphosis provides a unique experimental opportunity. The hormone thyroxin triggers the appearance of new adult-specific structures and the selective destruction of larval tissues. These new cell types differentiate in contact with a functioning larval immune system, and thus provide a unique model for the acquisition of tolerance to self-antigens.

It is not the intent of this chapter to review the current state of knowledge of amphibian immunity in its entirety. Information of this kind is provided in several recent reviews (DuPasquier, 1973; Cohen, 1976; DuPasquier, 1976; Cooper, 1976; Manning and Turner, 1976). Rather, this chapter will focus on a limited number of immunologic processes in which amphibian systems are currently being exploited to good advantage.

II. Serum immunoglobulin class heterogeneity

It is generally accepted that all vertebrate species below the level of Class Amphibia synthesize and secrete only high molecular weight (18-19S) "IgM-like" immunoglobulin in response to antigenic stimulation. Possible exceptions to this generalization have been noted in elasmobranchs and cyclostomes where there is evidence for a monomeric (7S) IgM with a heavy chain that is antigenically identical to the 19S form (Clem and Small, 1967; Marchalonis and Edelman, 1968) and in lungfish (Dipnoi) which possess IgM and a low molecular weight antibody (122 000 d) with a heavy chain distinct from the μ chain (Marchalonis, 1969). Mice and humans have five major classes of immunoglobulin and several subclasses within these. Distinct roles in the immune response have been assigned to most of these subclasses. It is important to examine those species in which multiple classes of immunoglobulin first appear. In this way it may be possible to determine which cell types and lymphoid organization correlate with their emergence and what specific role(s) each newly evolved class may play in immunity.

Immunoglobulin classes with antigenically distinct heavy chains make their first appearance in the primitive anura (exceptions noted above). Urodeles that have been tested produce only 19S IgM-like serum immunoglobulins. A number of representative urodele species have been subjected to single and multiple dose injections of soluble and particulate antigens, both with and without adjuvant (Marchalonis and Cohen, 1973; Tournefier and Charlemagne, 1975). In all cases only 2-mercaptoethanol-sensitive 19S antibodies were found, even after prolonged immunization schedules. An exception has been reported in the adult axolotl, *Ambystoma mexicanum*, by Ching and Wedgewood (1967). Immunization with bacteriophage ϕX174 initially elicited only 19S antibody, while 7S antibody began to appear later in the response. Both the 19S and 7S forms had μ-like heavy chains and both were sensitive to inhibition by 2-mercaptoethanol.

Members of anuran species representing the Piped, Bufid and Ranid families (*Xenopus laevis, Bufo marinus, Rana pipiens, R. catesbeiana, R. clamitans, R. esculanta, R. temporaria*) have been tested and all possess at least two distinct classes of immunoglobulin. A 19S IgM-like class is nearly always predominant over the low molecular weight (7S) class in both normal and immune serum. The 7S heavy chain is physiochemically and antigenically distinct from the 19S μ chain and has been denoted "IgG-like" primarily because it approximates the molecular weight of mammalian gamma chains. The differences between the 7S immunoglobulin of frogs and the classical IgG of mammals have been enumerated (Marchalonis and Cone, 1973; Atwell and Marchalonis, 1975). The anuran Ig is more similar to the 7S Ig of birds and reptiles than it is to mammalian IgG. Both Ig classes are also present in immunocompetent larvae and no obvious changes in Ig pattern have been observed as a result of metamorphosis. This is rather surprising, considering the gross cellular and molecular alterations that characterize anuran metamorphosis (Weber, 1967; Frieden, 1968). Steiner *et al.* (1975) have combined immunochemical analyses with polyacrylamide gel electrophoresis in the presence of sodium dodecyl sulfate to identify three classes of serum Ig in larval and adult *R. catesbeiana, R. clamitans,* and *R. pipiens*. One class is high molecular weight and corresponds to the previously described predominating IgM-like class. The other two immunoglobulins are 7S, and while they are structurally similar, each has its own unique antigenicity.

It is quite clear that, at least in the case of Ranid frogs, two distinct classes of immunoglobulin are present in the serum of both pre- and post-metamorphic animals. Based on molecular weights and subunit composition they correspond roughly to mammalian IgM and IgG. The situation in the more primitive anuran *X. laevis* is less certain. As in Ranid frogs, a 19S IgM predominates in *X. laevis* serum. There is also a 7S immunoglobulin component, but the gamma-like nature of its heavy chain is debatable. Hadji-Azimi (1971) has reported a rather high molecular weight (64 480 d) for *X. laevis* 7S heavy chain, while Marchalonis' (1970) molecular weight data (52 700 d) are more in line with mammalian gamma chain size estimates. More definitive data (amino acid sequences, carbohydrate content) are required to determine the true relationship among amphibian immunoglobulins and mammalian μ and γ heavy chains.

If multiple classes of immunoglobulin first evolved among the anura, then it follows that these organisms provide a fruitful system for determining the relative role(s) of high and low molecular weight serum antibodies. It is of particular interest to compare specific immune functions in species (urodela) lacking IgG-like antibody with those of the IgG-endowed anura. Comparative studies might reveal what, if any, new cell types and lymphoid tissue organization accompany the emergence of new classes of Ig, and what further refinements of immune function are attributable to low molecular weight immunoglobulin.

In mammals 7S IgG has been implicated in, among other things, feedback regulation of antibody synthesis and the generation of anamnestic responses. It has been difficult to demonstrate true immunologic memory in amphibian humoral immune responses, although cellular alloimmune memory is firmly established in both urodela and anura. Many antigens tested (some bacterial forms and foreign erythrocytes) elicit exclusively IgM-like serum antibody, and in these cases a second antigenic challenge usually fails to produce a true anamnestic response. Other antigens, such as serum proteins and bacteriophage, generate secondary responses in which a second challenge results in a shorter lag period and higher peak antibody titers. These anamnestic responses in anura are usually accompanied by the appearance of 7S antibody and a gradual increase in the ratio of 7S to 19S. *Bufo marinus* injected with *Salmonella* flagellar protein had both 19S and 7S immunoglobulins in their sera, but specific agglutinating antibody against flagellin was found only in the 19S fraction as late as 65 days post-immunization (Diener and Marchalonis, 1970). In contrast, bacteriophage f2 elicits IgG-like and 19S antibodies in larval and adult *R. catesbeiana* (Marchalonis and Edelman, 1966). The 7S class constitutes up to 90% of the specific antibody by 58 days post-immunization. Pross and Rowlands (1975) demonstrated modest increases in 7S antibody in larval and adult *R. catesbeiana* following booster injections of three different phages and two different hapten-carrier conjugates.

One might speculate that humoral memory parallels acquisition of low molecular weight immunoglobulins. Although immunologic memory for cell-mediated responses is well established in urodeles, the evolution of humoral response memory may have occurred later, in the primitive anura. Whether IgG-like serum antibodies in anura are accompanied by the appearance of a second type (non-IgM) of membrane receptor (analogous to IgD in mouse and human) remains to be seen.

III. Immunoglobulin as antigen receptor on amphibian lymphocytes

Cell surface receptor molecules provide the molecular basis for antigen recognition and binding by immunocytes. Recognition and binding are prerequisites, although not always sufficient, to initiate cell activation and differentiation (Moller, 1970; Gershon, 1974). In human B cells both 7S IgM and IgD may function as antigen-specific receptors (Vitetta and Uhr, 1975). Thymocytes and thymus-derived cells of mammals also have antigen-specific receptors (Binz and Wigzell, 1975). In contrast to B cells, the evidence demonstrating endogenous receptor Ig on mammalian T cell membranes is controversial (Vitetta *et al.*, 1972; Marchalonis, 1975). In studies that purport to demonstrate T cell Ig, the heavy chain is distinguishable from B cell and serum μ chain on antigenic, physiochemical, and functional grounds (Hammerling *et al.*, 1976; Hauston *et al.*, 1975; Feldmann *et al.*, 1975). Phylogenetic studies of lymphocyte receptors from lower vertebrates having B and T cell functions analogous to those of birds and mammals should clarify the question of T cell receptors and the possible significance of the relationship between cell surface IgM and IgD.

Charlemagne and Tournefier (1975) have studied membrane-associated Ig in the urodele *Pleurodeles waltii*. Indirect immunofluorescence (using rabbit anti-Pleurodeles IgM and FITC goat anti-rabbit) revealed membrane Ig on spleen and thymus cells of both larvae and metamorphosed juveniles; adult spleen cells were tested and also found positive. The use of two different dilutions of rabbit anti-IgM revealed the presence of two distinct populations of lymphocytes with respect to the intensity of fluorescence. With dilute anti-IgM, 65% of splenic lymphocytes from larval, juvenile and adult stages were intensely labeled while 35% remained unlabeled. Application of a more concentrated anti-IgM exposed patchy fluorescence on 20% of the previously unlabeled lymphocytes while 10% remained negative. Thymocyte membrane Ig was easily detectable, as even dilute anti-IgM resulted in patchy fluorescence on 98% of the cells. Therefore, in contrast to mammals, thymocyte membrane Ig is readily detectable by indirect immunofluorescence. The majority of positive staining thymocytes and splenocytes underwent capping following brief incubation at 37°C. The authors suggest that the two spleen cell populations distinguished by differential staining may represent B cell (intense stain) and T cell (patchy stain) equivalents. The effect of thymectomy on the distribution of lightly staining lymphocytes in the spleen might clarify this point.

Membrane Ig on lymphocytes of the anuran *X. laevis* has also been reported (DuPasquier *et al.*, 1972; Jurd and Stevenson, 1976). Ig-positive cells are first detected by immunofluorescence in larval thymus 6-8 days post-fertilization (Nieuwkoop and Faber stage 45), prior to spleen colonization. It is noteworthy that Ig synthesis in *X. laevis* embryos may be initiated as early as 2-3 days post-fertilization (stage 34-36) when the embryo hatches from its jelly and prior to the formation of thymus and spleen. Immunoglobulin light chain determinants were detected first in stage 35 embryos by radioimmune assays of whole-embryo homogenates. It is not known if this material represents functional antibody (Moyer *et al.*, 1977).

The percentage of Ig-positive thymocytes increases during embryogenesis and is maintained at 80% throughout larval life. Beginning one month after metamorphosis the thymus begins to involute and the percentage of intensely staining Ig-positive thymocytes drops to 1-10%, where it persists throughout adulthood. Membrane Ig becomes detectable on larval splenocytes approximately three days after the appearance of Ig-positive cells in the thymus. Unlike the thymus, splenic levels of Ig-positive cells remain constant at 40-60% in the adult. Induced capping, shedding and resynthesis experiments have verified the endogenous nature of these immunoglobulins for both thymus and spleen. As was found in *P. waltii*, membrane fluorescence of Ig-positive spleen cells is always more intense than that of thymocytes. Jurd and Stevenson (1976) have examined membrane Ig on lymphocytes from thymus, spleen, adult kidney, and larval ventral cavity bodies (lymphoid accumulations in the pharyngeal region of larvae that disappear during metamorphosis). Peripheral blood leucocytes from larvae, metamorphic larvae and adults were also examined. The level of Ig-positive cells in larval peripheral blood was 40%, increasing to 60-80% in adults. Ventral cavity body cells were 30-40% Ig-positive and 50% of adult kidney cells were IgM-positive. The proportion of cells staining positive for IgG was usually less than 1% and IgM and IgG were never detected together on the same cell.

Electron microscope studies using ferritin-labeled anti-*Xenopus* Ig indicate that Ig molecules are randomly distributed on the surface of adult spleen cells (Hadji-Azimi, 1976). The quantitative results matched those obtained earlier with indirect immunofluorescence. When treated at 4°C, 67% of adult splenic lymphocytes displayed ferritin-immune complexes, and variations in ferritin grain counts suggested the presence of two subpopulations of Ig-bearing splenocytes.

Michea-Hamzehpour (1976) has reported the presence of Ig-positive cells in the intestinal lamina propria of *X. laevis*. Duodenal lymphocytes stained positively for membrane-bound IgM by indirect immunofluorescence; the heavy chains were determined to be of the 19S H type. It is not known if these Ig-positive cells participate in antigen binding.

A direct link between the presence of membrane Ig and the ability to bind specific antigen has been established for *R. pipiens* (Edwards *et al.*, 1975). Injection of foreign erythrocytes generated antigen-binding cells (ABC) in the thymus, spleen and jugular bodies of adult frogs. The effect is time and dose dependent, and readily quantitated by immunocytoadherence assays. The Ig nature of the antigen-binding receptor has been confirmed by blocking experiments with rabbit anti-*Rana* IgM. Spleen cells from animals immunized against horse erythrocytes (HRBC) were prevented from binding antigen by preincubating these cells with anti-IgM. A similar result was obtained with *R. pipiens* jugular body lymphocytes sensitized *in vivo* to trinitrophenyl-HRBC (Edwards and Ruben, 1977). When cultured for 24 hours, dispersed jugular body cells released antigen-binding molecules into the culture medium; their binding activity was also blocked by anti-IgM.

It has been established that Ig-positive cells are plentiful in most, if not all, lymphoid organs of larval and adult amphibians. There is suggestive, albeit limited, evidence that monomeric IgM-like molecules serve as antigen recognizing and binding units in specific immune responses. The isolation and partial characterization of surface Ig has been accomplished in only a few lower vertebrates: two teleost fish (goldfish and carp) and one reptile, the tortoise (Fiebig and Ambrosius, 1976; Ruben *et al.*, 1977). In these three cases thymocyte surface Ig was shown to differ antigenically and physiochemically from spleen cell Ig. In addition, a second class (not IgM) of membrane Ig has been isolated from tortoise spleen and peripheral blood and has been termed IgY. Tortoise IgY has some properties similar to the 7S Ig of anuran amphibians and mammalian IgD (Fiebig and Ambrosius, 1976).

Developing amphibia provide unique opportunities to study the ontogeny of cells and receptors involved in antigen recognition and binding. The majority of cells in a number of lymphoid organs possess readily detectable membrane Ig. The thymus and spleen become lymphoid sequentially and in many anura antigen-specific binding cells can be elicited in very young larvae possessing fewer than one million lymphocytes. Isolation and characterization of surface Ig from thymus, spleen and other lymphoid organs of naive and immune animals should clarify the nature and role of T cell receptors and perhaps reveal a predecessor to human IgD on B cell equivalents.

IV. Physiology of antigen-binding cells

A. GENERAL FEATURES

Humoral responses following *in vivo* immunization of amphibia have been quantitated by immunocytoadherence, local hemolysis (plaque formation), microtiter hemagglutination, and bacteriophage neutralization assays. The immunocytoadherence (ICA) assay has been particularly useful for monitoring the earliest stages of response, since antigen-specific ABC can be readily detected 2-10 days post-immunization. Significant levels of PFC are not usually detectable until 10-14 days and serum antibodies usually require 15-20 days to reach titers measurable by micro-hemagglutination. The kinetics and intensity of amphibian humoral responses depend on the usual array of variables that also affect higher vertebrates: (1) injection route, (2) antigen dosage and schedule, (3) nature of antigen (soluble, particulate, with or without adjuvant). In addition, environmental temperature plays a vital role in the immune response of poikilotherm organisms.

Amphibians are capable of generating ABC to viruses, bacteria, foreign erythrocytes and serum proteins. Both T-dependent (hapten-carrier conjugates) and T-independent (bacterial lipopolysaccharide, polymerized flagellin) responses have been quantitated by ICA assays (Diener and Marchalonis, 1970; DuPasquier, 1970; Kidder *et al.*, 1973; Ruben, 1975). For the purpose of reviewing some aspects of ABC physiology, discussion will be restricted to ABC generated against foreign erythrocytes (RBC) and RBC haptentated with the trinitrophenyl moiety (TNP-RBC). It is assumed that the physiologic and biochemical characteristics of these ABC are representative of ABC generated against most other antigens.

The amphibian anti-RBC responses have been most extensively characterized in a urodele (*Notopthalamus viridescens*), a primitive anuran (*Xenopus laevis*), and a more advanced anuran (*Rana pipiens*) (Ruben *et al.*, 1973; Ruben, 1975; Edwards *et al.*, 1975; Edwards and Ruben, 1976). These three species offer an interesting evolutionary progression for comparative studies of the ontogeny and phylogeny of the vertebrate immune system.

B. SECRETORY AND NON-SECRETORY ANTIGEN-BINDING CELLS

Relatively low doses of RBC (2×10^4 RBC g^{-1} body weight) elicit peak levels of ABC in the thymus and spleen between 2 and 4 days (25°C) after intraperitoneal injection. The number of ABC declines to background level by 10-12 days. Higher doses (2×10^8 RBC g^{-1} body weight) also generate ABC at 2-4 days in the thymus, while in the spleen ABC peak at 8 days. A detailed accounting of anti-RBC cytodynamics in *N. viridescens* and *R. pipiens* is available (Ruben, 1975). What is of prime interest with regard to amphibian lymphocyte physiology is that ICA assays reveal two distinct populations of ABC. When lymphocytes from immune animals are incubated with the appropriate RBC antigen, sensitized lymphocytes bind either a single layer or multiple layers of RBC onto their surfaces. Secretory (S+) ABC are those cells which bind more than one layer of adherent RBC onto their surfaces. Non-secretory (S-) ABC bind only a single layer of RBC. The RBC to RBC binding necessary to form multilayered S+ ABC is believed to result from the release of antibody of the same specificity as the surface Ig of the ABC. As mentioned previously, *R. pipiens* spleen cell preparations rich in S+ ABC secrete IgM-like molecules in culture that specifically agglutinate the sensitizing RBC.

ICA assays of immune amphibian cells reveal three important aspects of the ABC response. The ratio of S+/S- depends on the antigen dose and the organ source of lymphocytes. Secretory ABC can form even at low (5°C) temperatures. Secretory and non-secretory ABC may be differentially affected by drugs and metabolic inhibitors.

ICA assays of thymocytes invariably yield only S- ABC regardless of the immunizing dose (none, 2×10^4, 2×10^8 RBC g^{-1} body weight) or time of assay (2 or 8 days post-injection). Only S- cells are found in the spleens of naive animals. Non-secretory ABC also predominate 70-80%) in the spleens of animals two days after low or high dose immunization. Secretory ABC increase with time after high dose immunization and constitute 45-60% of the total ABC population in the spleen by day eight, the time when the total number of ABC is maximal. Warming the assay mixture to 25°C prior to incubation at 4°C increases the proportion of S+ ABC (Ruben, 1975). The generation of S+ ABC in mammals requires 37°C while S- ABC are very fragile and are best demonstrated at 4°C (Haskill *et al.*, 1972). The appearance of S- ABC following a low dose stimulation parallels the kinetics of "helper cell" activity in anti-hapten responses and thus may represent T helper cells in a T/B collaborative response.

C. EFFECTS OF INHIBITORS AND ADRENERGICS ON ABC

In an effort to further characterize and differentiate between S- and S+ ABC, immune spleen cells from *R. pipiens* were treated *in vitro* with selected inhibitors and blocking agents prior to ICA assay (Edwards *et al.*, 1975). It has already been noted that pre-incubation with anti-IgM prevents antigen binding by immune cells. Antigen binding is also reduced 60-80% by 10^{-3}M sodium azide and by a mixture of 10^{-4}M colchicine and 2·5 ug ml^{-1} cytochalasin B. Secretory and non-secretory ABC were affected equally. Both inhibition of protein synthesis with emetine-HCL and gentle fixation of cell membranes with buffered paraformaldehyde selectively inhibited the formation of S+ ABC. Apparently neither protein synthesis nor receptor mobility is required for binding of antigen to form S- ABC.

Recent studies on the properties of ABC membranes include the effects of α- and β-adrenergic agonists and their respective antagonists on the splenic ABC of representative urodeles and anura (Hodgson *et al.*, 1977). Spleen cells from RBC-immunized newt, *X. laevis*, or frog were incubated *in vitro* at 22°C for 3 hours with drugs (10^{-6}M) and assay RBC. The resulting number of S- and S+ ABC were compared to drugless controls. Drug effects were blocked when the appropriate antagonists were included in the assay.

The β-adrenergic agonist isoprenaline decreased both S- and S+ ABC in the urodele while increasing the number of S+ ABC in the two anuran species. Isoprenaline had no effect on *X. laevis* S- ABC generated by a low dose of SRBC when assayed at 2 or 8 days post-injection. Thus, the population stimulated by low immunogen dose is different from that generated by high doses. The α-adrenergic agonist phenylephrine caused a marked decrease, particularly of S+ ABC in binding cells of both newt and frog. It appears that newt lymphocytes, while possessing receptors for both α- and β-adrenergic agonists, cannot distinguish between them. Anuran lymphocytes, on the other hand, respond differentially to these two agents. It may be of interest that both affect antibody secretion. This in itself may suggest an approach toward understanding the physiology of antibody secretion.

In summary, incubation of sensitized lymphocytes with antigen at 4°C allows direct visualization of S- and S+ ABC. The relative proportion of S- and S+ cells depends on antigen dose, interval between immunization and assay, and on the source of cells assayed. S+ ABC are antibody producing cells (APC) capable of active secretion of specific antibody even at low temperatures. Active metabolism and protein synthesis are required for release of antibody. The S- ABC population probably includes T "helper" cells, memory cells, and precursors to APC.

D. TEMPERATURE EFFECTS ON AMPHIBIAN IMMUNE RESPONSES

The effects of ambient temperature on the ability of immunized poikilotherms to generate specific antibodies and reject foreign tissues has been investigated in several amphibian species (Hildemann and Haas, 1959; Cohen, 1966; Ching and Wedgewood, 1967; Diener and Marchalonis, 1970; Lin and Rowlands, 1973). The general finding is that lower temperatures retard and may even completely inhibit immune responses, at least as measured by the synthesis and secretion of serum antibodies. Experimental temperature shifts during the course of an immune response have provided some indications of which particular phase(s) may be temperature sensitive.

There appears to be a temperature sensitive event or events that normally occur during the first 2 to 3 days following *in vivo* immunization. The available evidence indicates that antigen-binding by precursor cells, antibody synthesis and secretion by APC, agglutination of antigen by antibody, and binding and lytic activity of amphibian complement all readily occur at low temperatures (Wright *et al.*, 1975; Ruben *et al.*, 1977a). The temperature sensitive phase seems to involve the proliferation and/or differentiation of the initial population of antigen sensitive cells (Wright *et al.*, 1975; Avtalion *et al.*, 1976). Priming of immunocompetent cells and the eventual synthesis and release of antibody seem not to be temperature sensitive.

The temperature sensitivity of poikilotherm physiology provides a valuable tool for the dissection of immune responses. The potential for exploiting temperature effects in poikilotherms is well illustrated by temperature studies on teleost fish (Avtalion *et al.*, 1976). Among the findings are that helper cells generated at warm temperatures can co-operate with potential APC in the cold, and that specific tolerance can be induced by exposure to antigen at low temperatures.

Since primary responses can be elicited in amphibian spleen fragments *in vitro* it should be possible, by employing temperature shifts, to expose discrete events which would otherwise remain obscured within the complexity of the overall response.

V. Effects of mitogens and anti-immunoglobulin on lymphocyte activities

A. MITOGENESIS

Lymphocytes of both urodela and anura can be induced to undergo blast transformation by classical T cell (PHA, soluble Con A) and B cell (LPS, PPD) mitogens (Collie *et al.*, 1975; Goldstine *et al.*, 1975; Reddy and Wright, 1975; Collins *et al.*, 1976; Wright *et al.*, 1975). As in mammals, mitogen-induced DNA synthesis provides a useful model for antigen-induced blastogenesis. Mitogens specific for mammalian T and B cells have been used in amphibian systems in attempts to demonstrate lymphocyte heterogeneity and the presence of functional equivalents to mammalian T and B lymphocytes.

Splenic and peripheral blood lymphocytes of a urodele, *A. mexicanum,* were stimulated to proliferate by Con A, PHA, and LPS (Collins *et al.*, 1976; Collins and Cohen, 1976). The activities differed markedly from mammalian systems in that responses were generally lower, slower to develop (7-11 days at 26°C) and occurred over a wide range of mitogen concentrations. For example, stimulation indices (SI) for Con A were generally less than 5 for 6-25 ug ml^{-1} mitogen. The B cell activator LPS generated stimulation indices of approximately 20, albeit at relatively high concentrations (200-600 ug ml^{-1}).

An intriguing finding was that *A. mexicanum* thymocytes failed to respond to PHA, Con A, or to LPS under a variety of culture conditions. Tests on the level of binding of these mitogens by thymocytes have not been reported. Mixing thymocytes with spleen cells did not suppress the normal response of mitogen-reactive spleen cells. Thymocytes also failed to respond to allo-antigens in mixed lymphocyte cultures. The possibility that adult urodele thymocytes are a post-mitotic population has not been ruled out.

Anuran responses to B and T cell mitogens are generally more rapid than in urodeles and result in higher stimulation indices. *R. pipiens* splenic lymphocytes and peripheral blood cells can be induced to synthesize DNA by Con A, PHA, LPS, and PPD (Wright *et al.*, 1975; Goldstine *et al.*, 1975; Reddy and Wright, 1975). Heterogeneity of the responding populations is indicated because different culture conditions alter the efficacy of the mitogenic stimulation. The response to PHA or Con A peaks at 3-4 days (SI-16-36), occurs in the presence of fetal calf serum (FCS), and is poteniated by 10^{-5}M mercaptoethanol. Responses to LPS or PPD peak at 2 days (SI-5-13) fail to occur in FCS-supplemented medium, and are not affected by mercaptoethanol. The T cell mitogenic response is further enhanced by 10^{-4}M hypoxanthine or sodium bicarbonoate. These additives have no effect on LPS mitogenicity. Thus, *R. pipiens* spleen houses at least two biochemically distinct populations discernible by T and B cell mitogens and selective media. Similar tests on thymocytes, larval lymph glands, and jugular body cells are needed to clarify the role of these physiologically distinct populations. It would be of interest to see if there are B cell mitogen responsive cells in the thymus since there are reports of plasma cells and plaque forming cells in the anuran thymus (Moticka *et al.*, 1973; Minagawa *et al.*, 1975).

Manning *et al.* (1976) have combined larval thymectomy with differential mitogenesis in an attempt to demonstrate T and B cell equivalents in *X. laevis*. Larvae were bilaterally thymectomized 7-8 days post-fertilization, when the thymus contains less than 10^3 cells and the spleen is not yet colonized by lymphocytes. Mitogen responsiveness was tested nine months later in adult toadlets. Spleen cell responses to PPD and LPS were identical in thymectomized and sham-operated controls. In contrast, thymectomy caused a significant (90%) reduction in the Con A response. The low residual Con A activity in thymectomized toadlets was a consistent finding and represents a persisting population of Con A sensitive cells in thymusless animals. Thymocytes from normal adult *X. laevis* have a low but measurable response to Con A and PHA (SI-3-4) but not to LPS or PPD (Donnelly *et al.*, 1976).

In amphibia, as in higher vertebrates, mitogens provide a powerful tool for studying lymphocyte activation and for distinguishing functionally diverse cell populations. Mitogen-induced blastogenesis should be particularly useful in amphibia for investigating lymphocyte differentiation in the developing embryo. *In vivo* administration of mitogens and isotopically labeled thymidine, followed by autoradiography of whole body sections of developing larvae might pinpoint the tissue origin, time of differentiation and migratory paths of B and T cell equivalents.

B. LIGAND BINDING AND LYMPHOCYTE RECEPTOR MOBILITY

Observations at the light microscope level suggest that amphibian lymphocyte surface immunoglobulins can be induced to move and aggregate in the plane of the plasma membrane similar to mammalian lymphocytes. When *X. laevis* spleen cells are treated at 4°C with FITC-rabbit anti-*Xenopus* Ig or with rabbit anti-*Xenopus* Ig followed by FITC-goat anti-rabbit, Ig-positive cells display a uniform ring fluorescence. Raising the temperature to 20-32°C shifts the fluorescence to discrete patches followed by aggregation of label at one pole of the cell. The "capped" material is internalized and the cell surface becomes temporarily refractory to anti-Ig binding until its complement of surface Ig has been resynthesized (DuPasquier *et al.*, 1972; Jurd and Stevenson, 1976).

Time-dependent changes in the morphologies of ABC from *R. pipiens* jugular body cells also suggest antigen-induced receptor mobility (Edwards and Ruben, 1977). Immunocytoadherence assay of jugular body cells following *in vivo* immunization with TNP-RBC shows TNP-specific binding cells ranging from minimal non-secretory (3-4 TNP-RBC bound directly to a lymphocyte surface) to heavily secretory ABC (25-50 TNP-RBC bound in multiple layers and often localized at one pole of the cell). When assayed early (3-6 hours after mixing lymphocytes with the TNP-RBC antigen) the majority of ABC are of the non-secretory "ring" type. As incubation time increases there is a shift towards "horseshoe" and "polar" configurations. By 24 hours the majority of secretory ABC are highly polar. The multiple hapten determinants on the carrier RBC surface provide sufficient cross-linkage to induce receptor mobility and aggregation. All of this occurs at 5°C, demonstrating that membrane immunoglobulin mobility as well as secretion of antibody may occur in amphibia at low ambient temperatures. As mentioned above, raising the incubation temperature to 25°C increases the proportion of secretory ABC and allows aggregation of receptors to be visualized after only 20-30 minutes.

Hadji-Azimi (1976) has investigated the surface immunoglobulin distribution on *X. laevis* splenic lymphocytes by immuno-ferritin electron microscopy. When prepared at 0-4°C immune complexes were located uniformly all around the spleen cell membranes.

Unfortunately, comparable data were not provided for thymocytes. Raising the temperature to 15-32°C caused a rapid internalization of the immune complexes into micropinocytotic vesicles. It is interesting that rapid endocytosis apparently occurred without prior aggregation or capping of immunoglobulin. A similar phenomenon has been described for human B lymphocytes (Ault *et al.*, 1973). Thus the "capping" observed by low resolution light microscopy may in fact be due to rapid local endocytosis rather than aggregation of cross-linked receptors in the plane of the plasma membrane. The use of metabolic and structural inhibitors (e.g. sodium azide, cytocholasin B) and careful manipulation of temperature coupled with high resolution microscopy is needed to clarify the causal relationships among receptor mobility, cross-linking, receptor aggregation and endocytosis.

Urodele lymphocytes can also be induced to undergo apparent capping by anti-Ig (Charlemagne and Tournefier, 1975). Since urodele lymphocytes are relatively large (their surface area may exceed 10× that of mammalian lymphocytes) it is of interest to know how the density and distribution of their surface Ig compare with the smaller Ig-bearing lymphocytes of anura and mammals.

VI. Specificity of antigen binding

A. THE PROBLEM OF FEW LYMPHOCYTES AND MANY ANTIGENS

The immune system of anuran embryos matures very rapidly and is capable of synthesizing antibodies against a large number of antigenic specificities while possessing less than 1×10^6 lymphocytes (DuPasquier, 1970; DuPasquier, 1973). Spontaneous ABC (but not PFC) are found in unimmunized *A. obstetricans* larvae and as their total number increases the proportion of ABC decreases from 1% to 0·1% as the spleen lymphocyte population increases (DuPasquier, 1970). Since immunological competence does not consistently parallel chronological age or external morphology of larvae, a more accurate indicator of immune maturity is the number of lymphocytes present in the spleen. Larvae acquire the ability to respond to injections of foreign RBC when the number of splenic lymphocytes reaches $1\text{-}2 \times 10^4$, and the total number of lymphocytes in a single larva is estimated to be only 5×10^5 cells (DuPasquier, 1976). At this stage of development (*c.* 20 days post-fertilization at 22°C), the number of spontaneous ABC in the spleen of a non-immune larva reaches a plateau that is maintained through adulthood. It is noteworthy that the number of splenic lymphocytes necessary for an *in vivo* larval response (1-2 × 10^4) matches the estimated minimum number of cells necessary for *in vitro* stimulation of adult spleen fragments (Auerbach and Ruben, 1970).

It is estimated that of the 1-2 × 10^6 lymphocytes present in a young larva, only 10^4 represent potentially active antigen-sensitive clones (Haimovich and DuPasquier, 1973). If each clone is unipotential with respect to the specificity of antibody produced, then it is difficult to see how such a system could synthesize sufficient antibody specificities to cope with the estimated 10^6-10^7 antigenic specificities that are thought to exist. It should be remembered that these organisms develop from the outset in direct contact with an antigenically hostile environment.

It may be that young larvae simply fail to recognize a large percentage of the potential antigenic determinants as foreign material. If such is the case, then their range of defenses would be limited to the specificities of a relatively few lymphocytes. The existence of pluripotential lymphocytes is an alternatively possibility. Amphibian lymphocytes may display either more than one distinct receptor specificity per cell, or a single molecular species of receptor capable of binding a wide range of structurally distinct determinants. "Polyfunctional" antibodies have been described that bind structurally dissimilar molecules such as DNP and menadione. Such multispecificity could provide a limited number of cells with the ability to respond to a greater number of determinants (Konigsberg and Richards, 1972; Richards *et al.*, 1975).

It is also possible that a given cell or its progeny may express different specificities during development and differentiation. If this occurs, then one would expect that the number of response capabilities would increase in the maturing animal. Pross and Rowlands (1975) compared *R. catesbeiana* larvae and adults against a panel of antigens and concluded that the humoral responses are qualitatively similar but may differ quantitatively.

Because of the accessibility of its early developing immune system the larval amphibian is a model system that lends itself well to experiments on the maturation of antibody repertoire and the question of pluripotential lymphocytes.

B. BINDING SPECIFICITY OF LARVAL SERUM ANTIBODIES

Many antigens have been tested in larval amphibians and *in vivo* humoral responses have been elicited by viruses, bacteria, allogeneic and xenogeneic serum proteins, foreign erythrocytes and hapten-(DNP and TNP) carrier conjugates (DuPasquier, 1976). Thus, within the limits of the antigens tested to date, larvae appear to match the qualitative immune capacity of adults. It also appears that larvae do not gradually acquire the ability to respond to different types of antigen during development (Pross and Rowlands, 1975). Once immunocompetence is acquired it is acquired for the complete range of specificities for which that organism has the appropriate immune response genes.

Miniaturization of the plaque assay in liquid medium and of the bacteriophage neutralization assay for serum antibodies has provided the sensitivity necessary for assaying larvae weighting less than 1 gram and having only 1-2 $\times$ 10^6 lymphocytes. The larvae of many anuran species are transparent enough to permit injection of 1-2 μl of antigen directly into the heart of larvae under light anesthesia. Splenic ABC and PFC can be assayed 5-8 days post-injection while serum antibody can be detected by 20 days.

The specificity of larval responses has been evaluated by measuring the degree of cross-reactivity between selected antigen pairs. Very little cross-reactivity was obtained between human erythrocytes (HRBC) and sheep erythrocytes (SRBC) in *A. obstetricans* (DuPasquier, 1970) or between mouse RBC and SRBC in *X. laevis* (Auerbach and Ruben, 1970). Tobacco mosaic virus, phage T_4, T-uneven phages, and *Salmonella* did not cross-react in *R. catesbeiana* tadpoles (DuPasquier, 1973). Thus, at a gross level of specificity with multi-determinant antigens, larval responses show a considerable degree of discrimination.

More definitive tests of antibody specificity have been performed by immunizing with a hapten-carrier such as DNP-keyhole limpet hemacyanin or TNP-T_4 (Haimovich and DuPasquier, 1973). Inhibition of phage neutralization by various concentrations of strucurally related haptens allows an estimate of relative affinities and cross-reactivity of antibodies.

Immunization with DNP-KLH elicits a different group of antibodies than does TNP-KLH. Anti-DNP antibodies are inhibited more effectively by competition with DNP-lysine and less so by TNP-lysine. Anti-TNP antibodies are inhibited equally well by DNP-lysine *and* TNP-lysine. In both cases MNP-lysine was the least effective inhibitor. Furthermore, the degree of specificity of the anti-DNP and anti-TNP antibodies from larvae equalled that of adult frogs and the anti DNP IgM antibody from goat (DuPasquier, 1976). It appears that larval immunocytes can distinguish between structurally similar determinants and that larvae are capable of producing a wide variety of antibodies, even when their lymphocyte complement is relatively small.

C. BINDING SPECIFICITY AT THE CELL LEVEL

The question of amphibian antibody specificity has also been approached at the level of the lymphocyte receptor for antigen. Adult *R. pipiens, X. laevis,* and *N. viridescens* were immunized with TNP-RBC and the resulting splenic ABC were tested for binding specificity in an ICA assay (Edwards and Ruben, 1976). Immunized spleen cells were pre-incubated with various concentrations of TNP-glycine, DNP-glycine, or dansyl-L-lysine prior to assay with TNP-RBC. The effective blocking concentration of each competitive ligand was determined. *R. pipiens* ABC were able to discriminate among all three ligands, while binding by *X. laevis* cells was blocked equally well by TNP-glycine *and* DNP-glycine. Even at high concentrations, the structurally dissimilar danslyl-L-lysine failed to block anuran lymphocyte binding of TNP-RBC. In contrast, all three ligands were equally effective at blocking *N. viridescens* ABC. Therefore, the receptor specificity on immune cells is greatest in *R. pipiens*, intermediate in *X. laevis*, and lowest in *N. viridescens*. The gradation of discriminatory ability correlates with the phylogenetic positions of these three species. It is not known if the specificities of the splenic lymphocyte receptors are the same as those of serum antibodies produced against TNP-RBC.

Further studies of *N. viridescens* ABC specificity suggest the interesting possibility of bipotential binding cells. When newt spleen cells immunized against TNP-HRBC are treated with TNP-glycine and assayed against HRBC and TNP-HRBC it is found that 50% of the resulting ABC carry receptors for both TNP *and* a determinant on HRBC (Ruben and Edwards, 1976). Preliminary tests of serum antibody against TNP-HRBC failed to detect bispecific antibody. The generality of this lack of phenotypic restriction by urodele ABC awaits further investigation with other hapten-carrier combinations and additional urodele species.

VII. The role of the thymus in amphibian immunity

A. CELL MEDIATED AND HUMORAL RESPONSES TO ANTIGEN

The thymus is the first organ to become lymphoid in developing amphibia and, as will be discussed below, there is evidence that thymic epithelium may be the embryonic source of most, if not all, lymphocytes. Larval amphibia provide ideal material for analysis of thymic function by extirpation experiments. Thymic buds are superficially located and can be surgically removed at a very rudimentary stage prior to seeding out of lymphocytes to peripheral locations. Successful larval thymectomies have been achieved in representative urodele (*Pleurodeles waltii, Triturus alpestris*) and anuran (*Alytes obstetricans, Xenopus laevis, Rana catesbeiana, Rana pipiens*) species (Horton and Horton, 1975).

The thymus of *X. laevis* has received the most attention for several reasons. The larvae have a single pair of thymic buds (pharyngeal pouch endoderm) which can be destroyed by microcautery at 7-8 days post-fertilization. At this stage (stage 48 of Nieuwkoop and Faber, 1967) thymuses measure approximately 100 μm in diameter and contain less than 2×10^3 cells; few, if any, are small lymphocytes. At stage 48 the spleen contains less than 1×10^3 cells. The survival rate of thymectomized embryos is very high and regeneration of thymus tissue rarely occurs. Microsurgical thymectomies have been performed on larvae as early as 4-5 days post-fertilization using glass needles (Tochinai and Katagiri, 1975). Incidences of both regeneration and lethality seem to be higher with this technique. Microcautery thymectomized *X. laevis* do not suffer from runting or wasting diseases and thus lend themselves to long-term studies on the effects of thymectomy. The high incidence of mortality following surgical thymectomy may result from wasting, and if so, would suggest that this technique provides for more complete elimination of T cell function.

Microcautery larval thymectomy appears to have little effect on the overall development and growth of the animal. Larval growth, metamorphosis, and maturation of the adult proceed as in sham-operated controls, although changes in the lymphoid system have been noted (Manning, 1971). In *A. obstetricans* thymectomy decreases spontaneous SRBC-binding cells in the spleen by 25-50%, increases the percentage of splenic Ig-positive cells and causes a doubling of serum immunoglobulin concentration. Similar changes have been reported for *X. laevis* (DuPasquier, 1970). In addition, early thymectomy results in a depletion of lymphocytes in larval ventral cavity bodies and reduction in adult spleen size; fewer cells are found in the red pulp region.

Normal *X. laevis* reject allogeneic skin grafts from non-sibling donors with mean survival times (MST) of 15-30 days. Thymectomy at 7-8 days of age greatly diminishes but does not completely abrogate the allograft response and grafts are eventually rejected in a chronic fashion (Horton and Manning, 1972). Toadlets grafted one year after early thymectomy showed the same degree of chronic rejection as those grafted at a shorter interval post-thymectomy. Apparently there is no restoration of the alloimmune response with time. If thymectomy is delayed until after the third week of life, subsequent allografts are invaded and rejected in a normal acute fashion. Therefore, the thymus is required only during the first two weeks of larval life in order to establish alloimmune responsiveness. The ability to reject allografts can be correlated in time with the histological development of the thymus into cortex and medulla (Horton and Horton, 1975).

It is interesting that following chronic rejection of a first-set allograft, a thymectomized toadlet can subsequently reject a second-set graft from the same donor in an acute fashion. The nature and specificity of this restorative ability have not yet been fully investigated. Acute rejection ability is also restored to thymectomized larvae by implants of allogeneic thymus tissue two weeks post-thymectomy (Horton and Horton, 1975). These animals were also shown to be rendered tolerant to skin grafts from the thymus donors. In contrast, spleen implants did not alleviate chronic rejection by thymectomized animals.

Other functions associated with T cell activities have been tested in thymectomized *X. laevis*. Spleen and blood leucocytes from larvae thymectomized at 7-8 days were tested for PHA responsiveness and MLR activity (DuPasquier and Horton, 1976). Both functions were abrogated by early thymectomy. Manning *et al.* (1976) have described a residual responsiveness to Con A in thymectomized animals and it is of interest to know if this population is responsible for the chronic rejection of first-set allografts and the restoration of acute rejection of second-set grafts. The residual activity suggests that either microcautery fails to destroy all T cells, or T cells seed out in small numbers before seven days of embryonic development. A third possibility is that lymphocytes with T cell functions may arise from an alternative non-thymic pathway (Turpen and Cohen, 1976a). The population which provides "residual" T function appears to exhibit two unique characteristics. Since no increase in their function occurs with developmental time (Manning and Collie, 1977), they probably are not stem cells, but rather represent some differentiation state along the "T" pathway. Also, they are clearly less antigen-sensitive than cytotoxic T cells since a single exposure to allogeneic antigens only serves to initiate memory. A second exposure to antigen is required to provide acute "killer" activity.

Larval thymectomy also abrogates the humoral response to T-dependent antigens such as SRBC and human gamma globulin, but on a different time scale than the allograft effect (Manning, 1975; Horton *et al.*, 1977). Whereas the thymus must be removed within the first two weeks to delete the allograft response, antibody production against

SRBC can be prevented by thymectomy as late as three weeks. A more prolonged thymic influence seems necessary to establish what may be T-helper cells required for a cooperative humoral response. Both *in vivo* and *in vitro* responses to the T-independent antigens LPS and PVP remain unimpaired by early thymectomy (Manning and Collie, 1975; Manning *et al.*, 1976; Tochinai, 1976). This suggests that stem cells for B cell functions are either extra-thymic in origin or are seeded out from the thymus prior to 7 days post-fertilization.

The effects of adult thymectomy on specific immune functions have not been investigated extensively in amphibia. *X. laevis*, thymectomized as young adults, generate a normal level of anti-SRBC ABC and PFC when immunized between 7 and 240 days post-thymectomy (Horton *et al.*, 1977). Preliminary results, also with adult *X. laevis*, indicate that thymectomy has no effect on the anti-TNP response (which requires T/B cooperation) when tested 0, 14, or 28 days post-thymectomy (Gruenwald, personal communication).

In contrast to most anura, the thymus of the urodele *T. alpestris* does not become lymphoid until 9-10 weeks after fertilization. This presents the interesting possibility of exposing an organism to antigens prior to thymic differentiation. Early exposure to antigens in this system might be a useful model for establishing specific unresponsiveness in a developing organism. It should be noted, however, that recent reports (Charlemagne and Tournefier, 1977a,b) suggest that *Pleurodeles waltii* thymectomized at 5 weeks do not lose their capacity to respond normally to *Salmonella* H and O antigens or to heterologous erythrocytes. In fact, *P. waltii* thymectomized at 5 weeks and immunized with SRBC as adults produced a higher titer of anti-SRBC thymuc may exert a suppressor-like regulator effect on Ig synthesis in this species.

In order to elicit a serum antibody response, what appears to be a rather high dose of flagellar H antigen, which in mammals is a partially thymus-dependent antigen, was administered in Freund's complete adjuvant. This is unfortunate since so high a dose could easily overcome the need for T cells in what is normally a cooperative response. Furthermore, it is possible that the presence of adjuvant decreases the necessity for T-helper function in this system. The question of whether "helper" activity, demonstrable in urodeles, involves T cells is crucial to our understanding of the evolution of cooperative immunity. We hope that these experiments with T-dependent antigens in urodeles will be performed with antigen doses likely to elicit helper T cell function.

Cells of thymic origin or thymic factors have been implicated in the phenomenon of sequential antigenic competition (Ruben, 1978). Spleen cells of adult *X. laevis* fail to respond either *in vivo* or *in vitro* to immunogenic doses of HRBC if SRBC are administered 4 days prior to attempted immunization with HRBC. The ability to respond to HRBC can be restored to SRBC-competed spleens by including thymus tissue from naive animals in the culture. Thymuses from animals undergoing competition by SRBC do not restore responsiveness to HRBC. The mechanism underlying antigenic competition and the possible roles of thymocyte sub-populations is currently under investigation in this system.

B. THE THYMUS AND EMBRYONIC LYMPHOPOIESIS

There is an impressive body of experimental evidence that strongly suggests that all lymphocytes of anura (*R. pipiens* in particular) arise *in situ* from the thymus gland (Turpen *et al.*, 1975; Volpe and Turpen, 1975). This is in direct and unexpected contrast to the situation in birds and mammals where it is believed that blood-borne stem cells originate in the yolk sac and migrate to the thymus where inductive interactions further their differentiation (Moore and Owen, 1967; Metcalf and Moore, 1971). Later, the embryonic liver and then bone marrow become the repositories for lymphopoietic stem cells. Unique features of amphibian embryogenesis have been exploited in attempts to trace the source of lymphocytic stem cells. The paired thymic primordia (endoderm of the second pharyngeal pouch) of *R. pipiens* can be surgically removed and transplanted at 72 hours after fertilization. The embryo is completely avascular and the thymus is embryonically determined but undifferentiated at this stage. Therefore, presumptive thymus tissue can be removed prior to any possible entry of stem cells and before the thymus itself becomes lymphoid. It retains the ability to self-differentiate into a definitive thymus gland when transplanted to a heterotopic site in a host embryo (Turpen *et al.*, 1975). Furthermore, triploidy can be induced immediately following fertilization, providing a permanent nuclear marker to follow the fate of transplanted cells.

When thymic primordia were removed at 72 hours and reciprocally exchanged between diploid and triploid embryos the chimeric animals developed normally through metamorphosis. The ploidy (and therefore origin of cells was determined by cytophotometry of Feulgen-stained cell preparations. When cells from bone marrow and spleen of adult chimeras were analyzed, greater than 80% of them were of donor origen (*i.e.* diploid cells from transplanted thymus populated lymphoid organs of triploid host and vice versa). Additional studies established that donor cells originated from the thymic epithelium itself (endoderm) and not from mesenchyme carried along in the transplant (Turpen and Cohen, 1976a). In transplants of triploid blood island tissue orthotopically to diploid hosts, contribution of donor tissue was minimal (7-12%). Ventral blood islands are the source of erythroid stem cells in anura (Turpen and Cohen, 1976b).

A combination of thymectomy and parabiosis has established that lymphocytes migrate out from surgically undisturbed thymus tissue and colonize other sites (Volpe and Turpen, 1976). A diploid embryo was joined in parabiosis at the gill region with a triploid embryo, establishing a common circulation. The paired thymic rudiments of the triploid embryo were surgically removed prior to lymphopoiesis. Later analysis showed lymphocytes in the thymuses and spleen of the non-thymectomized diploid larva to be almost exclusively diploid. The spleen of the thymectomized triploid larva was also populated almost entirely (90%) by diploid cells. Therefore, the thymectomized ($3n$) larva contributed few or no lymphocytes to its partner, while the diploid larva with intact thymuses was able to populate the spleen of the triploid larva.

A more drastic surgical technique has strengthened the position that thymic tissue is the primary source of all lymphocytes in *R. pipiens*. Two 72-hour embryos (one $2n$ and one $3n$) were cut in half transversely and their anterior halves interchanged (Volpe and Turpen, 1975). Perfect alignment of anterior and posterior halves resulted in normal adult frogs. Cell suspensions from adult thymus, spleen, kidney, and bone marrow from the humerus and femur were tested for ploidy in animals with diploid anteriors and triploid posteriors. Both thymus glands were at least 95% diploid, again suggesting minimal contribution from ventral blood islands ($3n$). The anteriorly located humerus bone marrow and posteriorly located spleen and femoral bone marrow were greater than 80% diploid. The kidney was approximately 25% diploid and 75% triploid. The kidney contains about three times as many erythroid cells as lymphoid cells. The erythroid contribution is primarily from the blood islands ($3n$ in this case), so it is likely that the 25% diploid cells found represent the majority of lymphoid cells in the kidney. Thus, posterior structures located in a triploid environment are populated by diploid lymphocytes. The most likely source of these cells is the thymus.

In spite of a strong case for the thymic origin of all lymphocytes, the results of recent experiments indicate that the situation may be more complex. Reciprocal orthotopic transplants of 72-hour thymus tissue between diploid and triploid *R. pipiens* larvae suggest that the majority of peripheral lymphocytes are derived from the thymus, with a possible minor contribution from the ventral blood islands. However, in thymectomized larvae the ventral blood islands become a major source of lymphocytes (Turpen and Cohen, 1976). Thymectomy may trigger compensatory homeostatic mechanisms which invoke an alternative pathway of lymphopoiesis.

When diploid thymic primordia were transplanted heterotopically to the ventral surface of a triploid host, both donor and host thymuses became chimeric (Turpen *et al.*, 1977). Host thymuses contained 70-80% host-derived cells and 20-30% diploid donor cells. The grafted thymus was also populated by a high proportion (*c.* 50%) of host cells. Although orthotopically transplanted thymuses received insignificant contributions from the host, heterotopic transplants became heavily populated by lymphocytes from some extrinsic source. These findings do not rule out a strictly thymic origin of lymphocytes since the chimerism observed in heterotopic transplants could be accounted for by thymus-to-thymus migration between donor and host primordia.

Recent studies with anuran species other than *R. pipiens* support an extra-thymic origin of lymphocytes. When gill arches were orthotopically exchanged between diploid and triploid embryos (stage 21; 36 hours at 18°C) of *X. laevis*, developing thymuses were populated solely by host lymphocytes. This result is in direct contrast to that obtained in identical experiments with *R. pipiens* in which orthotopically transplanted donor thymuses appear to be the primary source of lymphocytes. Transplant experiments using labeled thymus and ventral blood island tissues also revealed that *R. pipiens* larval liver is a site of lymphopoiesis (primarily of plasma cells) and is *not* populated by lymphoid cells immigrating from the thymus or ventral blood islands (Turpen *et al.*, 1977).

The formation of lymphoid stem cells is such a basic embryological function that it is difficult to believe that the germ layer origin or the pathways of differentiation should differ drastically among amphibians, birds and mammals. Some of the differences described to date may have their origin in the extirpation and transplantation procedures used to investigate thymic differentiation. Surgical intervention in which tissue and organ microenvironments are altered may trigger "abnormal" alternate paths of differentiation and migration by pluripotent embryonic cells.

VIII. Metamorphosis as a model for self-sufficiency

Among vertebrates the phenomenon of metamorphosis is unique to the class Amphibia. It is particularly dramatic in the anura where, under the influence of the hormone thyroxin, profound biochemical and morphological changes occur in all tissues and organs. During the transition period new adult-specific structures, cells, and macromolecules differentiate in the presence of a functioning larval immune system. Many new antigens arise during development without stimulating larval immune responses and providing a unique system for studying the acquisition of self-tolerance. Aspects of the system can be regulated in that precocious metamorphosis can be induced by exogenous thyroxin and persistent larvae can be obtained by thyroidectomy or thyroid-inhibiting drugs such as thiourea. It should be noted that at the onset of metamorphosis larvae have a fully competent immune system. Thymus, spleen, ventral cavity bodies, and lymph glands are well developed and are capable of mediating responses to a wide range of cellular and soluble antigens. Whether or not these functions are depressed or shut down completely during the emergence of new adult-specific antigens remains to be seen.

Metamorphosis is characterized by regression and rearrangement of larval tissues balanced and coordinated with the emergence of adult-specific structures. The tissues and organs of the lymphoid system are among those subject to change. Growth of thymus and spleen are interrupted during metamorphosis. The thymus actually loses 80-90% of its cells before undergoing a renewed growth period after metamorphosis (DuPasquier, 1976). Although the percentage of thymic Ig-positive cells remains constant, comparison of "spot" fluorescence assays with the more sensitive "cap" assay for surface immunoglobulins indicates that the percentage of intensely staining Ig-positive cells falls precipitously during metamorphosis and remains low in adulthood (Jurd and Stevenson, 1976). Other lymphoid accumulations do not make their appearance until after metamorphosis. Lymphopoietic bone marrow, GALT, and the lymph node-like jugular bodies are adult-specific features of the immune system.

It has been suggested that tolerance to adult-specific antigens is induced by interactions between antigen and the larval immune system. Maniatis *et al.* (1969) have shown that *R. catesbeiana* larvae injected with adult type hemoglobin from the same species produce antibody against the hemoglobin. In normal development tolerance to adult hemoglobin is acquired as the system differentiates and larval RBC switch to adult hemoglobin synthesis (Jurd and Maclean, 1970) or new adult-specific RBC arise (Hollyfield, 1966). An elegant investigation of this problem has been performed by Triplett (1962). An entire pituitary gland was removed from one larva and transplanted to another, where it continued to grow. After a period of time in the new host, the pituitary gland was placed back into the original donor larva where it was rapidly rejected as if it were an allograft. As a control, only one half of a pituitary gland was removed, transplanted, and then returned to the original larval donor. This graft was *not* rejected, showing that rejection in the first case was not due to passive acquisition of alloantigens from the host larva. It is clear that rejection was due to the new organ-specific antigens expressed by the pituitary during differentiation and growth. Normally these antigens are acquired while interacting with the larval immune system and are recognized as "self".

Attempts to detect stage-specific changes in immune responsiveness have been made by comparing reaction capacities before, during, and after metamorphosis. Metamorphic *R. pipiens* (Bovbjerg, 1966) and *R. catesbeiana* (Hildemann and Haas, 1959) reject allografts on a par with pre-metamorphic larvae, although invasion of the grafts may be slightly delayed. On the other hand, there is a report that tumor grafts into *X. laevis* are more readily accepted when performed during metamorphosis (Ruben, 1970). Responsiveness of MLR between genetically unrelated individuals is not depressed during metamorphosis (DuPasquier and Weiss, 1973). Suppression of cell mediated responses is suggested by allograft studies between sibling *X. laevis* (Chardonnens and DuPasquier, 1973; Chardonnens, 1975; DuPasquier, 1976). Grafts between siblings made during metamorphosis result in 25-50% cases of tolerance, whereas pre-metamorphic larvae and adults show rejection in 100% of the cases. The major variables which influence the balance between tolerance and immunity seem to be graft size and the genetic relationship between host and donor.

There is one report that the serum response to RBC antigens in *R. catesbeiana* may be suppressed during metamorphosis (Moticka *et al.*, 1973). On the other hand, Nagata reported that metamorphic *X. laevis* larvae and thiourea-treated (metamorphosis inhibited) persistent larvae generated equivalent serum responses to rabbit RBC (Nagata, 1976). Nagata's results are difficult to interpret because larvae were given multiple injections of RRBC over a period of time, and 5 weeks elapsed between initial exposure to antigen and assay. A more accurate indicator of humoral immune capacity during metamorphosis is obtained by monitoring splenic ABC 7-8 days after a single injection of antigen. Preliminary studies with SRBC-immunized *X. laevis* larvae showed that the number of ABC per 10^6 spleen cells increases gradually with age and size of larvae and is not affected by metamorphosis (Edwards, 1977). It should be noted that while metamorphosis may not depress the recognition capacity of the immune system, the ultimate expression of serum antibodies may be inhibited by general physiological depression during this period. Analysis of more specific immune functions such as helper cell activity in an anti-hapten response are currently being investigated (Jones, 1978).

Recent *in vitro* studies have shown that spleens of mid-metamorphic *X. laevis* respond to antigen just as well as pre- and post-metamorphic spleens. Spleens from all three stages produce lytic antibody specific for SRBC when stimulated in culture by sonicated SRBC (Ruben *et al.*, 1977). On the other hand, thymuses from mid-metamorphic donors were less effective at restoring the lytic response to spleens when combined in culture with spleens from thymectomized larvae. Whether this deficiency is due to the reduced number of cells in metamorphic thymuses is not known at this time.

Information to date on the effects of metamorphosis on amphibian immune capacity is scarce and at times contradictory. What is clear is that amphibia traverse two distinct periods during which self-tolerance is acquired; first as embryos when the larval immune system differentiates and then again during metamorphosis as adult-specific antigens arise. This system provides a unique opportunity to study the acquisition of tolerance to self-antigens in an immunologically competent organism.

References

Atwell, J. L. and Marchalonis, J. J. (1975). *J. Immunogen.* 1, 367-391.

Auerbach, R. and Ruben, L. N. (1970). *J. Immun.* **104**, 1242-1246.

Ault, K. A., Karnovsky, M. J. and Unanue, E. R. (1973). *J. clin. Invest.* **52**, 2507-2516.

Avtalion, R. R., Weiss, E. and Moalem, T. (1976). *In* "Comparative Immunology" (Ed. J. J. Marchalonis), pp. 227-238. Blackwell, Oxford.

Binz, H. and Wigzell, H. (1975). *J. exp. Med.* **142**, 197-211.

Bovbjerg, A. M. (1966). *J. exp. Zool.* **161**, 69-80.

Chardonnens, X. and DuPasquier, L. (1973). *Eur. J. Immun.* **3**, 569-573.

Charlemagne, J. and Tournefier, A. (1975). *In* "Advances in Experimental Medicine and Biology" (Eds W. H Hildemann and A. A. Benedict), vol. 64, pp. 251-256. Plenum Press, New York.

CHARLEMAGNE, J. and TOURNEFIER, A. (1977a). *Eur. J. Immun.* **7**, 500-502.
CHARLEMAGNE, J. and TOURNEFIER, A. (1977b). *In* "Developmental Immunobiology" (Eds J. B. Solomon and J. D. Horton), pp. 267-276. Elsevier North Holland, Amsterdam.
CHING, Y-C. and WEDGEWOOD, R. J. (1967). *J. Immun.* **99**, 191-200.
CLEM, L. W. and SMALL, P. A. (1967). *J. exp. Med.* **125**, 893-920.
COHEN, N. (1966). *J. exp. Zool.* **163**, 157-172.
COHEN, N. (1976). *In* "Comparative Immunology" (Ed. J. J. Marchalonis), pp. 209-226. Blackwell, Oxford.
COLLIE, M. H, TURNER, R. J. and MANNING, M. J. (1975). *Eur. J. Immun.* **5**, 426-427.
COLLINS, N. H. and COHEN, N. (1976). *In* "Phylogeny of Thymus and Bone Marrow-Bursa Cells" (Eds R. K. Wright and E. L. Cooper), pp. 143-151. North Holland, Amsterdam.
COLLINS, N. H., MANICKAVEL, V. and COHEN, N. (1975). *In* "Advances in Experimental Medicine and Biology" (Eds W. H. Hildemann and A. A. Benedict), vol. 64, pp. 305-314. Plenum Press, New York.
COOPER, E. L. (1976). "Comparative Immunology" Prentice-Hall, Inc., New Jersey.
DIENER, E. and MARCHALONIS, J. J. (1970). *Immunology,* **18**, 279-293.
DONNELLY, N., MANNING, M. J. and COHEN, N. (1976). *In* "Phylogeny of Thymus and Bone Marrow-Bursa Cells" (Eds R. K. Wright and E. L. Cooper), pp. 133-141. North Holland, Amsterdam.
DUPASQUIER, L. (1970a). *Immunology,* **19**, 353-362.
DUPASQUIER, L. (1970b). *Transplant. Proc.* **2**, 293-295.
DUPASQUIER, L. (1973). *In* "Current Topics of Microbiology and Immunology" (Eds W. Arber *et al.*), vol. 61, pp. 37-88. Springer-Verlag, Berlin.
DUPASQUIER, L. (1976). *In* "Comparative Immunology" (Ed. J. J. Marchalonis), pp. 390-418. Blackwell, Oxford.
DUPASQUIER, L. and HORTON, J. D. (1976). *Immunogenet. Lett.* **3**, 105-112.
DUPASQUIER, L., WEISS, N. and LOOR, F. (1972). *Eur. J. Immun.* **2**, 366-370.
EDWARDS, B. F. (1978). Unpublished observations.
EDWARDS, B. F. and RUBEN, L. N. (1976). *In* "Phylogeny of Thymus and Bone Marrow-Bursa Cells" (Eds R. K. Wright and E. L. Cooper), pp. 153-159. North Holland, Amsterdam.
EDWARDS, B. F., RUBEN, L. N., MARCHALONIS, J. J. and HYLTON, C. (1975). *In* "Advances in Experimental Medicine and Biology" (Eds W. H. Hildemann and A. A. Benedict), vol. 64, pp. 397-407. Plenum Press, New York.
ELSON, C. J., ALLAN, D., ELSON, J. and DUFFUS, W. H. P. (1972). *Immunology,* **22**, 291-300.
FELDMANN, M., BOYLSTON, A. and HOGG, N. M. (1975). *Eur. J. Immun.* **5**, 429-431.
FIEBIG, H. and AMBROSIUS, H. (1976). *In* "Phylogeny of Thymus and Bone Marrow-Bursa Cells" (Eds R. K. Wright and E. L. Cooper), pp. 195-204. North Holland, Amsterdam.

FRIEDEN, E. (1968). *In* "Metamorphosis: A Problem in Developmental Biology" (Eds W. Etkin and L. I. Gilbert), pp. 349-398. Appleton-Century-Crofts, New York.

GECZY, C. L., GREEN, P. C. and STEINER, L. A. (1973). *J. Immun.* **111**, 1261-1267.

GERSHON, R. T. (1974). *Contemp. Top. Immunobiol.* **3**, 1-40.

GOLDSTINE, S. N., COLLINS, N. H. and COHEN, N. (1975). *In* "Advances in Experimental Medicine and Biology" (Eds W. H. Hildemann and A. A. Benedict), vol. 64, pp. 343-351. Plenum Press, New York.

GREEN, P. C., EPSTEIN, S. M., EPSTEIN, K. A. and STEINER, L. A. (1974). *Fedn Proc. Fedn Am. Socs exp. Biol.* **33**, 735.

HADJI-AZIMI, I. (1971). *Immunology,* **21**, 463-473.

HADJI-AZIMI, I. (1976). *J. exp. Zool.* **201**, 115-126.

HAIMOVICH, J. and DUPASQUIER, L. (1973). *Proc. Acad. Sci. U.S.A.* **70**, 1898-1902.

HAMMERLING, U., MACK, C. and PICKEL, G. (1976). *Immunochemistry,* **13**(6), 525-531.

HASKILL, J. S., ELLIOT, B. E., KERBEL, R. and AXELRAD, M. A. (1972). *J. exp. Med.* **135**. 1410-1415.

HENRY, M. and CHARLEMAGNE, J. (1977). *Dev. Comp. Immun.* **1**, 23-32.

HILDEMANN, W. H. and HAAS, R. (1959). *J. Immun.* **83**, 478-485.

HOLLYFIELD, J. G. (1966). *J. Morph.* **119**, 1-5.

HORTON, J. D. and HORTON, T. L. (1975). *Am. Zool.* **15**, 77-84.

HORTON, J. D. and MANNING, M. J. (1972). *Transplant Bull.* **14**, 141-154.

HORTON, J. D., RIMMER, J. J. and HORTON, T. L. (1977). *Dev. Comp. Immun.* **1**, 119-132.

HAUSTEN, D., MACK, J. J. and HARRIS, A. W. (1975). *Biochemistry,* **14**, 1826-1834.

JONES, R. (1978). Thesis.

JURD, R. and MACLEAN, N. (1970). *J. Embryol. exp. Morph.* **23**, 299-309.

JURD, R. and STEVENSON, S. T. (1976). *Comp. Biochem. Physiol.* **53A**, 381-387.

KIDDER, G. M., RUBEN, L. N. and STEVENS, J. M. (1973). *J. Embryol. exp. Morph.* **29**, 73-85.

KONIGSBERG, W. H. and RICHARDS, F. F. (1972). *Proc. natn. Acad. Sci. U.S.A.* **69**, 877-881.

LIN, H. H. and ROWLANDS, D. T. (1973). *Immunology,* **24**, 129-133.

MANIATIS, G. M., STEINER, L. A, and INGRAM, V. M. (1969). *Science,* **165**, 67-69.

MANNING, M. J. (1971). *J. Embryol. exp. Morph.* **26**, 219-229.

MANNING, M. J. (1975). *Am. Zool.* **15**, 63-71.

MANNING, M. J. and COLLIE, M. (1975). *In* "Advances in Experimental Medicine and Biology" (Eds W. H. Hildemann and A. A. Benedict), vol. 64, pp. 353-362. Plenum Press, New York.

MANNING, M. J. and TURNER, R. J. (1976). *In* "Comparative Immunobiology", pp. 79-115. John Wiley, New York.

MANNING, M. J., DONNELLY, N. and COHEN, N. (1976). *In* "Phylogeny of Thymus and Bone Marrow-Bursa Cells" (Eds. R. K. Wright and E. L. Cooper), pp. 123-132. North Holland, New York.

MARCHALONIS, J. J. (1969). *Aust. J. exp. Biol. med. Sci.* **47**, 405-419.

MARCHALONIS, J. J. (1975). *Science,* **190**, 20-29.

MARCHALONIS, J. J. and COHEN, N. (1973). *Immunology,* **24**, 395-407.

MARCHALONIS, J. J. and CONE, R. E. (1973). *Aust. J. exp. Biol. med. Sci.* **51**, 461-488.

MARCHALONIS, J. J. and EDELMAN, G. M. (1968). *J. exp. Med.* **127**, 891-914.

MARCHALONIS, J. J., ALLEN, R. B. and SAARNI, E. S. (1970). *Comp. Biochem. Physiol.* **35**, 49-56.

METCALF, D. and MOORE, M. A. S. (1971). *In* "Haemopoietic Cells". Elsevier, Amsterdam.

MICHEA-HAMZEHPOUR, M. (1976). *J. exp. Zool.* **201**, 109-114.

MINAGAWA, Y., OHNISHI, K. and MURAKAWA, S. (1975). *In* "Advances in Experimental Medicine and Biology" (Eds W. H. Hildemann and A. A. Benedict), vol. 64, pp. 257-266. Plenum Press, New York.

MOYER, C., ARMENTROUT, R. W. and BROWN, R. D. (1977). *Devl. Biol.* **61** 338-345.

MOLLER, G. and SJOBERG, O. (1972). *Transplant. Rev.* **8**, 26-49.

MOORE, M. A. S. and OWEN, J. J. T. (1967). *J. exp. Med.* **126**, 715-726.

MOTICKA, E. J., BROWN, B. A. and COOPER, E. L. (1973). *J. Immun.* **110**, 855-861.

NAGATA, S. (1976). *J. Fac. Sci. Univ. Tokyo.* **20**, 183-191.

PROSS, S. H. and ROWLANDS, D. T. (1975). *In* "Advances in Experimental Medicine and Biology" (Eds W. H. Hildemann and A. A. Benedict), vol. 64, pp. 373-382. Plenum Press, New York.

REDDY, A. L. and WRIGHT, R. K. (1975). *In* "Advances in Experimental Medicine and Biology" (Eds W. H. Hildemann and A. A. Benedict), vol. 64, 335-342. Plenum Press, New York.

RICHARDS, F. F., KONIGSBERG, W. H., ROSENSTEIN, R. W. and VARGA, J. M. (1975). *Science,* **187**, 130-137.

RUBEN, L. N. (1970). *Devl. Biol.* **22**, 43-58.

RUBEN, L. N. (1975). *Am. Zool.* **15**, 93-106.

RUBEN, L. N., VAN DER HOVEN, A. and DUTTON, R. W. (1973). *Cell. Immun.* **6**, 300-314.

RUBEN, L. N. and EDWARDS, B. F. (1976). *In* "Phylogeny of Thymus and Bone Marrow-Bursa Cells" (Eds R. K. Wright and E. L. Cooper), pp. 143-151. North Holland, Amsterdam.

RUBEN, L. N. and EDWARDS, B. F. (1978). *Dev. Comp. Immun.* **2**, 175-180.

RUBEN, L. N. and RUBEN, J. (1978). Personal communication.

RUBEN, L. N., EDWARDS, B. F. and RISING, J. (1977a). *Experientia,* **33**, 1522-1523.

RUBEN, L. N., WARR, G. W., DECKER, J. M. and MARCHALONIS, J. J. (1977b). *Cell. Immun.* **31**, 266-283.

RUBEN, L. N., HODGSON, R., CLOTHIER, R. H. and BALLS, M. (1977c). *In*

"Developmental Immunobiology" (Eds J. B. Solomon and J. D. Horton), pp. 277-282. Elsevier/North Holland, Amsterdam.

Steiner, L. A., Mikoryak, C. A., Lopes, A. D. and Green, C. (1975). *In* "Advances in Experimental Medicine and Biology" (Eds W. H. Hildemann and A. A. Benedict), vol. 64, pp. 173-184.

Tochinai, S. (1976). *Immunology,* **31**, 125-128.

Tochinai, S. and Katagiri, Ch. (1975). *Dev. Growth Diff.* **17**, 383-394.

Tournefier, A. and Charlemagne, J. (1975). *In* "Advances in Experimental Medicine and Biology" (Eds W. H. Hildemann and A. A. Benedict), vol. 64, pp. 161-172. Plenum Press, New York.

Triplett, E. L. (1962). *J. Immun.* **89**, 505-510.

Turpen, J. B. and Cohen, N. (1976a). *Cell. Immun.* **24**, 109-115.

Turpen, J. B. and Cohen, N. (1976b). *Ann. Immun.* (Inst. Pasteur), **127C**, 841-848.

Turpen, J. B., Volpe, E. P. and Cohen, N. (1975). *Am Zool.* **15**, 51-62.

Turpen, J. B., Clair, L. and Carpenter, K. L. (1977). *In* "Developmental Immunobiology" (Eds J. B. Solomon and J. D. Horton), pp. 115-122. Elsevier/North Holland, Amsterdam.

Vitetta, E. S., Bianco, C., Nussenzweig, V. and Uhr, J. W. (1972). *J. exp. Med.* **136**, 81-93.

Vitetta, E. S. and Uhr, J. W. (1975). *Science,* **189**, 964-969.

Volpe, E. P. and Turpen, J. B. (1975). *Science,* **196**, 1101-1103.

Volpe, E. P., Tompkins, R. and Reinschmidt, D. (1977). *In* "Developmental Immunobiology" (Eds J. B. Solomon and J. D. Horton), pp. 109-114. Elsevier/North Holland, Amsterdam.

Weber, R. (1967). *In* "The Biochemistry of Animal Development" (Ed. R. Weber), vol. 2, pp. 227-301. Academic Press, New York.

Wright, R. K., Reddy, A. L. and Cooper, E. L. (1975). *In* "Advances in Experimental Medicine and Biology" (Eds W. H. Hildemann and A. A. Benedict), vol. 64, pp. 325-334. Plenum Press, New York.

Subject Index

A

Adjuvant granuloma, 125-126
Allograft rejection, 4
 afferent lymph, changes in, 125
 amphibians, 273-275, 281
 obese mouse, 162
Amino acid sequences of immunoglobulins, 9, 11, 13, 15-16
Amphibian immunity, 255-282
Antibody-dependent cell mediated cytotoxicity (ADCC) reaction, 3
Antibody-mediated suppression of immune responsiveness, 154-155
Antigen-binding cells, amphibian, 263-267, 270, 273
 adrenergics, effects of, 265-266
 inhibitors, effects of, 265-266
 secretory and non-secretory, 264-265
 specificity, 273
Appendix, 167, 168
 anti-sheep red blood cell plaque-forming cells, 183-184
 cytokinetic studies, 172
 extirpation studies, 180-182
 functional morphology, 169-173
 irradiation and Ig formation, 182
 ontogeny, 175
 shielding during sublethal irradiation, 182
 suppressor cells, 189
 T cell function in TDA, 188
 thymus and post-natal development, 175
Asplenic mouse
 bone marrow function, 141-142
 immune response ontogeny, 141-142, 163
 T cell function, 142
 thymus function, 141-142
Athymic mouse, *see also* Nude streaker mouse, 138-141, 163
 B cells, 139, 140
 lymphocyte recirculation in, 44
 T cells, 139, 140
 thymus grafts, 140
 thymus ontogeny, 138-139
Autoimmune disease
 dogs, 19-21
 NZB mice, 151
Autoimmune hemolytic anaemia (AIHA), 19, 20

B

B lymphocytes, *see also* Lymphocytes, 3, 26
 amphibians, 256
 antigen-binding activity, 26
 athymic mouse, 139, 140
 C3H/He mice, 152

complement (C_3) receptor, 3
deficiency in in CBA/N mouse, 153, 163
differentiation, 46-47, 190-192, 203
efferent lymph after antigenic challenge, 104
GALT, 173, 203
during immune response, 87, 104
inflamed tissue, 84
lamina propria, 193
lymph node, 64, 87, 89
lymph node transit time, 74
maturation, 46-47
mitogenesis in amphibians, 268-269
mitogenesis in GALT, 179
NZB autoimmune mice, 164
Peyer's patches, 80
recirculation, 27
spleen, 77
surface immunoglobulin receptors, 3, 260
thoracic duct, 100
Beige mouse
natural killer cell deficiency, 162
Blood-thymus barrier, 54-56
Bone marrow, 52-53
amphibians, 256, 280
asplenic mouse, 141-142
B cell differentiation in, 191
irradiation and Ig formation, 182
osteopetrotic mouse, 162
Bronchus-associated lymphoid tissue (BALT), 168, 200, 205
antigen transport in lympho-epithelium, 196
cytokinetic studies, 198
IgE responses, 187-188
mitogenesis experiments, 199-200
ontogeny, 198
surface immunoglobulin on, 199

C

C3H mice
immune response ontogeny, 155
C3H/He mice
immune response ontogeny, 151-152, 164
C3H/HeJ mice
Lps gene, 164
CBA/N mice
B cell maturation, 163, 164
immune response ontogeny, 153-154
T cell deficit, 163
Capping, *see* Lymphocyte capping
Cell mediated immune (CMI) response, *see also* T lymphocytes, 4, 25-27
Complement
C_3 receptor on B cells, 3
conglutinin, reaction with, 224-225
immunoconglutinins, reaction with, 230-231, 248, 249
Conglutinating complement absorption test, 222, 246-247
as serological test, 222-223
Conglutination reaction, 221
detection of antibody, 221-222, 245-249
direct, 245-246
as serological tool, 245-249
Conglutinin, 221-249
adsorbed complement, reaction with, 224-225
antimicrobial activity, 239-243, 249
assay for complement-fixing immune complexes, 247-248
biological significance, 236-245
chromatographic purification of, 226-227
colostrum, 229
foetal levels, 229
infection and serum titer, 237-238
milk, 229, 237
molecular characteristics, 223-224
protection of RBC from lysis by streptolysin O, 247
seasonal fluctuation in, 227-228, 249

serum levels, 227-229, 236-237, 249
zymosan purification of, 225-226

D

Diabetic mouse
lymphokine production, 163
T cell function, 163
Dominant hemimelia, *see* Asplenic mouse
Dystrophic mouse
immune response ontogeny, 147-148
T cell function, 148
thymus, 148

G

Gut-associated lymphoid tissue (GALT), 169-192
amphibians, 256, 280
antigen-specific killer T cells, 188
antigen stimulation in development, 176
B cell differentiation and proliferation in, 191, 203-205
as bursal equivalent, 167, 168, 190-192, 204
extirpation studies, 179-182
functional morphology, 169-174
graft versus host reaction, 188
"helper" T cells, 188
IgA precursors, 184-186, 192
IgE responses, 186-188
immunocompetence, 179-190
lymphocyte circulation, 127
mitogenesis, 179
ontogeny, 174-176
physiological characteristics, 176-190
post-natal development, 126, 130
reconstruction experiments, 182-184
suppressor cells, 189
surface immunoglobulin on, 177-179
thymic markers on, 176-177

H

Ha/ICR mice
immune response ontogeny, 152-153
Hairless mouse
T cell function, 162
High endothelial venules (HEV), 66-69, 71
appendix TDA, 172-173
BALT, 197, 198, 207
homing receptor, 36-39, 71-72
lymph node development, 48
lymphocyte homing to, 36-44, 71-72, 73, 86, 89
lymphocyte transit through, 72, 73, 74
MALT, 206
Peyer's patches, 80, 152
unidirectional permeability, 74
High responder mouse strains, 152
Humoral immune response, 4-5, 8-9 11, 13, 15-18, 25-27

I

Immune response ontogeny, 135-164
amphibians, 257-263
strain differences in mice, 137
Immunoconglutinins, 221-249
antimicrobial activity, 239-243, 249
autostimulation of, 233
biological significance, 236-245, 249
complement, reaction with, 230-231, 248, 249
experimental production, 231-234
heterostimulation of, 231-233
infection and serum titer, 238-239, 249
molecular characteristics, 229-230
persistence in serum, 234
phagocytosis enhancement, 243-244, 249
purification, 234-236
red blood cell destruction, 248
saliva, 237

serological activity, 248
serum, 237
viral infections, 244-245
Immunodeficiency disorders, 21
Immunoglobulin, *see also* specific immunoglobulins
amino acid sequence studies, 9, 11, 13, 15-16
amphibians, 257-260
antigen receptor on amphibian lymphocytes, 260-263, 269-270
constant region sequences, 15-16
evolution of subclasses, 1
on foetal liver cells, 136
framework region structures (FRI), 13
GALT cell markers, 177-179
heavy chain sequences in dog, 11, 13, 15-16
immunologic memory and, 259, 260
J polypeptide chain, 16-17
light chain sequences in dog, 9, 11, 15
lower vertebrate surface Ig, 262-263
in lymph, 113-114
myeloma paraproteins, 5
secretory component (SC) polypeptide chain, 17-18
subclasses, 5
variable region sequences, 9, 11, 13, 15
Immunoglobulin A (Ig A)
amino acid sequence studies, 11, 13
appendix, 177
B cell differentiation, 192
bile, 201
BALT, 198
GALT extirpation studies, 181
immunoconglutinins, 230, 249
intestinal lymph, 113-114, 117, 127
J polypeptide chain, 16-17
lamina propria, 193, 195
milk, 201
mucosal immune system, 81, 83, 168, 177, 208-209
myeloma paraprotein, 5
Peyer's patches, 80-81, 179, 185
precursor cells, *see* Ig A precursor cells
saliva, 201
secretory, Ig A, 78
secretory component (SC) polypeptide chain, 17-18
solitary lymph node, 185
Immunoglobulin A (Ig A) precursor cells
appendix, 183, 184
BALT, 184
GALT, 184-186, 203-204, 209
lamina propria, 183, 184, 193
MALT, 207-208
migratory pathway, 185-186
Peyer's patches, 82, 87, 127, 183, 184
Immunoglobulin D (Ig D), 3, 46-47, 260
Immunoglobulin E (Ig E),
B cell differentiation, 192
BALT, 187-188
cellular distribution, 186
GALT, 186-188, 192
mast cells, 187
mesenteric lymph nodes, 187
parasitic infections, 186, 187
post-natal antibody production, 188
precursor cells in GALT, 192, 203-204
precursor cells in Peyer's patches, 187
Immunoglobulin G (IgG)
amino acid sequence studies, 11, 13
amphibians, 258-259, 262
appendix irradiation and, 182, 183
BALT, 198

bone marrow irradiation and, 182, 183
canine B cells, 3
efferent lymph after antigenic challenge, 113
GALT extirpation studies, 181
immunoconglutinins, 230, 231, 233, 249
intestinal lymph, 127
myeloma paraprotein, 5
Peyer's patches, 185
precursor cells in GALT, 203-204
precursor cells in Peyer's patches, 209
tonsil tissue, 200
Immunoglobulin M (IgM)
amino acid sequence studies, 11, 13, 15-16
amphibians, 256, 258, 259, 260, 262
appendix, 177
B cell differentiation, 46-47, 192
canine B cells, 3
cryoimmunoglobulin, 9
efferent lymph after antigenic challenge, 113
GALT, extirpation studies, 181
GALT, reconstitution experiments, 182
immunoconglutinins, 230, 231, 233, 249
intestinal lymph, 100, 127
irradiation of bone marrow versus appendix and, 182
J polypeptide chain, 16
myeloma paraprotein, 5, 8-9
Peyer's patches, 179, 183, 185
precursors in GALT, 203-204
secretory component (SC) polypeptide chain, 18
Immunologically mediated nephritis, 20
Inflammation, acute, 102-104
Inflammatory lesions, chronic, 83-86, 123-124, 125-126
lymphocyte migration in, 128-130
Intestinal lamina propria and epithelium, *see* Lamina propria

J

J chain, 78
Jugular bodies, frog
antigen-binding cells, 262

L

Lamina propria, 205
amphibian membrane Ig, 262
cytotixic activity, 194
lymphoid tissue, 193-195
macrophage migration inhibition factor (MIF), 189
mitogenic response, 195
Larval antibodies, amphibian, 271-272
Lethal mouse mutants, 136
Lethargic mouse, 147
Liver
as bursal equivalent, 45
foetal cell-mediated immune reactions, 136
lymphopoiesis in amphibian larva, 279
LSP responsiveness
mouse strain differences, 151-152
Lung
lymphocyte accumulation, 98-99
Ly antigens
T cell differentiation, 46
after antigenic challenge, 90
Ly cells
hairless mouse, 162
Lymph, afferent
allogenic reactions, 124-125
arachidonic acid, 122
cellular composition, 116-121
chronic inflammatory reactions, 123-124
coagulation, 122-123
formation, 112-115
from pathological sites, 121-125
phospholipase A, 122

PMNs in acute reactions, 121-122, 123
prostaglandins in, 114-115, 122
Lymph, efferent
antibody-forming cells, 105-107
after antigenic challenge, 104
arachidonic acid metabolites in, 114-115
blast cells, 105-107
cellular composition after antigenic challenge, 105-110
coagulation and fibrinolysis, 115-116
factors modulating lymphocyte and macrophage functions, 114
immunoglobulins, 113-114
interferon, 116
phospholipase, 114-115
plasma proteins, 112-116
prostaglandins in, 114-115
sensitised cells in, 107-110
Lymph, intestinal, 126-127
Lymph, lymph node
after antigenic challenge, 111-112
passage through nodes, 59-63
Lymph nodes, 56-74
amphibian, *see also* Jugular bodies, 256, 280
blood flow and prostaglandins, 114-115
development, 48
enlargement during antigenic challenge, 87, 90, 104
functional comparison with adjuvant granuloma, 125-126
high endothelial venules, *see* High endothelial venules
hyperemia following antigenic challenge, 104-105
lymph transit, 99-100
lymphocyte emigration into, 71-74, 86
lymphocyte output after antigenic challenge, 101-110
protein and immunoglobulin synthesis during immune response, 113
reticular cells, 56, 59
"specific recruitment" of lymphocytes, 89
structure, 63-64
subcutaneous, 128-130
vasculature, 64-71
Lymphocyte
afferent lymph, 117
amphibians, 260-263, 267-270
antigen, binding specificity, 270-273
B, *see* B lymphocytes
blood, 98-100
capping, 29, 31, 33, 269-270
cervical lymph, 101
chemotaxis, 33-36
circulation, *see* Lymphocyte migration
cytoskeleton, 33, 41-42
differentiation during development, 44-52
differentiation during immune response, 86
genetic factors in homing behaviour, 42-44
locomotion, *see also* Lymphocyte migration, 29, 31, 33-36
lung, 98
lymph node output after antigenic challenge, 101-110
migration, *see* Lymphocyte migration
motility and homing behaviour, 39, 41-42
null cells, 3, 117, 178, 193
Peyer's patches, 126
proliferation in thymus following peripheral antigen inoculation, 89-90
receptors for homing to HEV, 37, 71-72
recruitment following antigenic challenge, 104-105
recruitment and hyperemia, 114-115

shutdown following antigenic challenge, 103
T, *see* T lymphocytes
thoracic duct, 11-101
traffic through chronic inflammatory lesions, 84
Lymphocyte migration, 25-90, 97-98, 100
anti-lymphocyte antibody and, 110-111
into appendix lumen, 171
chronic inflammatory sites, 128-130
cycles associated with mucosal immunity, 81-83
foetal, 44-52, 130
GALT, 127
during immune response, 86-90
into lymph nodes, 71-74
mesenteric lymph nodes, 128-130
subcutaneous lymph nodes, 128-130
W mouse, 162
Lymphoid tissue, 25-90
central, 52-56, 190
chronic inflammatory lesions, 83-86
development, 47-52
obese mouse, 147
peripheral, 56-86
pituitary dwarf mouse, 147
thymus and post-natal development, 175
Lymphoproliferation mouse, 145

M

Macrophages
afferent lymph, 117-118
as antigen-binders for T cells, 26, 43
appendix follicles, 172
bone marrow, 53
cell products in chronic inflammatory reactions, 123-124
GALT, 179
lymph nodes, 56, 61, 63, 87
spleen, 74-75
thymic maturation, 45
thymus, 53-54
Major histocompatibility complex
immune response ontogeny and, 148-150
lymphocyte homing and, 42-44
mouse strain differences in immune response, 137-138
thymus epithelial cells, 53
T-locus and, 143, 144
Mammary gland, 200-202
Mast cells
W series mice, 162
Mesenteric lymph nodes, 126
cytotoxic activity, 194
IgE synthesis, 187
lymphocyte migration, 128-130
suppressor cells, 189
Metamorphosis, amphibian, 280-282
Mixed conglutination reaction, 247
Motheaten mouse
immune response ontogeny, 145-146, 163
spleen function, 146
thymus function, 146
Mucosa-associated lymphoid tissue (MALT), *see also* GALT and BALT, 200-203, 205-209
Mucosal immune system, *see also* BALT, GALT and MALT, 77-83, 167-209
structure, 78-81
Multiple myeloma, 19
Mutations, mouse, 138-155

N

Natural killer cells
beige mouse, 162
obese mouse, 162
Normal lymphocyte transfer (NLT) reactions, 124, 125
Nude mouse, *see* Athymic mouse
Nude streaker mouse, 140-141
Null cells
afferent lymph, 117

GALT, 178
lamina propria, 193
NZB autoimmune mice
immune response ontogeny, 151, 163-164

O

Obese mouse, 147, 162
natural killer cells, 162
skin graft rejection, 162
Ontogeny, *see* Immune response ontogeny
Osteopetrotic mouse
bone marrow development, 162

P

Peyer's patches, 167, 168
cytokinetic studies, 172
cytotoxic activity, 194
development, 51-52, 175
extirpation studies, 180-182
functional morphology, 78-81, 173-174
lymphocyte circulation, 81-82, 87
post-natal development, 126
purified tuberculin protein, response to, 189
suppressor cells, 189
T cell functions in TDA, 188
Peripheral lymph nodes
suppressor cells, 189
Pituitary dwarf mouse
immune response ontogeny, 147, 163
lymphoid tissue, 147
T cells, 147
thymic hormone activity, 147
thymus, 147
Primitive recognition mechanisms
T-locus and, 143-144
Prostaglandins
afferent lymph during acute inflammatory response, 122
lymph node blood flow and, 114-115

R

Rheumatoid arthritis, 20

S

SJL mice
immune response ontogeny, 152
Sacculus rotundus, 167, 168
anti-sheep red blood cell plaque forming cells, 183-184
cytokinetic studies, 172
extirpation studies, 180-182
functional morphology, 174
ontogeny, 175
suppressor cells, 189
Salivary gland, 202
Secretory component, 17-18
Self-tolerance
amphibian metamorphosis and, 280
Sequential antigenic competition, 276-277
Sjogren's-like syndrome, 20
Solitary lymphoid nodules
GALT, 174
Spleen, 74-77
amphibians, 256, 260-261, 268, 282
antigen-binding cells, 262, 264, 265, 270, 273
development, 48, 51, 150
lymphocyte emigration into, 77, 98
motheaten mouse, 146
shielding during sublethal irradiation, 182
structure, 75-77
suppressor cells, 189
Swiss Webster mouse
immune response ontogeny, 155
Systemic lupus erythematosus, 19, 20

T

T lymphocytes, *see also* Lymphocytes, 2-3, 26
afferent lymph, 117
amphibians, 256

antigen receptor, 26, 43
asplenic mouse, 142
athymic mouse, 139, 140, 141
brain tissue specific surface marker and, 3
CBA/N mice, deficit in, 163
colostrum and milk, 201
diabetic mouse, 163
differentiation, 44–46
dystrophic mouse, 148
efferent lymph after antigenic challenge, 104
GALT, 188–190, 192, 203
Ha/ICR low responder mice, 153
hairless mouse, 162
"helper" cells, 26, 46, 188, 266, 267, 276
during immune response, 87
in inflamed tissue, 84
killer cells, 162, 188
lamina propria, 193
Ly antigen, 46
in lymph nodes, 64, 87, 89
lymph node transit time, 74
maturation, 44–46
migration in GALT ontogony, 175
migration through subcutaneous and mesenteric lymph nodes, 128
migrations, mucosal, 208
mitogenesis in amphibia, 268–269
mitogenesis in GALT, 179, 188
motility, 29, 31
NZB mouse, 151
obese mouse, 162
Peyer's patches, 80, 189
pituitary dwarf mouse, 147
spleen, 77
suppressor cell function, 46, 189
thoracic duct, 100
Thy-1 antigen, 45, 46
thymectomy and, 275–276
Temperature
amphibian immune response and, 266–167
Teratomas
H-2 antigen expression, 149, 150
T-locus mutants, 144–145
Thy-1 antigen
bone marrow stem cells, 45
T cell differentiation, 46
Thymic hormone
pituitary dwarf mouse, 147
Thymus, 53–56, 190
amphibians, 256, 260–262, 268, 273–279, 282
antigen-binding cells, 262, 264, 265
and appendix development, 175
asplenic mouse, 141–142
blood-thymus barrier, 54–56
dystrophic mouse, 148
embryonic lymphopoiesis and, 277–279
extirpation in amphibian larvae, 273–275
lymphatic tissue development and, 47–48, 175
during metamorphosis, 280
motheaten mouse, 146
ontogeny, 45, 150
ontogeny in athymic mouse, 138–139
pituitary dwarf mouse, 147
Thymus lymphocyte antigen
BALT cells, 199
GALT cells, 176–177
Thrombocytopenic purpura, 21
T-locus mutations
immune response ontogeny, 142–145, 163
primitive recognition mechanisms and, 143–144
teratoma developmental studies, 144–145
Tonsil, 200

W

W series mice
lymphocyte circulation, 162
mast cell deficiencies, 162